# Basics of CANCER PAIN

A Comprehensive Guide for the Cancer Care Providers

# Basics of CANCER PAIN

## A Comprehensive Guide for the Cancer Care Providers


*Editors*

**Aparna Chatterjee** MD, FCARCSI (Dublin)
Professor and Head (Division of Pain)
Department of Anesthesiology, Critical Care and Pain
Tata Memorial Centre and Homi Bhabha National Institute, Mumbai, India

**Sumitra Bakshi** MD, DNB
Professor
Departmental Lead for Acute Pain Service
Department of Anesthesiology, Critical Care and Pain
Tata Memorial Centre and Homi Bhabha National Institute, Mumbai, India



CBSPD

**CBS Publishers & Distributors** Pvt Ltd

New Delhi • Bengaluru • Chennai • Kochi • Kolkata • Lucknow • Mumbai
Hyderabad • Jharkhand • Nagpur • Patna • Pune • Uttarakhand

*Disclaimer*

Science and technology are constantly changing fields. New research and experience broaden the scope of information and knowledge. The editors have tried their best in giving information available to them while preparing the material for this book. Although all efforts have been made to ensure optimum accuracy of the material, yet it is quite possible some errors might have been left uncorrected. The publisher, the printer and the editors will not be held responsible for any inadvertent errors, omissions or inaccuracies.

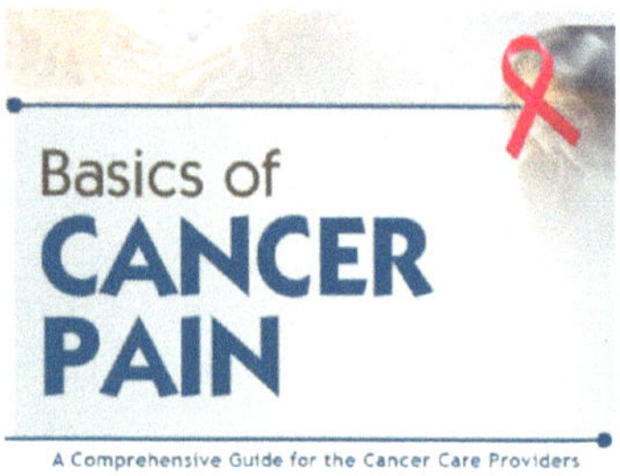


**ISBN:** 978-81-9798-221-7



**First Edition 2025**



Published by Satish Kumar Jain and produced by Varun Jain for
**CBS Publishers & Distributors Pvt Ltd**
4819/XI Prahlad Street, 24 Ansari Road, Daryaganj, New Delhi 110 002, India
Ph: 011-23289259, 23266838 Fax: 011-23243014
Website: www.cbspd.com e-mail: delhi@cbspd.com

*Corporate Office:* 204 FIE, Industrial Area, Patparganj, Delhi 110 092, India
Ph: 011-49344934 Fax: 011-49344935
e-mail: publishing@cbspd.com; publicity@cbspd.com

*Branches*

- Bengaluru: Seema House 2975, 17th Cross, KR Road, Banasankari 2nd Stage, Bengaluru 560 070, Karnataka, India
  Ph: +91-80-26771678/79 Fax: +91-80-26771680 e-mail: bangalore@cbspd.com
- Chennai: 18/8B, Subbarayan Street, Shenoy Nagar, Chennai 600 030, Tamil Nadu, India
  Ph: +91-44-42032115, 26681266 e-mail: chennai@cbspd.com
- Kochi: 42/1325, 1326, Power House Road, Opposite KSEB, Power House, Ernakulum 682 018, Kochi, Kerala, India
  Ph: +91-484-4059061–67 Fax: +91-484-4059065 e-mail: kochi@cbspd.com
- Kolkata: 147, Hind Ceramics Compound, 1st Floor, Nilgunj Road, Belghoria, Kolkata 700 056, West Bengal, India
  Ph: +91-33-25330055/56 e-mail: kolkata@cbspd.com
- Lucknow: Basement, Khushuma Complex, 7 Meerabai Marg (behind Jawahar Bhawan), Lucknow 226 001, UP, India
  Ph: +91-522-4000032 e-mail: tiwari.lucknow@cbspd.com
- Mumbai: PWD Shed, Gala No. 25/26, Ramchandra Bhatt Marg, Next JJ Hospital Gate No. 2, Opp. Union Bank of India, Noorbaug, Mumbai 400 009, Maharashtra, India
  Ph: +91-22-66661880/89 e-mail: mumbai@cbspd.com

*Representatives*

- **Hyderabad** 0-9885175004 • **Jharkhand** 0-9811541605 • **Nagpur** 0-8692091830
- **Patna** 0-9334159340 • **Pune** 0-9664372571 • **Uttarakhand** 0-9716462459

*Printed* in India

*to*

Our patients,
who have immense faith in all their care providers

# Contributors


**Ajeeta M Kulkarni**
BSc (Physiotherapy), MSc (Psychology), MPTh (Cardiopulmonary) Certified Lymphedema Therapist (UK)
Scientific Assistant 'F'
Department of Physiotherapy
Tata Memorial Centre and
Homi Bhabha National Institute, Mumbai

**Akankshya Sarangi** DNB (Anesthesiology)
Consultant Anesthesiologist
Department of Anesthesiology
Critical Care and Pain
Advanced Centre for Treatment, Research and Education in Cancer, Tata Memorial Center
Mumbai

**Amiya Agrawal** MD (Radiation Oncology)
Radiation Oncology
Navodaya Cancer Hospital, Bhopal

**Anil Tibdewal** MD (Radiation Oncology)
Associate Professor
Department of Radiation Oncology
Tata Memorial Centre and
Homi Bhabha National Institute, Mumbai

**Anjana Wajekar**
DNB, Fellowship in neuro-anesthesiology, FAIMER Fellow
Professor, Advanced Centre for Treatment, Research and Education in Cancer
Department of Anesthesiology
Critical Care and Pain
Tata Memorial Center
Homi Bhabha National Institute, Mumbai

**Anshita Sharma** MD (Palliative Medicine)
Senior Resident
Department of Palliative Medicine
Tata Memorial Centre and
Homi Bhabha National Institute, Mumbai

**Anuradha A Daptardar**
BSc (Physiotherapy), Certified Lymphedema Therapist (UK)
Officer-in-Charge
Department of Physiotherapy
Tata Memorial Centre and
Homi Bhabha National Institute, Mumbai

**Aparna Chatterjee** MD, FCARCSI (Dublin)
Professor and Head (Division of Pain)
Department of Anesthesiology, Critical Care and Pain
Tata Memorial Centre and
Homi Bhabha National Institute, Mumbai

**Ashwini Rane** DNB, Fellowship in Pediatric Anesthesia
Assistant Professor
Department of Anesthesiology
Critical Care and Pain
Tata Memorial Center and Advanced Centre for Treatment, Research and Education in Cancer
Mumbai

**Bhakti Trivedi**
MD Anesthesiology Pediatric Anesthesiology
Head, Clinical Anesthesia; OIC Academic Cell, Clinical Services
Department of Anesthesiology
Critical Care and Pain
Advanced Centre for Treatment, Research and Education in Cancer
Tata Memorial Center, Mumbai

**Bharti Veer** PhD Nursing
Nursing, Tata Memorial Centre and
Homi Bhabha National Institute, Mumbai

**Bindiya Salunke** MBBS, MD (Anesthesiology)
Professor
Department of Anesthesiology
Critical Care and Pain
Tata Memorial Centre and
Homi Bhabha National Institute, Mumbai

**Chandni Rana** MD Anesthesia
Senior Resident, Department of Anesthesiology
Critical Care and Pain
Tata Memorial Centre and
Homi Bhabha National Institute, Mumbai

**Chhaya Dhanve**
RNRM, Diploma in Oncological Nursing, Post Basic BSc. Nursing
Nursing Administration
Tata Memorial Centre and
Homi Bhabha National Institute, Mumbai

**Debashree Lahiri** MBBS, DNB
Assistant Professor
Department of Anesthesiology
Critical Care and Pain
Tata Memorial Centre and Homi Bhabha National Institute, Mumbai

**Dhanashri Kudal** MBBS, MD
Senior Resident
Department of Palliative Medicine
Tata Memorial Centre and
Homi Bhabha National Institute, Mumbai

**Gauri R Gangakhedkar**
DA, DNB (Anesthesiology), Fellowship in Neuro-anesthesia
Assistant Professor
Department of Anesthesiology
Critical Care and Pain
Advanced Centre for Treatment
Research and Education in Cancer
Tata Memorial Centre and Homi Bhabha National Institute, Mumbai

**Jayita Deodhar** MD, DNB, Diploma in Palliative Medicjne (Cardiff University) MRCPsych
Professor and Head
Department of Palliative Medicine
Tata Memorial Centre and Homi Bhabha National Institute, Mumbai

**Kunal Gala** DMRD, DNB (Radiology)
Professor Interventional Radiology
Department of Radiology
Tata Memorial Centre and Homi Bhabha National Institute, Mumbai

**Manju Sengar** MD, DM
Professor and Head
Department of Medical Oncology
Tata Memorial Centre and Homi Bhabha National Institute, Mumbai

**Manjusha Vagal**
PhD, MSc (Occupational Therapy), CLT (USA)
Professor and OIC, Occupational Therapy
Tata Memorial Centre and Homi Bhabha National Institute, Mumbai

**M Naga Sailaja** MD, DNB
Fellow in Onco-anesthesia and Pain
Department of Anesthesiology
Critical Care and Pain
Tata Memorial Centre and Homi Bhabha National Institute, Mumbai

**Monish GK** MD (Radiodiagnosis), DM (IR)
Fellow, Interventional Radiology
Department of Radiology
Tata Memorial Centre and Homi Bhabha National Institute, Mumbai

**Nitin Satish** MBBS, DNB, FNB
Fellow, Onco-anesthesia
Department of Anesthesiology
Critical Care and Pain
Tata Memorial Centre and Homi Bhabha National Institute, Mumbai

**Nitin S Shetty** MD, DNB (Radiology)
Head, Department of Radiodiagnosis
Advanced Centre for Treatment, Research and Education in Cancer
Tata Memorial Centre and Homi Bhabha National Institute, Mumbai

**Pankaj Singh Rana**
MBBS, MD, (Anesthesiology), PDCC (Critical Care Medicine)
Assistant Professor, Department of Anesthesiology
Critical Care and Pain
Advanced Centre for Treatment, Research and Education in Cancer
Tata Memorial Centre and Homi Bhabha National Institute, Mumbai

**Prasun P** MBBS, MD (Palliative Medicine)
Assistant Professor and Lead Consultant
Department of Palliative Medicine
Advanced Centre for Treatment
Research and Education in Cancer
Tata Memorial Centre and Homi Bhabha National Institute, Mumbai

**Pravin Dhakane** MD (Anesthesiology)
Assistant Professor
Department of Anesthesiology
Critical Care and Pain
Advanced Centre for Treatment, Research and Education in Cancer, Tata Memorial Centre and Homi Bhabha National Institute, Mumbai

**Savita Goswami** MA (Clinical Psychology)
Clinical Psychologist
Department of Psycho-Oncology
Tata Memorial Centre and Homi Bhabha National Institute, Mumbai

**Shamali Poojary** MD, Palliative Medicine
Assistant Professor
Department of Palliative Medicine
Tata Memorial Centre and Homi Bhabha National Institute, Mumbai

**Sheetal Gaikwad**
MD (Anesthesia), Fellowship in Difficult Airway and Regional Anaesthesia, Germany
Associate Professor
Department of Anesthesiology
Critical Care and Pain
Tata Memorial Centre and Homi Bhabha National Institute, Mumbai

**Shruti Gairola**
MD (Anesthesia) KGMU, Lucknow, DM (Onco-Anaesthesia) AIIMS, New Delhi
Assistant Professor
Department of Anesthesiology
Critical Care and Pain
Tata Memorial Centre and Homi Bhabha National Institute, Mumbai

**Sindhu Nair** MSc, Nursing
Nursing Superintendent
Nursing Administration
Tata Memorial Centre and Homi Bhabha National Institute, Mumbai

**Sukhada Savarkar** MD (Anesthesiology)
Associate Professor. Department of Anesthesiology
Critical Care and Pain
Tata Memorial Centre and Homi Bhabha National Institute, Mumbai

**Sumitra Bakshi** MD, DNB (Anesthesiology)
Professor, Department of Anesthesiology
Critical Care and Pain
Tata Memorial Centre and Homi Bhabha National Insitute, Mumbai

**Supriya Salunkhe** GNM, Certificate course in Palliative care, Certificate course in Pain management
Oncology Pain and Palliative Nurse
Senior Pain Nurse
Tata Memorial Centre and Homi Bhabha National Institute, Mumbai

**Suyash Kulkarni**
DMRD, DNB (Radiology)
Head, Department of Radiology
Tata Memorial Centre and
Homi Bhabha National Institute, Mumbai

**Veer Thakkar** MBBS, MD
Assistant Professor
Department of Anesthesiology
Critical Care and Pain
Tata Memorial Centre and Homi Bhabha National Institute, Mumbai

**Venkatesh Kapu**
MBBS, MD (Gen. Med), DM (Med.Oncology)
Assistant Professor
Department of Medical Oncology
Tata Memorial Centre and Homi Bhabha National Institute, Mumbai

**Virinchi Sanapala** MD (Anesthesiology)
Assistant Professor
Department of Anesthesiology
Critical Care and Pain
Tata Memorial Centre–Advanced Center for Treatment, Research and Education in Cancer
Navi Mumbai

# Foreword

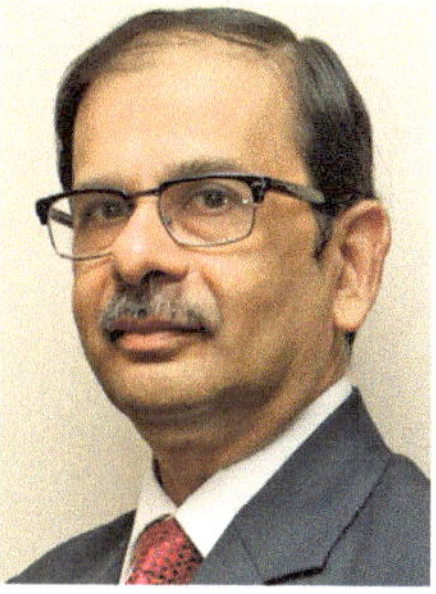

The Department of Anesthesiology, Critical Care and Pain (DACCP) at the Tata Memorial Hospital is recognized for its excellence in service, research and education. Over the years, it has spread its footprint to lead in academics by starting various educational activities directed towards students as well as advanced practitioners in anesthesiology [anesthesia review course (ARC), TMC Difficult Airway Conference (TMC-DAC)], critical care [Tutorials in Hemodynamic Monitoring and Therapy in Critical Care (THEMATICC), Case-Based Review in Critical Care Medicine for the Examinee (BRITE)] and pain management [Education in cancer and acute pain (ECAP)]. Several textbooks in anesthesiology and critical care have also been published under the aegis of the department.

The DACCP has a division of pain, with dedicated consultants and staff focussed on pain management that looks after the pain clinic and patients with acute postoperative pain and cancer pain. It is with immense pleasure that I welcome the initiative of putting together a book on cancer and acute pain by the Division of Pain, DACCP. *Basics of Cancer Pain: A Comprehensive Guide for the Cancer Care Providers* edited by Drs Aparna Chatterjee and Sumitra Bakshi is a comprehensive book catering to the Indian readership and is an amalgamation of inputs from authors from various departments across TMH, all of whom are excellent clinicians and academicians at the forefront of cancer care.

I am certain that this book will have extensive readership across India, both amongst trainee doctors and practising oncologists. I wish all the contributors and especially the editors and the DACCP all the very best.

**JV Divatia**
*Former* Professor and Head
Department of Anesthesiology, Critical Care and Pain
Tata Memorial Hospital, Mumbai
President, Indian Society of Anesthesiologists

# Foreword

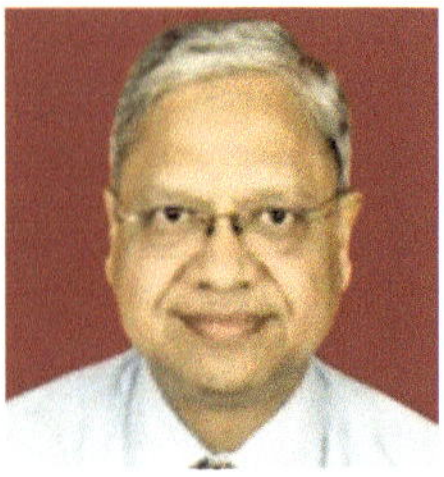

It is a matter of great pleasure and pride that the Division of Pain Medicine in the Department of Anesthesia, Critical Care and Pain, Tata Memorial Centre is publishing a book on cancer and acute pain.

The cancer pain clinic facilities were started at the Tata Memorial Centre way back in 1982 under the able guidance of Dr Sushila Shah, at a time when such services were restricted to a few pioneering medical institutions. Since then the service has steadily evolved. The acute pain service, one of its kind in India was started in 2002 with a dedicated team and protocols to ensure safe and effective postoperative pain relief. The formation of a pain division led to further development in clinical services, education and research.

The current endeavor of publishing a book on cancer pain medicine is praiseworthy. I am sure this book would serve as a milestone for reinforcing the knowledge and skills of budding pain physicians in the field of cancer pain.

I hope the readers find this book a useful practical and easy reference guide in the treatment of cancer pain.


**PN Jain**
*Former* Professor and Head
Department of Pain Division
Tata Memorial Centre and
Homi Bhabha National Institute, Mumbai

# Foreword

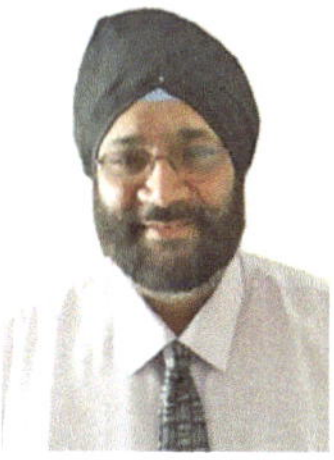

Pain medicine is a branch of medicine which uses a multidisciplinary approach for relieving the sufferings and improving the quality of life of the patients who are suffering with pain. Pain management team ideally includes pain physicians, anesthesiologists, occupational therapists, physiotherapists, clinical psychologists and pain nurses. An effective pain management team requires a coordinated effort of the pain management team.

Cancer pain is always a mild to severe type of pain, depending on the severity of the stage of the cancer in the patient. Treatment approaches to cancer pain includes pharmacological measures, such as non-narcotic and narcotic analgesics, tricyclic antidepressants and anticonvulsants, interventional procedures, physical therapy, psychological measures and palliative care. A standard strategy for improvement in cancer pain, palliative care as well as perioperative pain management includes guidelines and standards of practice such as written in this book. This book will be an important resource for ongoing training and as a reference for managing pain.

Overview in this book covers topics related to a wide range of treatments for pain management, including the anatomy of pain pathways, the pathophysiology of severe pain, pain assessment, therapeutic guidelines, analgesic options, organization of pain services, and the role of anesthesiologists, and nurses in providing optimal care. This book aims to provide an overall view on perioperative cancer pain management and overall pain management in an advanced cancer condition. It includes a compilation of various guidelines and procedures on different aspects of pain management namely acute postoperative pain in adults and children, as well as cancer pain management. It also included practical information about the cancer pain management in the daily practice, pharmacology of analgesics, neurolytic nerve and ganglion blocks, acute pain management in opioid tolerant patients and palliative care patients.

I have known the authors for more than 20 years, and their enthusiasm for teaching the residents and medical students. I am sure that all the readers of this book will benefit from the shared knowledge and experiences.


**RP Gehdoo**
*Former* Professor
Department of Anesthesia and Pain Medicine
Tata Memorial Center, Mumbai

# Preface

Pain is one of the most dreaded aspect of cancer and more often than not, crippling life. Emphasis on pain management has been found lacking across the globe as is the condition in the Indian scenario.

Tata Memorial Hospital (TMH) has been the lead pioneer in cancer care. This book on cancer pain management has been complied to amalgamate the immense knowledge at TMH from the years of experience and expertise. This book hopes to reach out to other practicing oncologists and health personnel and help them grow in cancer pain management.

Over the years, with better and improved diagnostics, the number of cancer patients has increased exponentially. With advances in cancer treatment, and favorable patient survival, many sub-types of cancer are now a well-controlled and stable disease condition. However, many patients continue to suffer from treatment related pain and hence we have approached the topic of pain in cancer survivors where we have delved on management of pain due to the treatment as opposed to that due to the disease.

The judicious use of opioids plays a very important aspect of cancer pain management. We have in this book included a chapter on how to not only use opioids safely but also emphasized on their storage, disposal and essential details on opioid policies across the hospitals in India.

Oncosurgical procedure too have become extensive and multi-visceral surgeries now predominate. Postoperative pain is a significant problem in such patients, which if not well managed could lead to chronic pain and debility. A well-planned multimodal pain management protocols in the immediate postoperative period goes a long way in overall well-being and better "Quality of Life (QoL)".

We hope that book will serve the purpose for which it has been complied and guide cancer care providers across India treat pain in cancer patients. We pray for a pain free future for all our patients.

**Aparna Chatterjee**
**Sumitra Bakshi**

# Contents

## SECTION III: PERIOPERATIVE PAIN



## SECTION IV: SUPPORT SYSTEMS AND PALLIATION IN CANCER PAIN

Section

I

# Cancer Pain Assessment and Diagnosis

Chapter 1

# Understanding Cancer Pain and the Indian Scenario

• Shruti Gairola

## Introduction

The revised definition of pain as given by the International Association for the Study of Pain (IASP) in 2020 characterizes pain as "an unpleasant combination of sensory and emotional sensations linked to, or resembling those linked to, real or possible tissue damage." Pain encompasses several dimensions, including the sensory-discriminative, affective-motivational, cognitive-evaluative, behavioral and physiological dimensions.

- *Sensory dimension:* Includes characteristics such as quality, intensity, site and duration of pain.
- *Affective dimension:* Reflects the emotional response to pain, including feelings of fear, anxiety, and distress.
- *Cognitive dimension:* Deals with the cognitive appraisal of pain, including its meaning, significance, and impact on the individual.
- *Behavioral dimension:* Deals with observable actions, reactions, and changes in behavior that individuals may exhibit in response to pain such as level of activity or analgesic intake, sleep disturbance and activity limitation.
- *Physiological dimension:* Deals with the organic etiology of the pain.

These components have been studied in great depth with respect to cancer-related pain. The physiological aspect of cancer-related pain typically arises from complications like bone metastases, nerve compression, obstruction, or the pressure exerted by a solid tumor on a hollow organ, diagnostic or therapeutic procedures, side effects, or toxicities of cancer treatment. Likewise the sensory component of cancer pain includes the physical quality or sensation associated with pain such as the perception of pain intensity, location, quality, and temporal characteristics. The cognitive component of cancer-related pain involves the thoughts, beliefs, and perceptions that individuals have about their pain experiences. One notable aspect of this cognitive component is the catastrophizing and the fear that pain signifies progression of cancer. This can have a profound effect on a person's psychological well-being leading to significant anxiety and distress.

Several scoring systems and questionnaires have been utilized to assess the multi-dimensional nature of pain. The sensory dimension can be evaluated through instruments such as the numerical rating scale (NRS), visual analog scale (VAS), and sensory McGill Pain Questionnaire (MPQ). Similarly, the affective dimension can be gauged using tools like the Beck Depression Inventory (BDI), State-Trait Anxiety Inventory (STAI), Symptom Checklist-90 (SCL-90), and affective component of the

McGill Pain Questionnaire (MPQ). For measuring the cognitive aspect of pain, various tools are available including the Pain Catastrophizing Scale (PCS), Pain Self-Efficacy Questionnaire (PSEQ), pain beliefs and perceptions inventory, and cognitive-behavioral assessment of pain (CBAP).[1]

## CLASSIFICATION OF CANCER PAIN

Categorization of cancer pain has been diverse, with considerations given to its etiology, pathophysiology, location, timing, intensity, and clinical attributes. Concepts such as breakthrough pain, neuropathic pain, nociceptive pain, and mixed pain require comprehensive understanding in order to effectively manage cancer-related pain. Moreover, particular pain syndromes have been identified in association with cancer-induced pain.

The IASP taxonomy of chronic pain is based on five axes:

1. Anatomical region or site of pain
2. Organ system involved
3. Temporal characteristics and pattern of pain occurrence
4. Pain intensity and time since onset
5. Etiology

### I. Based on Etiology

1. Caused by cancer—primary tumor or metastasis
2. Treatment related—surgical, chemotherapy, radiotherapy, and others
3. Concurrent pathology

A prospective study involving 2,266 cancer patients to assess localizations, etiologies and underlying physiological mechanisms of the pain syndromes found that, 17% had pain related to antineoplastic treatments and 9% had pain unrelated to cancer.[2]

### II. Based on Pain Characteristics

1. ***Severity:*** The intensity of pain serves as an important parameter in pain management strategies, as outlined in the World Health Organization (WHO) Analgesic Ladder. This framework provides a stepwise approach to pain management based on the severity of pain, with different analgesic interventions recommended for varying levels of pain intensity. Evaluating pain intensity allows healthcare providers to tailor treatment plans to effectively alleviate pain while minimizing side effects. One commonly used tool for assessing pain intensity is the Numerical Rating Scale (NRS)
2. ***Site of pain:*** Cancer can affect any organ, resulting in pain that may manifest in various sites. Broadly, these sites may include pain in the head and neck, chest wall, vertebrae and nerves (radicular pain), abdomen or pelvis, as well as the extremities.
3. ***Pain syndromes:*** Based on the recognition of a constellation of signs and symptoms and their association with specific type of cancers, certain pain syndromes have been identified. These syndromes provide valuable clinical insights into the underlying mechanisms of cancer-related pain and help guide diagnostic and treatment strategies.[3–5] These pain syndromes will be dealt in detail in the subsequent chapters.

### III. Timing and Temporal Classification

This refers to the categorization of pain based on its duration and onset, providing relevant information for understanding the nature of pain experiences. This classification system recognizes three main categories: Acute, subacute, and chronic pain.

Additionally, pain can manifest in different patterns, either continuous (also called as background pain) or intermittent. Breakthrough pain represents a distinct phenomenon within this framework, characterized by sudden and transient spikes in pain intensity amid an otherwise stable background pain level.

### IV. Based on Pathophysiology and Cancer Pain Mechanism

Nociceptive, neuropathic or mixed type of pain.

| **Nociceptive** | **Neuropathic** |
|---|---|
| *Somatic pain:* It is usually well localized and aching or throbbing in nature<br>*Visceral pain:* It is usually diffuse and difficult to localize | Nerve compression<br>Deafferentation nerve injury<br>Sympathetically mediated |

### *Does cancer-related pain constitute a unique entity?*

Cancer pain is a complex biological phenomenon which poses a multifaceted challenge in the domain of oncology, influencing patients' quality of life, treatment outcomes, and overall well-being. Its nature and mechanism is still not well understood. There lacks a well-established taxonomy for cancer pain[6] as can be seen by the various classifications elucidated before.

Cancer pain almost always affects the cancer patient at some point throughout the course of the illness. The concept of "total pain," was described by Dame Cicely Saunders, and is a fundamental principle in the field of palliative care, particularly in the context of cancer-related pain. Dame Cicely Saunders, a pioneer in the modern hospice movement and founder of the first modern hospice, St. Christopher's Hospice in London, emphasized the holistic approach to pain management, recognizing that pain extends beyond physical sensations to encompass psychological, social, emotional and spiritual dimensions.

Sometimes, it terrifies the patient as it can be a forerunner of disease progression or recurrence. Cancer pain can be the result of cancer *per se* or a part of the therapy such as chemotherapy related, radiation related or related to surgery. Cancer pain in the palliative setting is usually of moderate to severe grade.[7] It is usually at multiple sites and of varying intensity.

Complexity of cancer pain and its unique characteristics can only be understood by exploring its underlying mechanisms, varied clinical manifestations, and implications for management.

The updated ICD category for "chronic pain" includes cancer pain as one of the 7 independent groups. The other groups that are included in the new ICD category for "chronic pain" include primary pain, post-traumatic and postsurgical pain, neuropathic pain, headache and orofacial pain, visceral pain and musculoskeletal pain.[8]

## How Cancer Pain Affects QoL and Function?

Cancer-related pain has a profound impact on various facets of well-being, encompassing physical, emotional, and interpersonal dimensions. When not managed effectively it can have a range of adverse consequences, including disruptions in sleep patterns, feelings of depression, heightened distress, and a decline in overall quality of life (QoL).[9] The experience of pain extends beyond its physical manifestation and is intertwined with patient perceptions, which are influenced by mood, cultural background, psychological state, and individual beliefs.

Given the intricate nature of cancer pain, providing appropriate pain management is a challenging task. However, it is important as it plays a pivotal role in preserving the QoL. Effective pain management not only addresses the physical aspect of pain but also acknowledges and addresses the multifaceted nature of suffering experienced by patients. This holistic approach is essential for optimizing patient outcomes and enhancing their overall well-being amidst the complexities of living with advanced cancer.[10,11]

## Impact on Patients and Caregivers

The consequences of uncontrolled cancer-related pain extend beyond physical discomfort, affecting patients' functional status, psychological well-being, and social interactions. Persistent pain can lead to decreased mobility, sleep disturbances, anxiety, and depression, significantly impairing patients' quality of life. Moreover, unrelieved pain may contribute to treatment delays, dose reductions, and treatment discontinuations, thereby compromising therapeutic outcomes and potentially reducing survival rates. Caregivers and family members also experience emotional distress and caregiver burden as they witness the suffering of their loved ones.

## Cancer Pain as a Harbinger of the Disease

It is believed that a deeper understanding of cancer pain raises biological questions that, if addressed, could potentially alleviate not only the pain itself but also enhance survival rates.[12] Cancer pain is often perceived as a secondary outcome of cancer growth, tissue damage, and infiltration.

Cancers secrete algogenic mediators like proteases, endothelin-1 (ET-1), ATP, proteases, neurotrophic factors, bradykinin and tumor necrosis factor that subsequently sensitize or activate primary afferent neurons in the cancer microenvironment. Several of the pain-inducing mediators released by cancer cells share functional similarities with cancer-related pathways. An example of this is the proteases which are also involved in tissue invasion, metastasis and perineural invasion.[13]

## Variability in Cancer Pain Phenotype as a Result of Heterogeneity in Cancer Genomic

Cancer pain phenotype varies a lot according to factors such as histology. As an example melanomas are painless usually at primary as well as metastatic site unlike squamous cell carcinomas of the head and neck which present with pain as an initial complaint.

Same histology with similar location but different etiology can also have different phenotype. As in the case of oropharyngeal cancer with HPV as the etiological factor typically do not present with pain.[14]

Unlike other head and neck cancers which present with well-localized pain, adenoid cystic carcinoma which is a malignancy of the major and minor salivary glands with perineural invasion as a common pathologic feature presents with vague and dull pain.[15]

## Prevalence of Pain in Patients with Cancer Globally and in the Indian Subcontinent

The global annual occurrence of cancer reaches a staggering 10 million individuals, with a substantial portion experiencing pain as a primary concern.[16] Undertreated cancer pain remains a real problem in the current world. However, advancements in medical science over the past decade have led to decreased incidence of cancer pain, as well as enhanced understanding of its causes and the introduction of innovative treatment approaches.[17]

In India, cancer is not officially designated as a nationally notifiable disease, resulting in data collection primarily through Population-Based Cancer Registries (PBCRs). According to the National Cancer Registry Programme, the estimated number of cancer cases and crude incidence rate for the year 2020 stood at 14,61,427 (100.4 per 100,000), with a higher number of cases among females, totalling 749,251 (105.4 per 100,000), compared to males, which amounted to 712,176 (95.6 per 100,000). Projections indicate that the incidence of cancer cases is forecasted to increase from 1.46 million in 2022 to 1.57 million by 2025.

Examining incidence by site, the organs of the gastrointestinal system (288,054), breast (221,757), genital system (218,319), oral cavity and pharynx (198,438) and the respiratory system (143,062) bear the highest burden of cancer in both the genders. The combined likelihood of developing cancer throughout one's lifetime between ages of 0 and 74 years is approximately one in every nine individuals for all cancer types in both sexes, one in 67 for lung cancers in males, and one in 29 for breast cancer in females.

Among males, the leading sites of cancer include lung (10.6%), mouth (8.4%), prostate (6.1%), tongue (5.9%), and stomach (4.8%), whereas for females, they comprise breast (28.8%), cervix (10.6%), ovary (6.2%), corpus uteri (3.7%), and lung (3.7%). Lung cancer in males and breast cancer in females remain the predominant types of cancer. In the childhood age group, lymphoid leukemia, followed by brain neoplasms, emerge as the primary sites of cancer.[18]

In India out of the annual influx of the new cancer patients, between 60 to 80% are diagnosed in an advanced stage of the disease, with around 60% patients requiring only pain management and palliative care but, unfortunately, only 28% of the patients receive necessary palliative care and pain relief.[19–21]

According to the projections of the International Agency for Research on Cancer GLOBOCAN project, India is expected to experience a surge in its cancer burden, reaching 2.08 million cases by 2040, reflecting a 57.5% increase from the figures recorded in 2020.[18]

Significant findings emerged out of a recent comprehensive meta-analysis regarding the prevalence of cancer-related pain across various stages of the disease and treatment course. The study reported a prevalence of 39.3% for cancer pain following curative treatment, while during anti-cancer treatment, the prevalence increased to approximately 55.0%. For individuals with advanced, metastatic, or terminal disease, the prevalence soared to a striking 66.4%, with an overall average rate of 50.7% across all cancer stages.

Moreover, the severity of pain experienced by patients was notable, with 38% reporting moderate to severe levels of pain. These findings underscore the substantial burden of cancer-related pain on individuals undergoing treatment and those with advanced disease.

In a separate recent study, the prevalence of cancer pain was found to be even higher at 44.5%. This emphasizes the persistent need for ongoing attention and concerted efforts in the management of cancer pain throughout the continuum of care. Effective pain management strategies are essential to alleviate suffering and improve the QoL for individuals living with cancer.[22]

Another study looking at the quality of pain management, as assessed by the pain management index (PMI score), showed progressive improvement from 1994 to 2013. The proportion of patients with a negative PMI score fluctuated, with estimates averaging 46.6% during the latter years of the 1990s, decreasing to 31.8% in the most recent period. This reduction reflects a 32% decrease in undertreatment, equivalent to a 5% decline every 5 years.[23]

Cancers of genitourinary system, hematological and head and neck have a higher prevalence of pain. Breast and lung cancers are associated with highest incidence of neuropathic and chronic pain.[24]

## BARRIERS TO CANCER PAIN MANAGEMENT

Early and effective cancer pain management is foremost to ensure overall well-being of patients living with cancer. However, there are various barriers to effective pain treatment such as opiophobia (fear relating to the use of opioids), governmental restrictions on pain medications, financial constraints, etc. These barriers can be broadly classified into the following domains for the purpose of understanding.

### Patient-related Barriers

- *Communication barrier:* Under-reporting or misrepresentation of pain.
- *Stigmatization around use of opioids:* Fear of addiction, dependence, diminishing opioid efficacy, and side effects of pain medications.[25,26]
- Negative attitude towards effectiveness of analgesics.
- *Cultural and religious beliefs:* Fatalistic beliefs about cancer pain and its management can influence patients' willingness to seek and accept pain management interventions.
- *Psychological factors:* Anxiety, depression, and distress related to cancer diagnosis and treatment can exacerbate pain perception and interfere with pain management.

### Healthcare Provider-related Barriers

- *Inadequate assessment:* Healthcare providers may fail to conduct thorough pain assessments, leading to underestimation and thereby inadequate treatment of pain.
- *Lack of knowledge and skills:* Insufficient training in pain management among healthcare providers can result in suboptimal pain control strategies.
- Lack of patient referral systems.
- *Reluctance in prescribing opioid:* Concerns about misuse, addiction, regulatory scrutiny, or legal repercussions.[27]

### System and Regulatory Barriers

- *Limited access to healthcare services:* Geographic, financial, or logistical constraints may prevent patients from accessing comprehensive cancer care.
- *Resource constraints:* Inadequate availability of pain medications, supportive care services, or specialized pain management clinics can limit patients' access to effective pain relief.
- *Fragmented care:* Lack of multidisciplinary collaboration between physicians and pain specialists, can result in gaps or delays in pain management.
- *Over-rigorous pharmacovigilance around opioids:* Regulatory hurdles, such as stringent prescribing regulations for opioids, can restrict access to pain medications and complicate pain management practices.[28]

### Social and Environmental Barriers

- *Social support deficits:* Lack of adequate social support networks or caregiver burden can worsen patients' pain experiences.
- *Financial constraints:* High out-of-pocket costs for pain medications or supportive care services can act as a deterrent for the patients from seeking or adhering to pain management interventions.
- *Transportation and mobility issues:* Difficulty in accessing healthcare facilities due to transportation limitations or physical impairments can hinder patients' ability to receive timely pain management.

## CANCER PAIN AND NDPS ACT

The Narcotic Drugs and Psychotropic Substances Act, 1985 ("NDPS Act") inter alia provides for the legal framework relating to narcotic drugs, and sets out the mechanism for the control and regulation of narcotic drugs and psychotropic substances in India. The Act provides powers to Central and State Governments to prescribe the conditions and the manner in which narcotic drugs and psychotropic substances shall be supplied for medical necessity.

Cancer patients regularly complain of severe pain which may be attributed to chemotherapy, radiation therapy, or surgery. For effective pain management, cancer patients may be prescribed opioids, which are classified as narcotic drugs under the NDPS Act and are subjected to extensive regulatory scrutiny in India.

Section 2 (viiia) of the NDPS Act defines "essential narcotic drug" to mean "a narcotic drug notified by the Central Government for medical and scientific use", however, given the scope for potential misuse of the drugs, the Act provides for strict regulations on the production, prescription, and distribution of these drugs to prevent misuse for non-medical purposes.

Initially, when the NDPS Act came into effect, it only focused on preventing and combating abuse of narcotic drugs and psychotropic substances and the illicit traffic therein, however, in order to enable medical and scientific use of narcotic drugs and psychotropic substances, Section 4 of the NDPS Act was amended in 2014 and now the NDPS Act allows use of narcotic drugs and psychotropic substances for medical and scientific use subject to compliance with the various provisions of the NDPS Act.

## Conclusion

The repercussions of untreated cancer pain are severe and encompass functional limitations, loss of mobility, social seclusion, and emotional as well as spiritual turmoil. It negatively impacts a patient's performance status and can lead to anxiety, depression and a reduced quality of life.[29] In certain instances, inadequately managed cancer pain may result in the discontinuation of potentially curative treatments, thereby adversely affecting the patient's prognosis. Cancer patients often express heightened apprehension regarding suffering from pain rather than the prospect of death itself. Additionally, witnessing the pain and anguish endured by a loved one with cancer also takes a toll on family and friends.

## References

1. Ahles TA, Blanchard EB, Ruckdeschel JC. The multidimensional nature of cancer-related pain. Pain. 1983 Nov;17(3):277–288. doi: 10.1016/0304-3959(83)90100-8. PMID: 6657288.
2. Grond S, Zech D, Diefenbach C, Radbruch L, Lehmann KA. Assessment of cancer pain: a prospective evaluation in 2266 cancer patients referred to a pain service. Pain. 1996;64(1):107–14. doi: 10.1016/0304-3959(95)00076-3. PMID: 8867252.
3. Caraceni A, Weinstein SM. Classification of cancer pain syndromes. Oncology (Williston Park). 2001 Dec;15(12):1627–40, 1642; discussion 1642–3, 1646–7. PMID: 11780704.
4. Caraceni A, Shkodra M. Cancer pain assessment and classification. Cancers (Basel). 2019;11(4):510. doi: 10.3390/cancers11040510. PMID: 30974857; PMCID: PMC6521068.
5. Foley KM. Cancer Pain Syndromes. In: Stanley TH, Ashburn MA. (eds) Anesthesiology and Pain Management. Developments in Critical Care Medicine and Anesthesiology, 1994;29. Springer, Dordrecht. https://doi.org/10.1007/978-94-011-0816-4_23
6. Paice JA, Mulvey M, Bennett M, Dougherty PM, Farrar JT, Mantyh PW, Miaskowski C, Schmidt B, Smith TJ. AAPT Diagnostic Criteria for Chronic Cancer Pain Conditions. J Pain. 2017 Mar;18(3):233–246. doi: 10.1016/j.jpain.2016.10.020. Epub 2016 Nov 21. PMID: 27884691; PMCID: PMC5439220.
7. Wilkie DJ, Ezenwa MO. Pain and symptom management in palliative care and at end of life. Nurs Outlook. 2012 Nov-Dec;60(6):357–64. doi: 10.1016/j.outlook.2012.08.002. Epub 2012 Sep 14. PMID: 22985972; PMCID: PMC3505611.
8. Treede RD, Rief W, Barke A, Aziz Q, Bennett MI, Benoliel R, et al. A classification of chronic pain for ICD-11. Pain. 2015;156(6):1003–1007. doi: 10.1097/j.pain.0000000000000160. PMID: 25844555; PMCID: PMC4450869.
9. Katz N. The impact of pain management on quality of life. J Pain Symptom Manage. 2002 Jul;24(1 Suppl):S38–47. doi: 10.1016/s0885-3924(02)00411-6. PMID: 12204486.
10. Mollica MA, Smith AW, Tonorezos E, Castro K, Filipski KK, Guida J, et al. Survivorship for Individuals Living With Advanced and Metastatic Cancers: National Cancer Institute Meeting Report. J Natl Cancer Inst. 2022 Apr 11;114(4):489–495. doi: 10.1093/jnci/djab223. PMID: 34878107; PMCID: PMC9002286.
11. Porter LS, Keefe FJ. Psychosocial issues in cancer pain. Curr Pain Headache Rep. 2011 Aug; 15(4):263–70. doi: 10.1007/s11916-011-0190-6. PMID: 21400251.
12. Schmidt BL. What pain tells us about cancer. Pain. 2015;156 (Suppl 1):S32–S34. doi: 10.1097/j.pain.0000000000000099. PMID: 25789434; PMCID: PMC5215762.
13. Lam DK, Dang D, Zhang J, Dolan JC, Schmidt BL. Novel animal models of acute and chronic cancer pain: a pivotal role for PAR2. J Neurosci. 2012 Oct 10;32(41):14178–83. doi: 10.1523/JNEUROSCI.2399–12.2012. PMID: 23055487; PMCID: PMC3500608.
14. McIlwain WR, Sood AJ, Nguyen SA, Day TA. Initial symptoms in patients with HPV-positive and HPV-negative oropharyngeal cancer. JAMA Otolaryngol Head Neck Surg. 2014 May;140(5):441–7. doi: 10.1001/jamaoto.2014.141. PMID: 24652023.

15. Closmann JJ, Schmidt BL. Adenoid cystic carcinoma manifesting as maxillary jaw pain refractory to conventional treatment: a case report. Gen Dent. 2006 May-Jun;54(3):195–7. PMID: 16776413.
16. Henson LA, Maddocks M, Evans C, Davidson M, Hicks S, Higginson IJ. Palliative care and the management of common distressing symptoms in advanced cancer: Pain, breathlessness, nausea and vomiting, and fatigue. J Clin. Oncol. 2020;38:905–4. doi: 10.1200/JCO.19.00470).
17. Van den Beuken-van Everdingen MH, Hochstenbach LM, Joosten EA, Tjan-Heijnen VC, Janssen DJ. Update on prevalence of pain in patients with cancer: Systematic review and meta-analysis. J pain symptom manage. 2016;51(6):1070–90.e9. doi: 10.1016/j.jpainsymman.2015.12.340. Epub 2016 Apr 23. PMID: 27112310.
18. Ferlay J, Ervik M, Lam F, Colombet M, Mery L, Piñeros M, et al. Global cancer observatory: Cancer today. Lyon, France: International Agency for Research on Cancer; 2020.
19. Nair MK, Varghese C, Swaminathan R. Cancer: Current scenario, intervention strategies and projections for 2015. NCMH Background papers.
20. Rajagopal MR, Joranson DE. India: opioid availability. An update. J Pain Symptom Manage. 2007 May;33(5):615–22. doi: 10.1016/j.jpainsymman.2007.02.028. PMID: 17482057.
21. Portenoy RK. Cancer pain. Epidemiology and syndromes. Cancer. 1989 Jun 1;63(11 Suppl):2298–307. doi: 10.1002/1097-0142(19890601)63:11<2298::aid-cncr2820631140>3.0.co;2-a. PMID: 2655867.
22. Snijders RAH, Brom L, Theunissen M, van den Beuken-van Everdingen MHJ. Update on prevalence of pain in patients with cancer 2022: A systematic literature review and meta-analysis. cancers (Basel). 2023;15(3):591. doi: 10.3390/cancers15030591. PMID: 36765547; PMCID: PMC9913127.
23. Greco MT, Roberto A, Corli O, Deandrea S, Bandieri E, Cavuto S, Apolone G. Quality of cancer pain management: an update of a systematic review of undertreatment of patients with cancer. J Clin Oncol. 2014 Dec 20;32(36):4149–54. doi: 10.1200/JCO.2014.56.0383. Epub 2014 Nov 17. PMID: 25403222.
24. Jan F, Singh M, Syed NA, Wani D, Bashir M. Effectiveness of cognitive restructuring on intensity of pain in cancer patients: A pilot study in oncology department of tertiary care hospital. Asian Pac J Cancer Prev. 2022 Jun 1;23(6):2035–2047. doi: 10.31557/APJCP.2022.23.6.2035. PMID: 35763646; PMCID: PMC9587840.
25. Chen CH, Tang ST, Chen CH. Meta-analysis of cultural differences in Western and Asian patient-perceived barriers to managing cancer pain. Palliat Med. 2012 Apr;26(3):206–21. doi: 10.1177/0269216311402711. Epub 2011 Apr 7. PMID: 21474622.
26. Ward SE, Goldberg N, Miller-McCauley V, Mueller C, Nolan A, Pawlik-Plank D, Robbins A, Stormoen D, Weissman DE. Patient-related barriers to management of cancer pain. Pain. 1993;52(3):319–324. doi: 10.1016/0304-3959(93)90165-L. PMID: 7681557.
27. Jacobsen R, Sjøgren P, Møldrup C, Christrup L. Physician-related barriers to cancer pain management with opioid analgesics: a systematic review. J Opioid Manag. 2007 Jul-Aug;3(4):207–14. doi: 10.5055/jom.2007.0006. PMID: 17957980.
28. ACHEON Working Group; Kim YC, Ahn JS, Calimag MM, Chao TC, Ho KY, Tho LM, Xia ZJ, Ward L, Moon H, Bhagat A. Current practices in cancer pain management in Asia: a survey of patients and physicians across 10 countries. Cancer Med. 2015 Aug;4(8):1196–204. doi: 10.1002/cam4.471. Epub 2015 Apr 27. PMID: 25914253; PMCID: PMC4559031.
29. Cramer JD, Johnson JT, Nilsen ML. Pain in Head and Neck Cancer Survivors: Prevalence, Predictors, and Quality-of-Life Impact. Otolaryngol Head Neck Surg. 2018 Nov;159(5):853–858. doi: 10.1177/0194599818783964. Epub 2018 Jun 26. PMID: 29943677.

Chapter 2

# Genesis of Cancer Pain and Pain Pathways

• Debashree Lahiri

The incidence of cancer has significantly increased worldwide, so has the rate of cancer survival.[1] Hence, it is extremely important to address the ever increasing need for effective cancer pain management. Not every pain experienced by a cancer patient is related to cancer.[2] A large prospective trial[3] in cancer patients has shown that the incidence of pain due to unrelated etiology is approximately 10 percent. Thus, a mechanism-based approach is essential for adequate treatment of pain related to cancer. Cancer pain is a complex phenomenon, occurs due to interactions between cancer cells, host's central nervous system, peripheral nervous system and the immune system. Pain in cancer can be attributed to:[4]

1. Direct tissue damage by primary tumor or metastasis.
2. Damage as a result of cancer related procedures and treatment such as, diagnostic procedures, surgery, chemotherapy, radiotherapy, immunotherapy, molecular and hormone therapy.
3. Damage caused indirectly due to cancer and its treatment like metabolic imbalance, infections, myofascial pain.
4. Not related to cancer or its associated treatment.

The tumor itself can result in pain because of the following mechanisms:[4]

1. Necrosis of tumor within solid organs as in pancreatic malignancies
2. Tumor infiltration of hollow organs or encapsulated organs as in liver malignancies
3. Infiltration of bone and soft tissues by the tumor
4. Infiltration and inflammation of mucosa
5. Tumor infiltrating peripheral nerves
6. Occlusion of blood vessels by the tumor

Based on pathophysiology, cancer pain could be classified into nociceptive pain, neuropathic pain or mixed type.[4] Nociceptive pain is a consequence of nociceptor stimulation due to actual or threatened damage of the non-neural tissues[2] caused by infiltration of the cancer or metastasis or due to anticancer treatment. Nociceptive pain can further be classified as somatic and visceral pain depending on the location of these nociceptors. Somatic pain is defined as the pain originating from structures like soft tissues, skin and musculoskeletal tissues.[5] It is usually described as a sharp, localized pain. Classic example of somatic pain is pain due to bony metastasis.[6] Visceral pain usually arises from various organs of thorax, abdomen, pelvis.[5] It is usually expressed as dull aching and diffuse. Classic example is pain caused due to the stretch of the liver capsule.[6]

The International Association for Study of Pain Special Interest Group on Neuropathic Pain defines neuropathic pain as "pain arising as a direct consequence of a lesion or disease affecting the somatosensory system".[7] Thus, neuropathic pain can arise from various structures of somatosensory system such as the receptors, peripheral nerves, autonomic nerves and the central nervous system. In neuropathic pain, there is an abnormal functioning of the somatosensory nervous system which continues to function normally in those with nociceptive pain.[8] Neuropathic pain is usually expressed as burning with intermittent sharp stabbing pain and may be associated with tingling, numbness. Neuropathic pain can also manifest as hyperalgesia, i.e. exaggerated pain response to noxious stimuli or as allodynia, defined as pain due to a non-noxious stimulus or a stimulus which under normal circumstances would not be painful. In patients with malignancy, neuropathic pain is caused either due to direct nerve damage as a result of infections, infiltration or compression of the nerve by tumor or due to cancer related treatments like chemotherapy, radiotherapy, and surgery.[9] Therefore, neuropathic pain can further be classified as tumor related and treatment related.[8] Few examples of neuropathic pain are as follows:

*Tumor related*

1. *Involvement of central nervous system:* Metastatic vertebral collapse causing spinal cord compression, radicular pain caused by root compression, funicular pain caused by compression of long tracts of the spinal cord.
2. *Involvement of peripheral nervous system:* Thoracic tumors invading brachial plexus, abdominal and pelvic tumors invading lumbosacral plexus.

*Treatment related*

1. *Following surgery:* Post thoracotomy pain, post mastectomy pain as a result of damage to peripheral nerves.
2. *Related to radiation therapy:* Radiotherapy for lung and breast cancers leading to brachial plexopathy,[10] pelvic radiotherapy leading to lumbosacral plexopathy.[11] This type of pain can manifest much later[12] and can be progressive and irreversible.[13] It occurs mainly due to compression of the nerves caused by radiation induced fibrosis. Other reasons include, direct injury to nerves and blood vessels.[11] Large total doses (more than 50 Gy to plexuses, more than 60 Gy to cranial nerves), large doses per fraction (more than 2.5 Gy, stereotactic radiosurgery), radiotherapy volume involving a greater proportion of nerve fibers, heterogenous high dose distribution, hot spot high doses (field junctions), salvage radiotherapy of previously treated areas, intracavitary source of radium are considered high-risk factors for developing radiation induced fibrosis. Thus, radiation induced peripheral neuropathy can be minimized by reducing the total radiotherapy dose, the dose per fraction and radiotherapy volume each time if possible.[14]
3. *Chemotherapy induced peripheral neuropathy (CIPN):* It is usually reported as an "electric sensation" with a glove-and-stocking distribution, sensory loss and sensory ataxia. CIPN occurs as a result of direct neurotoxic effects of various chemotherapeutic agents on the dorsal root ganglion neurons and their axons.[14] The chemotherapeutic agents alter the amplitude of action potentials and the conduction velocity of nerve fibers. The cytotoxic agents produce changes in the intracellular calcium levels, activation of protein kinase C, production and release of nitric oxide, free radicals that give rise

to cytotoxicity in axons and cell bodies and thus, give rise to pain. Chemotherapeutic agents implicated are taxanes like Paclitaxel and Docetaxel, platinum based agents such as Oxaliplatin and Cisplatin, vinca alkaloids like Vincristine as well as Thalidomide and Proteasome inhibitor Bortezomib.[12–14] {Discussed in detail in Chapter 6}

4. *Musculoskeletal pain:*[15] Aromatase inhibitors are used in treatment and prevention of hormone receptor positive breast cancer. However, the Aromatase inhibitors are known to be associated with musculoskeletal adverse effects known as aromatase inhibitor associated musculoskeletal syndrome (AIMSS). AIMSS mainly includes symmetrical joint pain, stiffness which affects shoulder, hands, wrists, knees and ankles. It could also affect the spine and pelvis. AIMSS is also associated with reduced grip strength, myalgias and may have extra articular presentations such as carpal tunnel syndrome and trigger finger. Aromatase inhibitors induced bone loss, deprivation of estrogen are proposed as the causes of arthralgias.
5. Patients treated with granulocyte colony stimulating factors for neutropenia complain of headaches and bone pain. This occurs due to expansion of the hematopoietic matrix and also because of sensitization of the bone marrow nerve endings.

## PAIN PATHWAYS (Figs 2.1–2.3)

Somatic cancer pain originates as a result of invasion of skin, connective tissue, muscle, bone or joint by tumor. Visceral pain occurs due to distention, inflammation, ischemia, impaction of organs or traction on the mesentery. It is usually diffuse, poorly localized and may be difficult to identify the source of origin. Visceral pain is usually poorly localized due to lesser number of receptors involved in its pathway and its scarce representation in the primary somatosensory cortex.[4] Most of the visceral afferents are specific to the motor or reflex responses with only very few associated with pain transmission. The pain specific afferents are scantily distributed in the viscera. Diffuse, vague presentation of the visceral pain and it being referred to the superficial structures are secondary to

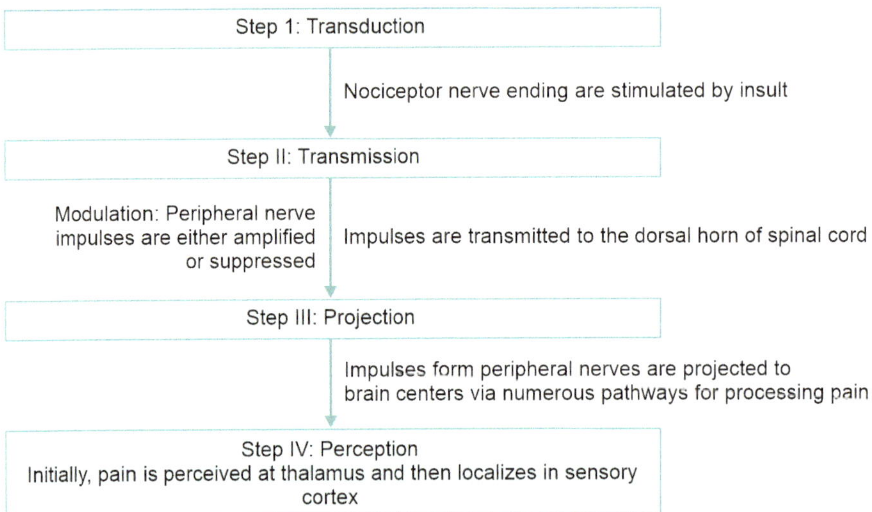


Fig. 2.1: Flowchart representing transmission of pain from tissue insult to perception

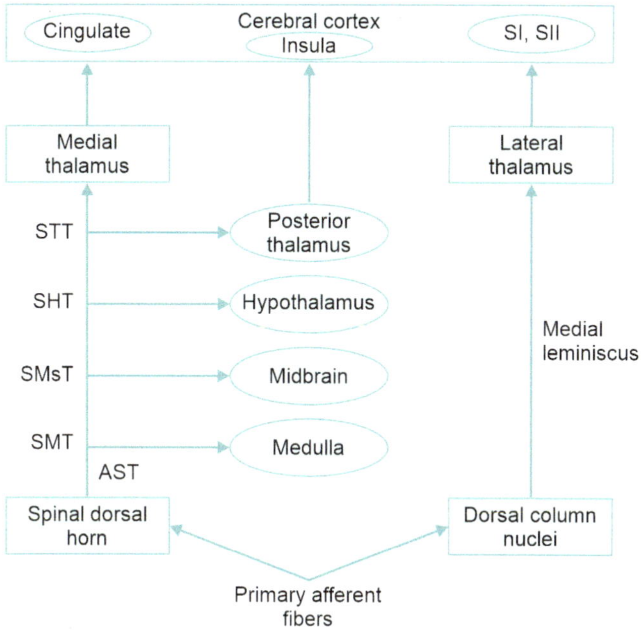


**Fig. 2.2:** Schematic representation of various pathways associated with somatic pain (AST: Anterolateral spinal tracts; SMT: Spinomedullary tracts; SMsT: Spinomesencephalic tract; SHT: Spinohypothalamic tract; STT:Spinothalamic tract

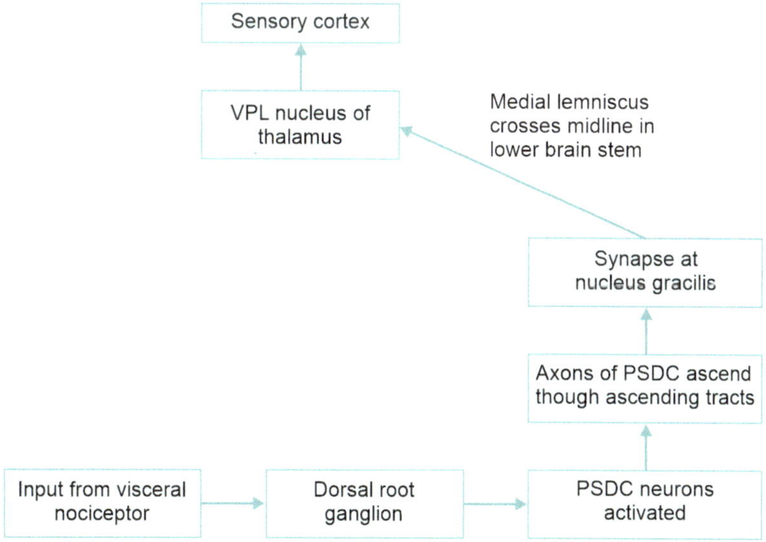


**Fig. 2.3:** Schematic representation of dorsal column pathway for pain transmission. (PSDC: Postsynaptic dorsal column; VPL: Ventral posterolateral)

viscerosomatic convergence, i.e. both the visceral and somatic afferents converge on same neurons at the dorsal horn of spinal cord. Visceral pain is often associated with autonomic reflexes such as nausea[18] due to inhibition of the dorsal motor neurons of vagus which leads to gastroparesis and nausea. As a result of the viscerosomatic convergence, any activity in ascending spinal pathways are misinterpretated as to be originating from the somatic structures and hence the term , "referred pain".[16]

The growing tumor stimulates local release of inflammatory mediators of the likes of bradykinin, histamine, prostanoids, cytokines, potassium ions and ATP which activate pain nociceptors located on afferent sensory neurons.[4] These nociceptors identify various mechanical, chemical and thermal stimuli, and convert them to electrochemical signals. Various experimental studies have shown that many of the visceral nociceptive afferents are silent.[18,19] In the presence of inflammation, tissue injury, ischemia, hypoxia, these silent afferents get sensitized and are stimulated.

Upon stimulation of the pain receptors, impulses are initially transmitted by thinly myelinated afferent A–δ fibers followed by the slower nonmyelinated C fibers.[16] Both these fibers terminate in the cell bodies of dorsal root ganglion of the spinal cord. This nociceptive stimulus is then transmitted from dorsal root ganglion to the higher centers through the anterolateral columns (Spinothalamic tract) of spinal cord.[17] Spinothalamic tract is the most important pathway for transmission of nociceptive stimulus to the ventroposterior nucleus of the thalamus and the periaqueductal gray matter. Majority of the spinothalamic tract cells project into contralateral thalamus. Those projecting into lateral thalamus, like the ventroposterolateral nucleus are involved in sensory discriminatory aspects of pain. The affective and motivational aspects of pain are transmitted by the spinothalamic tract projections to medial thalamus and also by spinoreticular and spinomesencephalic tracts. From the thalamus, these impulses are relayed to various regions of cortex via the somatosensory pathways. Complex interactions occur at cortical level involving the frontal cortex, somatosensory cortex, limbic system, locus ceruleus extending to the nucleus raphe magnus and dorsal horn of the spinal cord. The neurotransmitters commonly involved with ascending pathway are the glutamate (primary) and the substance P (secondary) within the spinal cord. Other neurotransmitters like gamma-aminobutyric acid (GABA), norepinephrine, dopamine, serotonin and endogenous opioids are involved within the cerebral cortex.

The viscerosensory information is transmitted by sympathetic and parasympathetic nerves.[20] Afferents from the thoracic nociceptors travel to thoracic splanchnics, converge into the paravertebral sympathetic trunks and then finally enter the dorsal horn. Afferents from abdominal nociceptors converge into the celiac plexus and the thoracic splanchnics before they enter into the sympathetic trunks and the dorsal horn. The pelvic visceral nociceptor afferents converge into the pelvic splanchnic nerves, which are mainly parasympathetic efferent fibers. Some pelvic afferents also pass through the lumbar sympathetic splanchnic nerves. In the dorsal horn, visceral afferents terminate over the spinal cord lamina I and V. It is said that these visceral afferents comprise only 10% of all the afferent inflow in spinal cord, which is relatively less compared to the large surface area of some visceral organs. However, there is a functional divergence of neurons in the dorsal horn so that 56 to 75% of dorsal horn neurons respond to visceral stimulation. There are no neurons that respond exclusively to only visceral afferents. There is evidence to suggest that viscerosomatic convergence occurs both at dorsal horn and supraspinal centers.[21] In the presence of active inflammation, spinal neurons alter their response to visceral stimulus. The exact cause for this is not known, however it is presumed that voltage-gated sensitization by the transient receptor potential vanilloid 1 (TRPV-1) and tetrodotoxin resistant (TTX-R) receptors may have a part to play.

Apart from spinothalamic and spinoreticular tracts, three new pain pathways are identified in the spinal cord. These are the dorsal column pathway, the spino-parabrachio-amygdaloid pathway and the spinohypothalamic pathway.[17] The difference between dorsal column pathway and spinothalamic neurons is that the former ascends ipsilaterally near midline and terminates in nucleus gracilis. From here, internal arcuate fibers relay the stimulus to ventroposterolateral nucleus of thalamus, then to the limbic centers, and further to the somatosensory cortex. Visceral pain is primarily represented in secondary somatosensory cortex and poorly represented in primary somatosensory cortex. Visceral pain is well represented in limbic system, anterior cingulate gyrus, insular cortex and amygdala. This forms base of the emotional component associated with visceral pain.

An important descending modulating pathway arises from the periaqueductal gray area, the locus ceruleus which descend to nucleus raphe magnus, dorsal horn of the spinal cord through the dorsal longitudinal fasciculus and terminates in laminae I, II, and IV.[17] At this level, inhibitory signals are sent by the interneuron, which inhibit pain signals ascending to brain by reducing the release of glutamate and substance P from presynaptic terminals of the primary afferent axons and also by reducing the postsynaptic excitatory signals of the secondary afferent axons. The periaqueductal gray area receives inputs from the thalamus, hypothalamus, cortex as well as from the spinothalamic tract. The neurotransmitters mainly involved in the descending pathways are serotonin, norepinephrine and endogenous opioids like enkephalins. The descending pain control can either be facilitatory or it can be inhibitory, though it cannot be fully dissociated anatomically. The descending pain facilitatory system consists of the anterior cingulate cortex, the rostral ventromedial medulla and the dorsal reticular nucleus of medulla. The descending inhibitory system comprises of the periaqueductal gray area, rostral ventromedial medulla and caudal lateral ventrolateral medulla. The descending control modulates pain circuitry at many levels. Numerous findings have identified that imbalance of descending pain modulation favoring pain facilitation contributes to chronic pain (Fig. 2.4).[22]

Nerve injury leads to stimulation of the C-fiber nociceptors and the low threshold Aβ-fiber mechanoreceptors.[23] This leads to accumulation of sodium channels at the site of injury and also along the length of axon.[24] All these sodium channels produce foci of hyperexcitability and produce an ectopic action potential in axon and cell body of nerve fibers. Also, nerve injury leads to expression of α-adrenoreceptor on the injured and uninjured axons making them sensitive to the circulating catecholamines. Nerve injury produces growth of sympathetic axons like a basket surrounding the sensory neurons of dorsal root ganglion.[25] Dorsal horn neurons receive both the excitatory input from sensory neurons as well as the inhibitory input from spinal cord and higher centers. It is said that peripheral nerve injury causes reduction of inhibitory control over the dorsal horn neurons.[26] This causes spontaneous firing of the dorsal horn neurons and an exaggerated response to a noxious stimuli.

In peripheral nerve damage, few neurons of spinal cord like Aβ fibers, which do not play any role in normal pain transmission sprout into the area of nociceptive afferent inputs, i.e. the lamina II of the dorsal horn. Thus, neurons from layer II to layer V combine together. As a result, there occurs hyperexcitability of other regions, greater neuronal activity and expansion of neuronal receptive field. This appears to be the central mechanism of allodynia.[27]

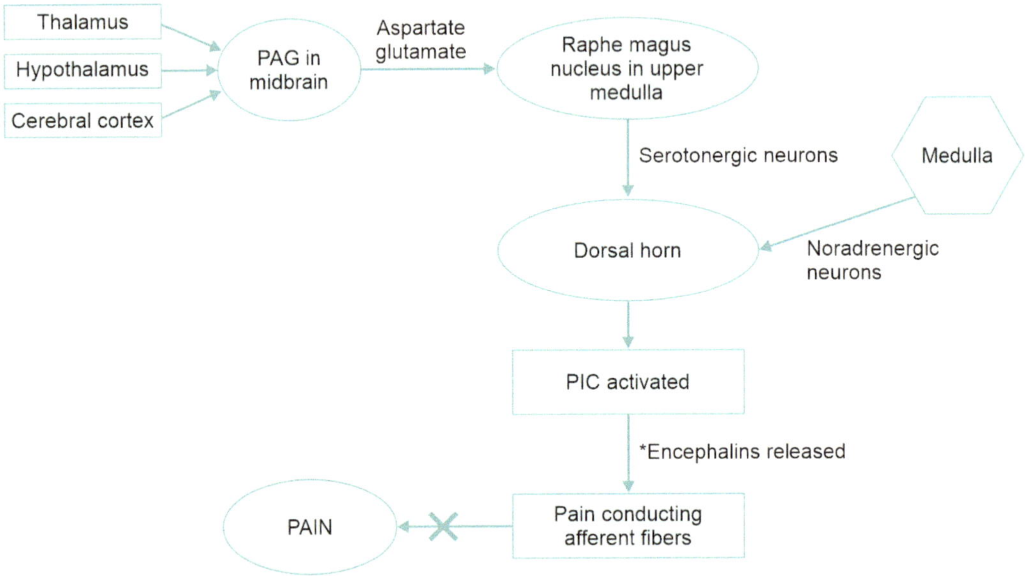


**Fig. 2.4:** Schematic representation of the descending modulating pathway. (PAG: Periaqueductal gray; PIC: Pain inhibitory complex. It comprises of multiple short enkephalinergic neurons which terminate on central endings of afferent pain fibers; *Encephalins prevent the release of substance P from pain nerve endings and thus produce pre and post synaptic inhibition)

Peripheral nerve injury leads to release of nociceptive neuropeptides like calcitonin-gene-related peptide and substance P in the Aβ fiber. This phenomenon known as phenotypic switch gives rise to a state of central hyperexcitability which is usually produced by a nociceptive input.

The tissue damage produced by the nociceptive stimulus leads to release of mediators such as substance P from primary afferent Aδ and C fibers along the antidromic pathway. This produces vascular bed dilatation and also increases the capillary permeability. This ultimately causes tissue edema and release of histamine from mast cells, serotonin and bradykinin from platelets, various other tissue mediators like nerve growth factor, prostanoids, and tumor necrosis factor-α. The mediators in turn also cause increased vascular permeability and release of substance P.[4]

1. *Bradykinin:* Bradykinin is a vasoactive peptide. In cancers like that of prostate, kallikrein is secreted which causes increase in the concentration of bradykinin. Bradykinin is also known to induce angiogenesis through the kinin B1 receptor.[28] Various animal studies have shown that bradykinin administration results in evoked response in the fibers.[29]
2. *Protons:*[29] Protons cause sensitization of the nociceptors to mechanical stimulus. The acidotic pH of the inflamed tissue giving rise to pain is associated with protons.
3. *Histamine:*[29] Histamine released by mast cells potentiates the action of bradykinin on nociceptors and also cause excitation of the polymodal visceral nociceptors.
4. *Adenosine and its derivatives:*[29] Activate nociceptors and thus pain.
5. *Arachidonic acid metabolites:*[29] Indirectly sensitise nociceptors located in skin and viscera to various endogenous chemicals.

6. *Nerve growth factor (NGF):*[4] It acts through the tyrosine kinase receptors and p74 receptors which are situated on neuronal membrane. Helps in growth and survival of the afferent sensory fibers. However, in the presence of inflammatory conditions, it facilitates cancer invasion and can also lead to development of thermal and mechanical hyperalgesia. Excessive NGF action leads to expression of acid-sensing ion channels (ASIC) and acid-sensitive receptors: vanilloid receptors (TRPV1) on the afferent sensory fibers. These lead to development of pain in cancer patient. NGF is also released by tumor cells which induce sprouting of primary afferent nerve fibers over the tumor-bearing bone. This can be blocked by administration of anti-NGF.
7. *Cytokines:*[29] Various inflammatory cytokines such as interleukin 6, interleukin 8, and tumor necrosis factor-α regulate the cancer microenvironment and are associated with excitation and sensitisation of nociceptors.
8. *Proteases:*[4,30] The cancer microenvironment contains ample amounts of proteases and proteolytic peptide products because they are produced as a result of tissue damage caused by infiltration of tumor cells. Proteases like trypsin activate protease-activated receptors located on cell surface of the primary afferent nociceptors either directly or via their peptide products. The release of serine proteases from both malignant and non-malignant cells leads to excitation of primary nociceptive afferents producing mechanical allodynia in cancer patients.

### Peripheral Sensitization

The above mentioned mediators and mechanisms produce neurogenic inflammation in the cancer microenvironment which leads to peripheral sensitization. Due to tissue injury, various chemical mediators of nociceptor origin like cholecystokinin, substance P and from non-nociceptive sources like prostaglandin, acetylcholine, bradykinin are released. This leads to activation and sensitization of the otherwise inactive nociceptors. They are triggered only due to stressful conditions like inflammation. Inflammation lowers the firing threshold of these afferents and increase the response to suprathreshold stimulus leading to peripheral sensitization.

Peripheral sensitization is also exacerbated due to the direct activation of nociceptors as well as extravasation of various algesiogenic and sensitizing factors. The peripheral sensitization of the nociceptors is essentially accountable for primary hyperalgesia which causes increased sensitivity of the injury site to noxious stimulus.

### Central Sensitization

In dorsal horn of the spinal cord, during transmission of nociceptive stimuli, excitatory amino acids, neurokinin A, substance P and other peptides are released which act as modulators or neurotransmitters. These mediators also activate receptors on other adjacent cells of the spinal cord. This leads to spread of the activation process which changes the properties of adjacent neurons. The N-methyl D-aspartic acid (NMDA) receptor does not participate in the normal pain circuit because its activation is a complex phenomenon.[17] Repeated and persistent stimulation of the nociceptive C fibers can stimulate the NMDA receptors. When stimulated, it results in a flux of calcium into the cell which produces massive depolarization of the neuron. Thus, the input signals to dorsal horn are prolonged and amplified. This sensitizes the wide, dynamic-range neurons in the dorsal horn. This results in touch input from Aβ fibers to activate nociceptive transmission to the higher centers.[17] These clinically manifest as hyperalgesia and allodynia. This process of central sensitization is most probably the cause of secondary hyperalgesia.[4]

The site and mechanism of actions of various analgesics are as follows:[31]

1. *Paracetamol:* Inhibit prostaglandin synthesis in central nervous system.
2. *NSAIDS:* Inhibit prostaglandin production by blocking cyclooxygenase both centrally and peripherally.
3. *Opioids:* In brain, they activate descending pain inhibitors, while in periphery, they reduce inflammation. Opioids also decrease the presynaptic calcium and sodium influx, production and release of excitatory amino acids like substance P and postsynaptic excitability in the spine.
4. *Anticonvulsants like pregabalin:* Inhibit high frequency neuronal firing by blocking the sodium channels.
5. *Ketamine:* Binds to NMDA receptor and inhibits glutamate activation in laminae I, II and III of dorsal horn of the spinal cord.
6. *Alpha-2 adrenergic agonists:* Act on descending pain pathways by stimulating release of acetylcholine. These drugs also act on ascending pain pathways by inhibiting substance P release from the primary afferent neurons, thus reducing transmission of pain.
7. *Antidepressants:* Act by inhibiting the presynaptic neuronal reuptake of norepinephrine and serotonin at descending pain pathway leading to inhibition of pain.

The mechanism and pathophysiology of bone pain are discussed in detail in Chapter 5.

*Triggering factors:*[17] Visceral pain is more related to the nature of the stimulus than to tissue injury. Adequate stimuli for visceral organs, i.e. one that produces a given sensation or pain, are distension, inflammation and ischemia. Hollow visceral organs like colon are extremely susceptible to luminal distension and inflammation but are insensitive to cutting and burning stimuli. Pain produced due to distension of colon is dependent on the distending pressure rather than the volume. A colonic tumor may continue to grow without causing any pain until the intraluminal pressure rises to 40 to 50 mm Hg and thus cause pain only when there is complete luminal obstruction. Serosal membranes of hollow organs are more sensitive than solid organs. Opioids, NSAIDs, and other adjuvants are the mainstay for treating visceral pain. If these are ineffective or have intolerable side effects, regional anesthesia techniques are considered. Regional techniques involve administration of local anesthetics, opioids or neurolytic agents to the neural axis as well as around the visceral plex. Continuous epidural or intrathecal infusion of local anesthetics with or without opioid may be used for abdominal or pelvic cancer pain. Selective blockade of certain pathways help provide relief from pain. This is the basis of sympathetic blocks with local anesthetics or neurolytic agents for visceral pain relief. The autonomic supply to pancreas, liver, spleen, kidneys, suprarenal glands and intestines arise from the celiac plexus. Thus, for visceral pain of pancreatic origin, neurolytic block of celiac plexus gives good relief. Neurolysis of superior hypogastric plexus gives good relief of pelvic pain due to tumor invasion. Similarly perineal pain caused by pelvic tumors can be treated by blocking the ganglion impar. Though uncommon nowadays, for refractory unilateral cancer pain, percutaneous cordotomy can still be beneficial.

Opioids may not be highly effective in treating neuropathic cancer pain. This is because peripheral nerve injury leads to destruction of presynaptic opioid receptors. Another reason for the reduced opioid sensitivity to neuropathic pain is the release of a neurotransmitter called cholecystokinin after nerve damage. Cholecystokinin selectively decreases the analgesic potency of morphine. Neuropathic pain treatment requires a combination of opioid with an adjuvant drug. Antidepressants are useful in treating neuropathic pain as these drugs enhance the descending inhibitory pathways, increase the release of serotonin and norepinephrine in the synaptic cleft at both spinal and supraspinal levels.[32] Anticonvulsants like Gabapentinoids decrease pain transmission in the spinal pathways and modulate the central descending inhibitory pathways. Thus they are extensively used for treatment of neuropathic pain.[33] Noxious stimulus causes release of excitatory neurotransmitter like Glutamate. Hence, NMDA antagonists can have a role in treatment of neuropathic pain.

Nerve injury causes axonal demyelination, retraction and fragmentation. Injury to peripheral nerves stimulates Schwann cells and produces myelin autophagy, macrophage recruitment and thus supports axonal regeneration. Thus there is emerging evidence supporting the use of Schwann cells in treatment of neuropathic pain.[34]

## Influence of Environmental and Genetic Factors on Cancer Pain

Pain is a multifaceted phenomenon. It arises from a complex interplay between the physiological, psychological, cognitive, social, genetic and many other factors. Environmental conditions such as natural light, music and artificial ambient lighting in hospitals have an impact on the pain experienced by hospitalized patients. Several studies have shown that environmental factors such as indoor plants, images of nature, view of nature from a window positively affect patients and decrease pain.[35] Psychosocial factors like sleep, smoking, social interaction, air pollution, environmental enrichment influence the perception of pain and the susceptibility to develop chronic pain conditions. Several studies have shown that there is a significant overlap between neuronal pathways, physiological and biological responses of stress and chronic pain.[36] Stress and anxiety are significantly associated with systemic inflammation which produce changes in pain perception and processing. Pain is also directly impacted by socioeconomic and psychosocial factors such as the individual's life history, goals, beliefs, expectations, fears and mood. Cancer patients with pain exhibit depressive symptoms and those suffering from depression are twice as likely to develop neuropathic pain. The exact physiological mechanisms of the connection between pain and depression remains unclear.[36]

There is a growing body of research to suggest that genetic factors alone as well as in combination with various environmental factors lead to different pain phenotypes as well as response to analgesics.[37] Genetic factors play a vital role in modulation of pain in both central and peripheral nervous system. There is evidence to suggest that genetic factors can alter the transmission of nociception as well as the central inhibitory signals which affect an individual's susceptibility to pain and their response to analgesics. Single nucleotide polymorphisms are closely linked with increasing or decreasing the risk of pain.[38] Various genetic biomarkers can be used to increase the understanding of an individual's sensitivity to analgesics which will aid in optimal control of cancer pain. Various studies have concluded that the polymorphism associated with ABCB1 gene can explain the interindividual differences in responses to opioids for treatment of cancer pain. Cancer patients who carry the homozygous minor allele experienced greater pain relief with Morphine therapy as compared to those with homozygous major allele.[39] Thus, modern genetics and genomics are powerful tools which help to predict treatment response and thus can help cancer patients with improved quality of life and reduced health care costs.[40]

## Summary

In cancer patients, pain is one of the commonest symptom for which they seek medical care. A thorough understanding of the pain physiology and its pathways are essential for treatment of cancer pain. The involvement of various brain centres, descending pathways, endogenous mechanisms and modulation theories highlights the complexity of pain perception and offers potential targets for therapeutic interventions.

## References

1. Haroun R, Wood JN, Sikandar S. Mechanisms of cancer pain. Front Pain Res. 2023;4(3):1030899.
2. Caraceni A, Shkodra M. Cancer pain assessment and classification. Cancers. 2019;11:510.
3. Grond S, Zech D, Diefenbach C, Radbruch L, Lehmann KA. Assessment of cancer pain: A prospective evaluation in 2266 cancer patients referred to a pain service. Pain. 1996;64:107–14.
4. Leppert W, Zajaczkowska R, Wordliczek J, Dobrogowski J, Woron J, Krzakowski M. Pathophysiology and clinical characteristics of pain in most common locations in cancer patients. J physiol pharmacol. 2016;67(6):787–99.
5. Kumar SP. Cancer pain: A critical review of mechanism-based classification and physical therapy management in palliative care. Indian J. Palliat. Care. 2011;17(2):116–26.
6. WHO Guidelines for the Pharmacological and radiotherapeutic management of cancer pain in adults and adolescents. Geneva: World Health Organization; 2018. Licence: CC BY-NC-SA 3.0 IGO.
7. Jensen TS, Baron R, Haanpaa M, Kalso E, Loeser JD, Rice ASC, Treede RD. A new definition of neuropathic pain. Pain. 2011;152:2204–05.
8. Edwards HL, Mulvey MR, Bennett MI. Cancer-related neuropathic pain. Cancers. 2019;11:373.
9. Shkodra M, Caraceni M. Treatment of neuropathic pain directly due to cancer: An Update. Cancers. 2022;14:1992.
10. Fathers E, Thrush D, Huson SM, Norman A. Radiation-induced brachial plexopathy in women treated for carcinoma of the breast. Clin Rehabil. 2002;16:160–5.
11. Delanian S, Lefaix JL, Pradat PF. Radiation-induced neuropathy in cancer survivors. Radiother Oncol. 2012;105:273–82.
12. Naleschinski D, Baron R, Miaskowski C. Identification and treatment of neuropathic pain in patients with cancer. Pain Clin Updates. 2012;20:1–4.
13. Bennett MI, Kaasa S, Barke A, Korwisi B, Rief W, Treede RD. The IASP classification of chronic pain for ICD-11: Chronic cancer-related pain. Pain. 2019;160:38–44.
14. Staff NP, Grisold A, Grisold, W, Windebank AJ. Chemotherapy-induced peripheral neuropathy: A Current Review. Ann Neurol. 2017;81:772–781.
15. Hyder T, Marino CC, Ahmad S, Nasrazadani A, Brufsky AM. Aromatase inhibitor-associated musculoskeletal syndrome: understanding mechanisms and management. Front Endocrinol (Lausanne). 2021;12:713700.
16. Smith TJ, Saiki. Cancer pain management. Mayo Clin Proc. 2015;90(10):1428–39.
17. Regan JM, Peng P. Neurophysiology of cancer pain. Cancer Control. 2000;7(2):111–9.
18. Habler HJ, Janig W, Koltzenberg M. Activation of unmyelinated afferent fibers by mechanical stimuli and inflammation of the urinary bladder in the cat. J Physiol (Lond). 1990;425:545–62.

19. McMahon SB, Koltzenberg M. Silent afferents and visceral pain. Pharmacological approaches to the treatment of chronic pain: New concepts and critical issues. Progress in Pain Research and Management. Vol 1. Seattle, Washington: IASP Press; 1994:11–30.
20. Cervero F. Sensory innervation of the viscera: Peripheral basis of visceral pain. Physiol Rev. 1994;74:95–138.
21. Cervero F. Pathophysiology of referred pain and hyperalgesia from viscera. In: Vecchiet L, Albe-fessard D, Lindblom U, et al (eds). New Trends in Referred Pain and Hyperalgesia, Pain Research and Clinical Management. Vol 7. Amsterdam: Elsevier Science; 1993:35–46.
22. Tao ZY, Wang PX, Wei SQ, Traub RJ, Li JF, Cao DY. The role of descending pain modulation in chronic primary pain: Potential application of drugs targeting serotonergic system. Neural Plasticity. 2019;1389296:1–16.
23. Ochoa J, Torebjork HE, Culp WJ, Schady W. Abnormal Spontaneous activity in single sensory nerve fibers in humans. Muscle Nerve. 1982;5(9S):S74–S77.
24. Devor M. The pathophysiology of damaged peripheral nerves. In: Wall PD, Melzack R, eds. Textbook of Pain. Edinburgh, Scotland: Churchill Livingstone; 1994:79–100.
25. McLachlan EM, Jang W, Devor M, Michaelis M. Peripheral nerve injury triggers noradrenergic sprouting within dorsal root ganglia. Nature. 1993;363:543–6.
26. Woolf CJ, Mannion RJ. Neuropathic pain: Aetiology, symptoms, mechanisms, and management. Lancet. 1999;353:1959–64.
27. Baron R, Binder A, Wasner G. Neuropathic pain: Diagnosis, pathophysiological mechanisms, and treatment. Lancet Neurol. 2010;9:807–19.
28. Schmidt BL. What pain tells us about cancer. Pain. 2015;156(1): S32–S34.
29. Kocoglu H, Pirbudak L, Pence S, Balat O. Cancer pain, pathophysiology, characteristics and syndromes. Eur J Gynaec Oncol. 2002;23(6):527–32.
30. Schmidt BL, Hamamoto DT, Simone DA, Wilcox GL. Mechanisms of cancer pain. Molecular Interventions. 2010;10(3):164–78.
31. Manworren RC. Multimodal pain management and the Future of a personalized medicine approach to pain. AORN. 2015;101(3):308–18.
32. Dharmshaktu P, Tayal V, Kalra BS. Efficacy of antidepressants as analgesics: A Review J Clin Pharmacol. 2012;52:6–17.
33. Jordan RI, Mulvey MR, Bennett MI. A critical appraisal of gabapentinoids for pain in cancer patients. Curr Opin Supportive Palliat Care. 2018;12:108–17.
34. Zhang W, Liu S, Ming L, Yu J, Zuo C, Hu D et al. Potential role of Schwann cells in neuropathic pain. Eur J Pharmacol. 2023;956:175955.
35. Jamshidi S, Parker JS, Hashemi S. The effects of environmental factors on the patient outcomes in hospital environments: A review of literature. Frontiers of Architectural Research. 2019;9(2):249–63.
36. Sant'Anna MB, Kimura LF, Vieira WF, Zambelli VO, Novaes LS, Hosch GN et al. Environmental Factors and their impact on chronic pain development and maintenance. Physics of Life Reviews. 2024;48:176–97.
37. Yang GS, Barnes NM, Lyon DE, Dorsey SG. Genetic Variants associated with cancer pain and response to opioid analgesics: Implications of precision pain management. Semin Oncol Nurs. 2019;35(3):291–99.
38. Reyes-Gibby CC, Shete S, Yennurajalingam S, Frazier M, Bruera E, Kurzrock R et al. Genetic and nongenetic covariates of pain severityin patients with adenoicarcinoma of the pancreas: assessing the influence of cytokine genes. J Pain Symptom Manage. 2009;38:894–902.
39. Campa D, Gioia A, Tomei A, Poli P, Barale R. Association of ABCB1/MDR1 and OPRM1 gene polymorphism with morphine pain relief. Clin. Pharmacol. Ther. 2008;83:559–66.
40. Bell GC, Donovan KA, McLeod HL. Clinical implications of opioid pharmacogenomics in patients with cancer. Cancer Control. 2015;22:426–32.

Chapter 3

# Assessment of Cancer Pain

• Bindiya Salunke

## INTRODUCTION

Pain is considered as fifth vital sign. Pain is considered a complex experience and depends on emotional, cognitive, and educational influences. Cancer pain is one of the most common but not adequately addressed sector in majority of population. Pain could occur at various stages of cancer at diagnosis, during treatment, in an advanced stage where the incidence is as high as 60–80%,[1] and may persist even in cancer survivors which is reported as 5–10%.[2,3] Pain if not adequately addressed will affect the patient both physically and psychologically and will adversely affect their quality of life (QoL). Regular assessment to identify the type, intensity and mechanism of pain should be a mandatory practice during routine care of a patient with cancer, which could help minimize their suffering and improve their quality of life. Thus, pain assessment is not a one-time assessment, it is an ongoing process till the pain management continues.

A major barrier to good cancer pain management is its inadequate assessment resulting in undertreatment. Lack of training and development of skills in health care providers necessary to adequately assess pain is one of the major reasons.

A thorough understanding of the cancer status and treatment modalities, type of cancer, and identification of the type of pain is essential to implementing an effective pain management strategy. Hence detailed cancer pain assessment with a comprehensive clinical history not only of the pain but also associated conditions such as the other medical history, extent of disease along with in depth examination to come to a cancer pain diagnosis is a must for the successful management of cancer pain and improving quality of life. Repeated and regular assessment of pain is must to assess the treatment effectiveness and need of change in treatment modality.

## HISTORY

Detailed history at first visit plays a very important part in the correct identification of the cancer pain. Proper and thorough patient evaluation is needed as the first step in pain evaluation. Good communication with patient, thorough history of presenting complains as well as other medical conditions, medication history, cancer treatment modalities and quick but relevant examination of patient is essential and is the base of good patient assessment. Characteristics of pain such as site of onset, duration, radiation, intensity, spatial characteristics, temporal variation, associated factors, provocative factors and alleviating factors, have to be characterized for effective treatment. Thorough interview about the pain helps us reach the etiology, severity and type of pain.[4] Pain being subjective, should be believed whatever patients tells and grades it as different individual has varied pain threshold. We should allow patients to describe their pain in their own words and provide them with different examples if they need help in describing their pain. Different aspects of pain needs to be covered while having dialogue with patient which should help us to reach the final etiology of pain and provide strong basis for its treatment modality selection.

### Location of Pain

The exact anatomical site of initiation of pain and its radiation if any will help us to identify the body tissue or viscera which is involved by cancer. Patient may also complain of more than one site, which is not uncommon in cancer pain as it can be related to cancer metastasis. Even the pain related to the side effect of cancer treatment are very common like mucositis. A body map can be provided to patient like mentioned in some assessment tools like paindetect or brief pain inventory for anatomical pain site identification.

### Pain Intensity

One of the dominant factors determining the effects of pain on the patient is the severity of pain and is the one that helps the clinician determine the urgency of the treatment process. Also depending on intensity of pain the level of treatment modalities will change ranging from mild nonopioid analgesics to strong opioid analgesics or interventional procedure. Unidimensional and multidimensional pain scales are available for assessing the severity of pain. Measuring and recording of pain intensity also help us to gauge the effectiveness of prior treatment.

### Pain Character

Pain quality can be easily reported with the help of standardized questionnaires and it helps to determine the etiology of pain.[5] The treatment modalities can change depending on etiology of pain. Treatment recommended for each type of pain is completely different. Pain can be characterized as nociceptive or neuropathic pain or mixed. Nociceptive pain can be further divided into somatic or visceral pain. Somatic pain is commonly seen due to involvement of cancer invasion of bones, joints, muscles or subcutaneous tissues and mucosa whereas visceral pain is due to viscera involvement. Somatic pain is generally described as aching, throbbing, stabbing or dull pain whereas visceral pain is described as squeezing, cramping or stretching pain.

#### *Neuropathic Pain*

The pain arising as a direct consequence of a lesion or disease affecting the somatosensory system is referred as neuropathic pain.[6] Neuropathic pain can be due to either, disease involvement or compression of the peripheral or central nervous tissues or due to nerve injury which can occur as a cancer treatment side effect. It is characterized by the presence of sensory alterations with either hypersensitivity or hyposensitivity symptoms and signs such as burning, shooting, pricking, or electric shock-like. It is shown that around 19% of patients with cancer pain suffer from neuropathic pain and around 39% of patients suffer from mixed pain.[7] The clinical characteristics of neuropathic pain are different from nociceptive pain. It is not easy to identify the presence of neuropathic pain. Multiple screening tools are available trying to distinguish neuropathic from nociceptive pain. Some of these tools like the neuropathic pain questionnaire (NPQ), ID Pain and Pain DETECT[38] are only interview based tools whereas the Leeds assessment of neuropathic symptoms and signs (LANSS) scale[37] and douleur neuropathique 4 questions (DN4) questionnaire[36] assess both interview based questions and physical testing. The LANSS scale and DN4 questionnaire show higher diagnostic accuracy.

#### *Spatial Characteristics of the Pain*

Depending on the site, depth, exacerbating and relieving factors and radiation of pain, we get very valuable information of pain characteristic. Neuropathic pain like sciatica pain will be radiating along particular dermatome and this will help us to reach the eitiology of that particular pain.

### Duration of Pain

Depending on the time frame from when the patient is complaining of pain, it can be classified as acute or chronic pain.

- *Acute pain:* Pain of less than 3 months duration.
- *Chronic pain:*[8] Pain which is persistent or recurrent and persisting beyond three months, or the course of an acute disease or after completion of tissue healing.
- *Chronic post-surgical pain (CPSP):* It is due to chronic ongoing inflammation or due to surgical injury to major nerves. Criteria for identifying CPSP includes:
  1. The pain must develop following a surgical procedure
  2. The pain should be present for at least two months duration
  3. Exclusion of other causes for the pain
  4. Exclusion of the possibility that the pre-existing condition is responsible for the pain.

### Temporal Pattern of the Pain

Cancer pain commonly shows the temporal pattern of pain with varying intensity in 24-hour period. Multidimensional pain scales and home diary maintained by patient help to identify this characteristic of pain. Temporal pattern assessment of pain is very crucial to pick up factors affecting exacerbation of pain and incidents of breakthrough pain. Breakthrough pain is defined as transitory increase in pain occurring in the context of stable baseline pain.[9] This breakthrough pain is known to affect patients QoL and daily activity and therefore it is recommended to utilise rapidly acting or short-acting opioids with rescue doses to treat this pain.[10,11]

### Aggravating/Alleviating Factors

Questioning patient about the factors which aggravate or alleviate the pain will help to formulate the treatment plan. Factors like some medication, interventional therapy (including acupuncture) or nonpharmacologic approaches like massage, physiotherapy, music or heat or cold therapy may help in relieving the pain. However, factors like certain movement or physical activity, lack of sleep, bad news may intensify the pain. Also, there could be certain symptoms associated with pain or related to pain treatment modality like nausea, vomiting, sleepiness, confusion, constipation, urinary retention, and weakness. All these factors should be considered during optimal pain management.

## Sleep Disturbances

Patients in pain commonly have sleep disturbances with inadequate sleep time and sleep quality. Over 65% of patients with chronic pain complain of sleep disturbance.[12] Therefore, questioning patients about adequate sleep is very important. Disturbed sleep in turn will increase frequency and intensity of pain.[13] Sleep disturbance with cancer pain can be related to anxiety, mental disturbance or mood of patient and depending on this significant history can lead to significant change in the pharmacological management of cancer pain.

## Assessing Pain Impact

The impact of pain on patients day to day functioning and its psychological outcome is crucial to assess. Measurement of QoL, mood, and social support systems are the important component of pain impact assessment.

### *Quality of Life (QoL)*

QoL measurement is comprehensive evaluation of patients physical functioning and symptoms, psychological status and social relationships.[14–16]

Multiple tools and measurement scales are available to determine QoL of cancer patients will require adequate time by the patient for filling the questionnaire and by clinician to evaluate and to interpret the results. The BPI is multidimensional tool and it can also help in assessing the QoL in cancer pain patients.

### *Mood*

It has been proven that stress related to disease in cancer patient is well tolerated psychologically, whereas if pain in these patients is not treated appropriately than the reports of psychiatric illnesses like anxiety disorder or clinical depression is more often noticed.[17–21]

The most commonly used questionnaire to measure anxiety in cancer patients is the State–Trait Anxiety Inventory[22] and the Beck Depression Inventory[23] is used measure of clinical depression.

### *Social Support*

This is another important factor which needed to be addressed in pain assessment however, it is difficult to measure or quantify. Therefore, interaction and support from family members and friends is very important to support cancer patients to go through their treatment journey.

## Pain Medication Assessment

Assessment of any pain medications is utmost important aspect to note. Due to side effect of pain medication or fear of dependence, irregular analgesic intake is often seen. So patient education of need of medication, need of breakthrough medication and reporting if pain relief is not satisfactory requires to be a part of assessment of chronic pain. If any side effects of pain medication are noted or expected, it should be assessed for and treated accordingly.

### Assessment of Stage of Cancer

This aspect is given least important but depending on which phase of treatment, the pain treatment modality will change. If patient is having tumor related pressure effect causing pain and is opted for surgery, the pharmacological treatment till surgery will be sufficient but if patient presented in advanced stage of cancer then, offering the patient an option of interventional pain management could be preferable and effective. Also, what cancer treatment (chemotherapy/radiotherapy) patient is receiving presently and its implication on pain need to be assessed.

## PAIN MEASUREMENT TOOLS

### Pain Scales

Unidimensional and multidimensional scales.

Unidimensional and multidimensional pain scales are available for assessing the severity of pain. Unidimensional scales are used to identify only a single dimension of pain, namely the pain intensity. Multiple such scales are available for use but most commonly used scales are described below and listed in Fig. 3.1.

- *Verbal descriptor scale (VDS):* Here patient will describe the pain as none, mild, moderate and severe pain.
- *Numeric rating scale (NRS):* Is an eleven-point scale, with zero being no pain and 10 as the worst possible pain. The intensity of pain experienced is expected to be marked by the patient on the scale. It is a very good tool for serial evaluation of same patient and to know the effectiveness of treatment. Because of its ease of administration and scoring this scale is most commonly utilized.
- *Visual analogue scale (VAS):* This is a simple tool with a 10 cm line with extreme ends marked as "no pain" one side and "the worst pain imaginable" on other side. The position of the mark by patient on this scale will be help to determine the pain severity.
- *Wong-baker faces pain rating scale:* It helps for better communication of pain in extremes of ages. It comprises of a drawing that illustrate facial expressions of different levels of pain severity. Each face is allotted a number as per NRS. Patient

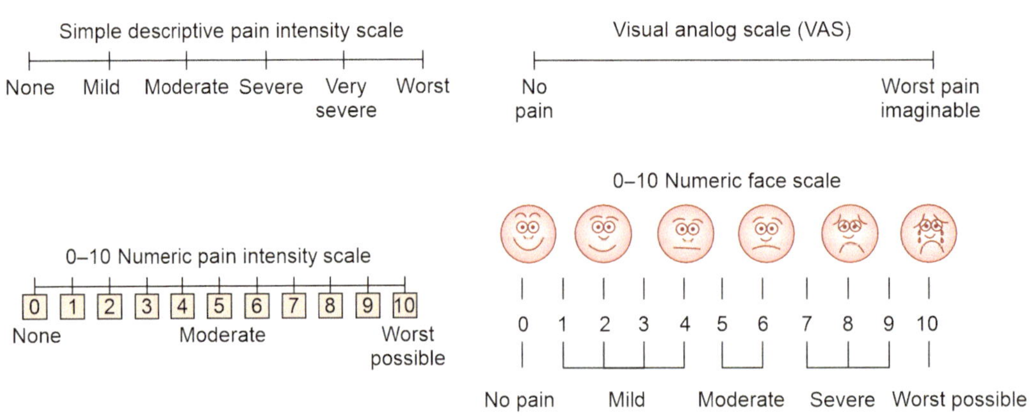


Fig. 3.1: Different unidimensional pain scales

will be selecting a facial expression which represents their pain experience. These scales are used to communicate with illiterate patients, children and old age patients who cannot adequately express their pain intensity.

- *FLACC scale:* This scale is very helpful in children, cognitive impaired and developmentally disabled patients who are unable to communicate verbally. This is an observational scale and clinician will observe the facial expression, activity/ mobility, cry of patient and how easily the patient can be consoled by caregiver. As per all these parameters, patient will be scored on the scale (Fig. 3.2).

The multidimensional pain scales provide information about the pain intensity and the other dimension of pain like sensory and affective components. Multiple questionnaires are available to provide multidimensional pain construct.

- *McGill pain questionnaire:*[24,25] This tool has three sections including sensory, affective, and evaluative scores. Maximum pain score measured by this tool is 78.
- *A short form of the McGill pain questionnaire (SF-MPQ):*[26] It includes 15 descriptors that are rated on verbal descriptive scale. Out of these 15 descriptors, 11 are sensory and 4 affective. This tool also includes the Present Pain Intensity (PPI) index and visual analogue scale. Both the original MPQ and the SF-MPQ have been proven highly reliable and gives adequate information about different types of clinical pain and the perceptual qualities of the pain.[27,28]
- *The memorial pain assessment card (MPAC)*[29] consists of a verbal descriptor scale and measures three characteristics of pain assessment: Pain intensity, pain relief, and mood.
- *Brief pain inventory:*[30] This is another useful tool for assessment of pain in cancer patients. This tool measures pain intensity using NRS over a period of past 24 hours at its worst, least and average as well as at the time of evaluation. It also assesses affective qualities of pain by measuring interference with general activity, walking, mood, sleep, relations with others, and enjoyment of life. This is also measured on 11-point NRS from "no interference" at one end and "interferes completely" at another end of scale. This tool also measures the patient's relief of pain on NRS if patient is on any pain medication, which helps us to identify and decide about the change

| | 0 | 1 | 2 |
|---|---|---|---|
| Face | No particular expression or smile | Occasional grimace or frown, withdrawn disinterested | Frequent to constant frown, clench jaw, quivering |
| Legs | Normal position or relaxed | Uneasy, restless, tense | Kicking or leg drawn up |
| Activity | Lying quietly, normal position, move easily | Squirming, shifting back and forth, tense | Arched, rigid or jerking |
| Cry | No cry (awake or asleep) | Moans or whimpers, occasional complaints | Crying steadily, screaming or sobs, frequent complaints |
| Consolability | Content, relaxed | Reassured by occasional touching, hugging or talking to distracted | Difficult to console or comfort |

Fig. 3.2: FLACC scale

in pain relief measures. The BPI has a has an outline of a body diagram so that the patient is able to mark out the exact site of pain.

- West Haven-Yale multidimensional pain inventory.
- Medical outcomes study 36 item short form (SF-36) health survey.

## INVESTIGATIONS/IMAGING

The metabolism and excretion of most most analgeiscs is via the liver and kidney. Also, the chemotherapy agents used for cancer treatment can cause alteration in renal and liver function of patient. Therefore, blood investigations like renal function and liver function tests are regularly requested in these patients. Most of the cancer patients have some imaging in the form of CT scan or MRI during the diagnosis of cancer. These images need to be evaluated during patient assessment to know the extent of disease as well as to identify possible neurological involvement. These imaging will also guide the physician with the possibility of interventional pain therapy.

### Neuroimaging Assessment of Pain

The newer concept of understanding of pain at the neuronal level is made possible with the help of neuroimaging technology. The term "pain matrix" is collectively referred for the areas in the brain activated by pain and these are primarily the primary somatosensory cortex, the secondary somatosensory cortex, anterior cingulate cortex, insula, prefrontal cortex, thalamus, and cerebellum.[31] Functional neuroimaging is used for objective evaluation of pain rather than depending on verbal reporting.

The alteration in metabolism and neurochemistry in the pain matrix is assessed using certain neuroimaging techniques.[31]

Metabolism alteration can be studied by studying the disturbances noted in the blood flow, brain volume, oxygen concentration, and glucose metabolism and neurochemistry alteration neurotransmitter precursor uptake and receptor binding.

These commonly used the neuroimaging techniques can be classified as:

- Techniques based on hemodynamic methods like magnetic resonance imaging (MRI), functional MRI (fMRI), near-infrared spectrum instrument (NIRS) and positron emission tomography (PET). These methods help us to broadly identify the pain processing areas of the brain and hence to pinpoint the site of pain.
- Techniques based on electrophysiological methods like electroencephalogram (EEG) and magnetoencephalography (MEG), and positron emission tomography (PET).[32] The time components of pain can be analyzed utilizing these methods.

The structural assessment of chronic pain can be done by assessing the gray and white matter changes in neuroimaging. Decrease in volume and density of regional gray matter is observed in chronic pain patients on neuroimaging. These changes in gray matter are attributed to changes in microstructures of gray matter or neuroimmune cell and are related to inflammation in gray matter. Alteration in white matter axonal integrity or axonal fiber pathways within the brain is also observed in patients with chronic pain. So any changes in structural integrity of white matter as suggested is due to pain in th eregions connected by these tracts.

In functional assessment of chronic pain fMRI and PET scans are very popular. fMRI works on the principle of differences in magnetic properties of oxygenated and deoxygenated blood where as PET scan identifies altered neurotransmitter/neuromodulator function in different brain regions in patients with chronic pain.

EEG displays the graphical representation of the voltage differences between different brain regions over time. The oscillatory activity of neurons between euphoria and low excitability is called neural oscillations, and changes in this oscillatory activity are used to assess the chronic pain activity. The expression of pain is represented by the alpha band and the theta band of EEG/MEG.

Different clinical trials are under process to evaluate neuroimaging-based therapies like transcranial direct current stimulation, transcranial magnetic stimulation, deep brain stimulation and real-time fMRI neurofeedback.

## Assessment of Pain in Cognitive Impaired/Critically Ill/Children

- In population who are not able to self-report their pain, the observational pain assessment tools are most useful. The observation of facial expression, how easily the patient can be consoled or distracted, verbal responsiveness and limb position are few of the observational findings used in such an assessment tool. Other tools used are nursing assessment of pain intensity (NAPI) or pediatric pain profile (PPP). Caregivers play important role in assessment of such patients.
- For critically ill patients who are not capable to self-report the pain, a behavioral pain scale (BPS) and a critical care pain observation tool (CPOT) are most commonly used in intensive care unit (ICU).[33, 34] Along with body movement, facial expression, and muscle tension, the compliance of patient with ventilator is also observed in these observational tools.

## Barriers to Adequate Assessment

1. *Patient factors:* The inability of patient to communicate and describe their pain due to language barrier, extremes of age, dementia or learning difficulty are common patient factors which act as major hurdle in pain assessment. Another major patient factor especially in cancer patients is the insecurity of patient that the cancer treatment may get sidelined if they keep complaining about their pain. Fear of becoming dependent/addicted to pain medication and fear of side effects of excess consumption of pain medication is very common in general public and this is another reason for underreporting of pain by cancer patients.
2. *Clinician/ healthcare professional factors:* Lack of knowledge and training regarding assessment of pain amongst the oncologist and nurses can be considered as one of the major barriers in cancer pain management. Early recognition and getting clear history of pain and treating it timely is the cornerstone of cancer pain management. Heavy workload and poor attitude are other factors which contribute towards inadequate pain assessment.[35]
3. *Lack of standardization:* Unavailability of standard pain protocols at the institution, lack of regular training of nurses and doctors in pain assessment, lack of regular documentation of pain assessment are few other reasons leading to inadequate pain assessment.

## Conclusion

Generally, inadequate and irregular assessment of cancer pain is the root cause undertreatment. Inadequate knowledge of pain assessment among clinicians and lack of self-reporting from patients are the two major reasons of suboptimal cancer pain assessment. Pain assessment need to take in account the severity and intensity of pain, characteristic of pain as well as its effect on QoL of patient and their caregivers. Interviewing patient with specific question about pain and taking help of available appropriate and validated questionnaires will help the clinician to reach the mechanism of pain and aid in management. Assessment of pain will be incomplete without a patient interview and medical–neurological examination along with questionnaires guided assessment tools. Regular and repeated assessment of cancer pain patient is an absolute necessity to assess the adequacy of treatment and to identify and manage the side effects of pain medication. Ideally "do you have any pain?" should be one of the routine questions to any cancer patient during each hospital visit and if pain is present, it should be assessed properly and treated.

## References


1. Van den Beuken-van MH, Hochstenbach LM, Joosten EA, Tjan-Heijnen VC, Janssen DJ. Update on prevalence of pain in patients with cancer: Systematic review and meta-analysis. J Pain Symptom Manag. 2016;51:1070–90.
2. Paul A Glare et al. Pain in cancer survivors. JCO 2014;32:1739–47.
3. Gallaway MS, Townsend JS, Shelby D, Puckett MC. Pain Among Cancer Survivors. Prev Chronic Dis 2020;17:190367.
4. Rayment C, Bennett MI. Definition and assessment of chronic pain in advanced disease. Oxf Textb Palliat Med. 2015;519–24.
5. Dworkin RH, Jensen MP, Gammaitoni AR, et al. Symptom profiles differ in patients with neuropathic versus nonneuropathic pain. J Pain 2007;8:118–26.
6. Treede RD, Jensen TS, Campbell JN, Cruccu G, Dostrovsky JO, et al. Neuropathic pain: Redefinition and a grading system for clinical and research purposes. Neurology 2008;70:1630–35.
7. Bennett MI, Rayment C, Hjermstad M, Aass N, Caraceni A, Kaasa S. Prevalence and aetiology of neuropathic pain in cancer patients: A systematic review. Pain 2012;153:359–65.
8. Bennett MI, Kaasa S, Barke A, Korwisi B, Rief W, Treede RD, IASP taskforce for the classification of chronic pain. The IASP classification of chronic pain for ICD-11: Chronic cancer-related pain. Pain 2019;160:38–44.
9. Portenoy RK, Payne D, Jacobsen P. Breakthrough pain: characteristics and impact in patients with cancer pain. Pain 1999;81:129–34.
10. Caraceni A, Davies A, Poulain P, Cortes-Funes H, Panchal SJ, Fanelli G. Guidelines for the management of breakthrough pain in patients with cancer. J Natl Compr Cancer Netw. 2013; 11:S29–S36.
11. Fallon M, Giusti R, Aielli F, Hoskin P, Rolke R, Sharma M, Ripamonti C, ESMO Guidelines Committee. Management of cancer pain in adult patients: esmo clinical practice guidelines. Ann. Oncol. 2018;29:iv166–iv191.
12. Finan PH, Goodin BR, Smith MT. The association of sleep and pain: an update and a path forward. J Pain. 2013;14:1539–52.
13. Duo L, Yu X, Hu R, Duan X, Zhou J, Wang K. Sleep disorders in chronic pain and its neurochemical mechanisms: a narrative review. Front Psychiatry. 2023;14:1157790.
14. Cella DF. Quality of life: concepts and definition. J Pain Symptom Manage 1994;9:186–92.
15. Gill TM, Feinstein AR. A critical appraisal of the quality of quality-of-life measurements. JAMA 1994;272:619–26.
16. O'Boyle CA, Waldron D. Quality of life issues in palliative medicine. J Neurol 1977;244(Suppl 4): S18–25.
17. Derogatis LR, Morrow GR, Fetting J, et al. The prevalence of psychiatric disorders among cancer patients. JAMA 1983;249:751–7.

18. Shacham S, Dar R, Cleeland CS. The relationship of mood state to the severity of clinical pain. Pain 1984;18:187–97.
19. Ahles TA, Blanchard EB, Ruckdeschel JC. The multidimensional nature of cancer-related pain. Pain 1983;17:277–88.
20. Glover J, Dibble SL, Dodd MJ, Miaskowski C. Mood states of oncology outpatients: does pain make a difference? J Pain Symptom Manage 1995;10:120–8.
21. Heim HM, Oei TP. Comparison of prostate cancer patients with and without pain. Pain 1993; 53:159–62.
22. Spielberger C. Manual for the State-Trait Anxiety Inventory. Palo Alto, CA: Consulting Psychologists Press, 2007.
23. Beck A, Steer R. Beck depression inventory manual. San Antonio: Harcourt Brace Jovanovich, 1987.
24. Melzack R. The McGill pain questionnaire: Major properties and scoring methods. Pain. 1975;1: 277–299.
25. Stein C Mendl G. The German counterpart to McGill Pain Questionnaire. Pain. 1988;32:251–255.
26. The short-form McGill pain questionnaire by Melzack, Ronald, 1. The short-form McGill pain questionnaire. Pain 1987;30(2):191–197.
27. Dworkin RH, Turk DC, Revicki DA, Harding G, Coyne KS, Peirce-Sandner S, Bhagwat D, Everton D, Burke LB, Cowan P, Farrar JT, Hertz S, Max MB, Rappaport BA, Melzack R. Development and initial validation of an expanded and revised version of the Short-form McGill Pain Questionnaire (SF-MPQ-2). Pain. 2009;144:35–42.
28. Katz JMR. The McGill Pain Questionnaire: Development, psychometric properties, and usefulness of the long form, short form, and short form-2. In: Turk, DCMR, (ed). Handbook of Pain Assessment. New York: Guilford Press; 2011.
29. Fishman B, Pasternak S, Wallenstein SL, et al. The memorial pain assessment card. A valid instrument for the evaluation of cancer pain. Cancer 1987;60:1151–8.
30. Cleeland CS, Ryan KM. Pain assessment: global use of the brief pain inventory. Ann Acad Med Singapore 1994;23:129–38.
31. Apkarian AV, Bushnell MC, Treede RD, Zubieta JK. Human brain mechanisms of pain perception and regulation in health and disease. European Journal of Pain (London, England). 2005;9(4):463–84.
32. Morton DL, Sandhu JS, Jones AK. Brain imaging of pain: state of the art. J Pain Res. 2016;9:613–24.
33. Gélinas C, Puntillo KA, Joffe AM, Barr J. A validated approach to evaluating psychometric properties of pain assessment tools for use in nonverbal critically ill adults. Semin Respir Crit Care Med. 2013;34(2):153–68.
34. Azevedo-Santos IF, DeSantana JM. Pain measurement techniques: spotlight on mechanically ventilated patients. J Pain Res. 2018;11:2969.
35. lotaibi K, Higgins I, Day J, Chan S. Paediatric pain management: knowledge, attitudes, barriers and facilitators among nurses–integrative review. Int Nurs Rev. 2018;65(4):524–533.
36. Bouhassira D, Attal N, Alchaar H, Boureau F, Bruxelle J, et al. Comparison pf pain syndromes associated with nervous or somatic lesions and development of a new neuropathic pain diagnostic questionnaire (DN4). Pain. 2005;114:29–36.
37. Bennett MI. The LANSS pain scale: the leeds assessment of neuropathic symptoms and signs. Pain. 2000;92:142–157.
38. Freynhagen R, Baron R, Gockel U, Tolle T. Pain DETECT: A new screening questionnaire to detect neuropathic components in patients with back pain. Curr Med Res Opin. 2006;22:1911–20.

Chapter 4

# Cancer Pain Syndromes: An Overview

• Sheetal Gaikwad

## INTRODUCTION

Chronic cancer pain presents a formidable obstacle in oncological management, contributing to compromised patient well-being and exacerbating the challenges associated with their disease. Despite advancements in cancer treatment, the undertreatment of cancer-related pain persists as a formidable issue, primarily attributed to inadequate pain assessment.[1] Effective management of chronic cancer pain necessitates a comprehensive understanding of the underlying pathophysiology, which can be elucidated through meticulous pain assessment.

Pain assessment serves as the cornerstone in the recognition and characterization of various pain syndromes associated with cancer. These syndromes encompass a constellation of symptoms, signs, and related findings, providing clinicians with invaluable insights into the nature and progression of disease. By identifying specific syndromes, clinicians can not only prognosticate disease trajectories but also facilitate informed decision-making regarding diagnostic evaluations and treatment strategies.

Moreover, the recognition of pain syndromes plays a pivotal role in patient counseling and education, enabling healthcare providers to effectively communicate disease progression and potential treatment outcomes to patients and their families.

In this context, it becomes imperative to explore the nuances of chronic cancer pain, delineating between syndromes associated with acute and chronic pain manifestations. By understanding the unique characteristics and implications of these syndromes, healthcare providers can tailor interventions to address the multifaceted needs of patients, thereby optimizing pain management strategies and improving overall patient outcomes.

## CLASSIFICATION

Cancer pain syndromes can be categorized into acute, characterized by sudden onset and short duration, and chronic, that persisting beyond the acute phase.

### Acute Pain Syndromes

These syndromes arise from anticancer therapy, diagnostic and therapeutic interventions or as a direct result of the cancerous tumor.

### *Acute Pain Syndromes due to Treatment*

*1. Mucositis:* The incidence of oral mucositis is particularly high in patients with primary tumors in the oral cavity, oropharynx, or nasopharynx, especially when receiving concomitant chemotherapy or a total radiation dose over 5,000 cGy, or treated with altered fractionation radiation schedules.[2] Mucositis is characterized by inflammation and ulceration of the mucous membranes lining the gastrointestinal tract, commonly affects the mouth, throat, esophagus, and intestines.

The onset of mucositis typically occurs within the first one to two weeks after initiating chemotherapy but this timing can vary based on the type of drugs used, their dosage, and the unique characteristics of each patient. Chemotherapeutic agents such as methotrexate, 5-fluorouracil, and doxorubicin are known to be strongly associated with mucositis. Additionally, various other chemotherapeutic agents, including other anthracyclines, alkylating agents, antimetabolites, taxanes, and targeted therapies like erlotinib, everolimus, and sorafenib, are also known to contribute to mucositis.

The pathophysiology of mucositis entails direct toxicity to mucosal cells, disrupting their rapid division and resulting in ulceration and inflammation. Moreover, treatment induced myelosuppression weakens the immune system, heightening susceptibility to mucosal infections.

Mucositis can manifest with symptoms ranging from mild discomfort to severe pain, and often accompanies other gastrointestinal symptoms. Severe pain can significantly impact a patient's ability to consume food, maintain proper nutrition,thus leading to further complications and treatment delays.

Preventive measures for mucositis include meticulous oral hygiene, hydration, and dietary modifications. Clinical practice guidelines recommend various interventions for prevention and treatment, including the use of anti-inflammatory agents like benzydamine mouthwash which is recommended specifically for patients with post radiation head, neck cancers with mucositis, salt and baking soda mouth rinses which is preferred following chemotherapy, photobiomodulation therapy, and cryotherapy.[3]

Management of mucositis-related pain involves a multimodal approach. Systemic analgesics such as nonsteroidal anti-inflammatory drugs (NSAIDs), opioids, and adjuvant medications may be prescribed to mitigate pain. Antimicrobial agents may also be necessary to prevent or treat secondary infections, particularly in neutropenic patients.

In cases of severe mucositis that is WHO grading as 3 (ulcers that require liquid diet) or 4 (ulcers where oral intake is not possible) and pain is intense, more aggressive pain management strategies may be required. This can include the use of transdermal fentanyl patches or patient-controlled analgesia (PCA) systems, allowing patients to self-administer analgesics as needed within prescribed limits.

Overall, effective management of mucositis requires a comprehensive approach aimed at reducing inflammation, controlling pain, preventing infection, and supporting the patient's nutritional and hydration needs.

*2. Radiation induced colitis and proctitis:* Acute radiation toxicity can result in inflammation and ulceration of mucous membranes within the radiation port, leading to various pain syndromes depending on the involved field. For example, radiation in the head and neck region may cause oral mucositis, pharyngitis, and esophagitis, while radiation in the pelvic area can lead to proctitis, enteritis, cystitis-urethritis, or vaginal ulceration.

Radiation therapy for pelvic and intra-abdominal tumors often encompasses the small bowel and colon within the treatment area. Over time, adjustments to radiotherapy techniques have aimed to reduce adverse effects, such as patient positioning , specialized treatment tables, dosage limitations, and multiportal delivery methods.[4]

Despite these improvements, radiation therapy can still adversely affect normal tissues, particularly the bowel, including small bowel and colorectum. At present, there are no targeted therapies available for acute radiation colitis, and management typically involves addressing symptoms such as diarrhea, abdominal pain, and tenesmus with supportive care.

The rectum is commonly impacted by pelvic radiotherapy, with a significant number of patients experiencing rectal symptoms during and after treatment. These symptoms may include loose stools, urgency, bleeding, pain, or tenesmus. Although acute symptoms often worsen throughout treatment, endoscopic and histologic findings typically peak around 2 weeks after start of radiation therapy and may stabilize or improve by treatment completion.[4]

Acute radiation proctitis (RP) is typically self-limiting and does not predispose patients to chronic RP. In about 20% of cases undergoing external beam radiation, a brief interruption of therapy may be necessary.[4] Management of acute RP primarily involves supportive care, including hydration, anti-diarrheal medications, and the use of butyrate enemas to facilitate tissue healing.

3. *Acute painful neuropathy:* Acute painful neuropathy is a common complication of chemotherapy, particularly associated with vinca alkaloids like vincristine, platinum-based agents such as cisplatin, thalidomide, and bortezomib. Symptoms typically arise following chemotherapy administration, characterized by burning pain, with or without accompanying paresthesia, and may include motor or sensory deficits like weakness or proprioceptive loss.

The mechanism of action involves inhibition of axonal transport, particularly with platinum-based agents and vinca alkaloids, while taxanes exert direct toxic effects on neuronal cell bodies and axons.[3] Acute pain may subside over weeks but can recur with subsequent chemotherapy cycles, occasionally evolving into chronic neuropathic pain.[1] Some patients experience symptomatic relief, yet exhibit long-term neurologic abnormalities.

Rarely, acute chemotherapy-related mononeuropathy, primarily associated with vincristine, may manifest as orofacial pain.[1]

In managing acute chemotherapy-induced neuropathy, clinicians evaluate the appropriateness of dose adjustments or discontinuation of chemotherapy for patients with severe neuropathy or functional disability. Duloxetine is currently the only agent supported by evidence for treating established painful chemotherapy-induced peripheral neuropathy (CIPN), although its benefits are often limited.[5]

4. *Diffuse bone pain /arthralgia and steroid pseudorheumatism:* Aromatase inhibitors (AIs) are often recommended for postmenopausal women diagnosed with hormone receptor-positive early-stage breast cancer. It can frequently cause AI-induced arthralgia characterized by morning stiffness and joint discomfort in various sites without signs

of inflammation, typically beginning around 2 months into treatment and peaking at around 6 months, attributed to the acute drop in estrogen; management involves education, counseling, physiotherapy, occupational therapy, and analgesics with or without anticonvulsants and antidepressants.[6]

Acute bone pain and arthralgia are also common adverse effects associated with therapies such as trans- retinoic acid, paclitaxel and colony stimulating factors. These pains are typically generalized in nature.

On the other hand, acute myalgia and arthralgia may occur following the abrupt cessation of steroid therapy, particularly with high doses and long-term usage. The pathogenesis of steroid pseudorheumatism is poorly understood, but it may involve the sensitization of joint and muscle mechanoreceptors and nociceptors.

Treatment usually involves restarting steroids and tapering them gradually to alleviate symptoms.

*5. Chemotherapy induced headache:*

- *Intrathecal methotrexate:* Can mimic meningitis with symptoms like headache, vomiting, and fever. Transretinoic acid: Can cause temporary headaches.
- *L-asparaginase:* May lead to cerebral thrombosis, presenting with severe headaches and other neurological symptoms often requiring intensive care.

*6. Cutaneous toxicities:*

- *Palmar–plantar erythrodysesthesia syndrome:* Hand-foot syndrome characterized by painful rash on palms and soles following chemotherapy with drugs like cytarabine, capecitabine, etc. It may progress to bullous formation and desquamation.
- *Other cutaneous toxicities:* Result from epidermal growth factor receptor inhibitors (e.g. erlotinib, sorafenib) manifesting as papulopustules, xerosis, paronychia, maculopapular rash, mucositis, and hyperpigmentation. Severe cases may require dose reduction and at times discontinuation of treatment.

*7. 5-Fluorouracil (capecitabine)–induced anginal chest pain:* Coronary vasospasm can occur, necessitating primary treatment of the cardiac event.

*8. Intravesical therapy:* Intravesical bacillus Calmette-Guérin or other local therapies for transitional cell carcinoma of the bladder may cause transient bladder irritability characterized by frequency and/or painful micturition.

*9. Hepatic artery infusion pain:* Severe abdominal pain during hepatic artery infusion chemotherapy may occur, often related to extrahepatic infusion and gastroduodenal ulceration. Intense abdominal pain has been observed specifically with oxaliplatin infusion without extrahepatic involvement. Oxaliplatin preparation time and hepatic artery diameter are potential influencing factors for pain during hepatic artery infusion chemotherapy (HIAC), as noted by Wu.[7] Pain treatment typically involves systemic analgesics, but intra-arterial lidocaine administered before and during the procedure may provide additional pain relief.

*10. Pain resulting from intravenous infusion:* Intravenous infusion pain may stem from various causes including chemical phlebitis, vesicant extravasation, venous spasm, and anthracycline-associated flares. Venous spasm, marked by brief pain without inflammation, can be alleviated by slowing the infusion rate. Extravasation, the most severe complication, may require local compresses and short-term analgesics for management. Anthracyclines like doxorubicin may elicit a venous flare reaction, manifesting as localized urticaria and transient discomfort at the infusion site.[1]

*11. Steroid-induced perineal burning:* This syndrome may develop shortly after the rapid intravenous administration of glucocorticoids. It occurs especially with dexamethasone. Its exact cause is uncertain.The patients may find reassurance in knowing that it typically resolves swiftly and is not linked to any injury.[1]

### *Acute Pain due to Direct Invasion of Tumor* (Table 4.1)

**Table 4.1: Acute pain syndromes due to tumor**

| Acute pain syndrome | Characteristics | Diagnosis and intervention |
|---|---|---|
| Pathologic fracture | Sudden onset of focal aching pain | Confirmation via radiography. Treatment is integration of analgesics with surgical, radiation, interventional, and pharmacologic therapies |
| Obstruction or perforation of a hollow viscus | Pain characteristics vary based on site and pathology. Prompt intervention such as stenting and symptom control therapies | Diagnosis usually straightforward, aiding in prompt intervention |
| Intratumoral hemorrhage | Presents with acute pain; imaging confirms diagnosis | Early intervention with transfusions and bleeding control essential to prevent life-threatening events |
| Superior vena cava obstruction | Dyspnea, facial swelling, and dilated neck veins. Acute neck pain or headache may occur | Effective treatment with vascular stenting or radiation therapy |
| Pain due to acute thrombosis | Acute pain and swelling in the affected extremity | Diagnostic evaluation warranted, even with minimal swelling |

## Chronic Pain Syndromes

Tumor related chronic pain:

*1. Bony metastatic pain:* The skeleton is a frequent site for metastasis for solid tumors, including breast, prostate, kidney, and lung cancers. Once bone metastasis occurs, it disrupts the balance of bone resorption, formation and remodelling. Common sites for bone metastasis include vertebrae, ribs, pelvis, and proximal humerus and femur. The mechanisms underlying chronic bony metastatic pain are varied, involving tumor implantation, alterations in bone metabolism, increased mechanical stimulation, activation and modification of peripheral nerves, peripheral nerve remodelling, and adaptive changes in the central nervous system.

Bone metastasis can manifest in various forms, including lytic, blastic, or mixed lesions. In lytic lesions, bone resorption surpasses bone formation, while in blastic lesions, the opposite occurs, resulting in a fragile bone structure.

Skeletal-related events (SREs) are common complications of bone metastasis, affecting approximately half of patients.[8,9] These events include pathological fractures, spinal cord compression, and severe pain, often necessitating emergency radiation therapy or surgery. SREs significantly impact patients' quality of life and contribute to morbidity associated with bone metastasis.

Vertebral metastasis can lead to compression of myeloradicular structures, such as spinal nerve roots and the spinal cord, resulting in neurological deficits or severe pain. These are emergency situations especially spinal cord compression where, immediate surgical intervention may be necessary. Concurrent therapy with corticosteroids can provide temporary relief from symptoms related to pressure and edema caused by the tumor deposit. The decision regarding the aggressiveness of surgical intervention depends on various factors, including preoperative neurological status, performance status, aggressiveness of the primary tumor, and patient's life expectancy. In advanced cancer scenarios, relieving compression and stabilizing the condition through palliative surgical measures, along with subsequent radiation therapy, can enhance the patient's well-being.

In addition to surgery, radiation therapy is an effective treatment option for achieving local tumor control and palliating painful bone metastasis. Radiation therapy enhances the ossification of osteolytic bone metastases and can provide pain relief by numbing small nerve endings, thus enhancing bone stability.[9]

For non-vertebral bone metastasis, surgical intervention with internal fixation is indicated for pathological fractures, even in advanced disease stages. In selected patients with impending fractures of long bones, prophylactic fixation followed by postoperative radiation therapy may be warranted. Initiating treatment with bone-targeted agents like zoledronate, denosumab upon diagnosis of bone metastases, regardless of symptomatic presentation, is advised to delay the time to first skeletal-related events (SRE) and reduce skeletal morbidity. Non-steroidal anti-inflammatory agents such as diclofenac as well as paracetamol are usually the mainstay of analgesic regimens for bone metastasis pain, which is predominantly somatic in nature. However, given the neuropathic component, the addition of strong opioids, adjuvants such as anticonvulsants, and antidepressants in small doses may be necessary for comprehensive pain management.

Other skeletal metastases may present as summarized in Table 4.2. Comprehensive management of plexopathy involves targeted radiation therapy, multimodal pain control measures, tailored chemotherapy, occasional neurolysis, interventions for dysesthesias, and lymphedema management, with a focus on preventive measures to preserve quality of life.

2. *Plexopathy:* Tumors have the capability to invade cervical, brachial, and lumbosacral plexuses either by direct infiltration from nearby organs or through metastasis to regional lymph nodes. In certain instances, tumors may follow the epineurium of the nerve plexus. Radiation-induced plexopathy is a significant concern in patients with a history of cancer treatment however, regional chemotherapy or fibrosis post-surgical resection of the primary tumor can also lead to plexopathy in some cases. The types of plexopathies that one may encounter are as mentioned (Table 4.3).

3. *Painful cranial neuralgias/head neck cancer pain syndrome:* Specific cranial neuralgias can occur from metastasis at the base of skull, leptomeningeal metastasis or due to invasive head and neck tumors.

a. ***Glossopharyngeal neuralgia:*** Presents with severe pain in the throat or neck triggered or aggravated by swallowing The pain may typically radiate to ear or mastoid region and triggered by various activities such as chewing, swallowing or speaking.
b. ***Trigeminal neuralgia:*** Pain is continuous with paroxysms of breakthrough pain which are severe and distressing. Head neck tumors invading foramen ovale, middle cranial

**Table 4.2: Skeletal metastasis and the pain pattern**

| Syndrome | Pain pattern |
|---|---|
| *Vertebral pain syndromes* | |
| Odontoid lesions | Base of the neck pain |
| Lower cervical and upper thoracic vertebral lesions | Interscapular pain |
| Lower thoracic or upper lumbar vertebral lesions | Pain iliac crest or buttock |
| *Pelvic and hip metastases* | |
| Pelvic metastases | Persistent localized discomfort; hip or groin pain exacerbated by walking; discomfort in the knee or thigh |
| Piriformis syndrome | Pain in the buttocks and/or radiating down the leg; worsened by internal hip rotation or painful plexopathy |
| Sacral syndrome | Intense localized pain spreading to the buttocks, back of the thighs, or perineum; worsened in supine or sitting position, relieved in orthostatic position or walking. Painful movement at the hip due to involvement of lateral hip rotators |
| *Base of skull metastases* | |
| Orbital metastasis | Retroorbital pain, proptosis, diplopia, visual distortion, chemosis of the involved eye, ophthalmoparesis, ipsilateral papilledema |
| Parasellar metastasis | Retroorbital and frontal pain; ophthalmoparesis with diplopia |
| Middle cranial fossa metastasis | Cheek or jaw pain; painful trigeminal neuropathy |
| Jugular foramen metastasis | Neck, ear or shoulder pain; glossopharyngeal neuralgia; syncope |
| Occipital condyle metastasis | Pain on one side of the back of the head, stiffness in the neck, tilting of the head, and shrinking of the tongue on one side due to tumor lateral to the foramen magnum |
| Metastatic deposits at clivus | Pain at the crown of the skull aggravated by bending the neck downward |

fossa or posterior fossa tumors can mimic trigeminal neuralgia, along with sensory disturbances involving ears, cheek, jaw and sometimes eyes.

***Treatment:*** The management of cancer-related pain in the head and neck region poses challenges due to the area's rich innervation and dynamic pain triggered by essential movements like talking and swallowing. In managing cancer-related pain in the head and neck, regional nerve blocks may be necessary when systemic therapy appears inadequate. A 3-stage approach involving diagnostic, prognostic, and therapeutic blocks is recommended. Diagnostic blocks with short-acting local anesthetics identify pain sources, prognostic blocks allow patients to experience block effects, and therapeutic blocks, either non-destructive or neurolytic, can provide pain relief. The interventions that can be offered are sphenopalatine, trigeminal and stellate ganglion block, glossopharyngeal nerve block and intrathecal implants.[10]

*4. Visceral pain syndrome:* Visceral pain, constitutes 28% of primary tumor-related pain, often coexists with neuropathic or somatic pain and may stem from treatment complications or concurrent illnesses.[12,13] Visceral pain can be due to hepatic metastases

Table 4.3: Types of plexopathies and their presentation

| Plexopathy | Anatomy and function | Pathophysiology | Clinical presentation |
|---|---|---|---|
| Cervical plexopathy[11] | Formed by C1–C4 nerve roots, innervating neck muscles and skin | Tumor invasion directly or via metastasis, commonly from head and neck cancers, lymphomas, lung adenocarcinomas | Neck, shoulder, or throat pain worsened by movement, swallowing, or coughing. Sensory loss may occur, along with potential motor dysfunction |
| Brachial plexopathy[11] | Originates from C5–C8 and T1 nerve roots, supplying arm muscles and skin | Often caused by direct extension or metastasis from lung or breast tumors. May affect lower (C8–T1) or upper (C5–C7) plexus | Shoulder and arm pain, reflex changes, and muscle weakness. Potential lymphedema if prior radiotherapy or surgery. Horner's syndrome possible with epidural involvement |
| Lumbosacral plexopathy[11] | Arises from L1–S4 nerve roots, controlling abdominal and leg muscles | Commonly invaded by pelvic tumors or metastases. May present as part of original tumor or due to direct compression or infiltration of nerves | Severe, constant leg pain exacerbated by movement. Followed by progressive numbness and weakness. Sensory disturbances, rectal involvement, and perineal symptoms may occur, particularly with colorectal or pelvic tumors |

causing capsular distension, biliary obstruction, pancreatic cancer, retroperitoneal adenopathy, and visceral organ obstruction such as colonic obstruction, mesenteric infiltration, and peritoneal implants of cancer. Intestinal obstruction leading to perforation, gangrene, mesenteric ischemia are some of the complications requiring surgical intervention.

Visceral pain is generally described as pressure-like, intermittently squeezing or cramping, with vague localization and difficulty in articulating its character. Nausea, vomiting, and sweating frequently accompany visceral pain, and in severe cases, the pain may radiate to superficial sites.

The management of visceral pain requires a distinct approach from somatic pain due to differences in pain processing. Adjuvant analgesics like gabapentinoids should be considered early in opioid therapy to prevent opioid-induced hyperalgesia and reduce opioid-related side effects. Interventional procedures targeting the sympathetic ganglia such as coeliac plexus or superior hypogastric plexus, tailored to the primary tumor and origin of pain, should be employed promptly to prevent the development of chronic, poorly responsive visceral pain.[12]

*5. Post-surgical chronic pain syndrome:* Post-surgical chronic pain often arises from nerve or plexus injury sustained during surgery. Symptoms typically manifest months after the surgical procedure and are neuropathic in nature. Patients may experience a spectrum of sensations including dull, burning, and aching pain, as well as allodynia and hyperalgesia. Treatment includes anticonvulsants, antidepressants along with opioids as recommended by WHO ladder.

i. ***Post-thoracotomy pain syndrome (PTPS),*** also known as chronic post-thoracotomy pain or post-thoracotomy neuralgia, is characterized by pain recurring or persisting along a thoracotomy incision for at least two months after the surgical procedure, as defined by the International Association for the Study of Pain (IASP). Post-thoracotomy pain syndrome (PTPS), involves a multifaceted treatment approach including conservative measures like anti-epileptics and antidepressants for neuropathic pain, analgesics for movement-related pain, and interventional options such as nerve injections and spinal cord stimulation, tailored to individual patient needs and pain severity to enhance comfort and quality of life.[14]

ii. ***Post-mastectomy pain syndrome (PMPS):*** It is a prevalent complication affecting a significant percentage of women post-mastectomy, yet research into its definition, causes, and treatment remains limited. Despite its high incidence (35.8% at our institution),[15] the exact etiology and pathogenesis of PMPS are not fully understood. PMPS significantly impacts patients' overall functional ability and quality of life. Treatment modalities encompass psychological interventions, pharmacotherapy, interventional therapy, physical therapy, and surgery. However, further research is needed to optimize treatment approaches and improve outcomes for patients experiencing PMPS.[16]

iii. ***Post-radical neck dissection pain:*** Neuropathic pain due to injury to cervical plexus along with musculoskeletal imbalance in shoulder girdle due to surgical removal of neck muscles can occur in few patients. It can rarely get complicated with suprascapular nerve entrapment with selective wasting of supraspinatous and infraspinatous muscle.

*6. Post-radiation chronic pain:* Post-radiation chronic pain syndrome encompasses various conditions that can manifest months to years after radiation therapy. Radiation-induced cervical, brachial or lumbosacral plexopathies may arise, presenting with less prominent pain compared to cancer-related plexopathy. Weakness, sensory changes, lymphedema, and skin alterations are common features. Distinguishing radiation-induced plexopathy from malignant plexopathy may be challenging, necessitating repeated imaging and biopsies. Chronic radiation myelopathy involves sensory symptoms, including burning dysesthesia, often preceding motor and autonomic dysfunction. Lymphedema, a frequent outcome of radiation, can also lead to pain, typically musculoskeletal, although neuropathic pain may occur due to nerve injury or entrapment.

***Chronic radiation proctitis:*** Patients with chronic radiation proctitis (RP) may experience symptoms ranging from rectal discomfort and passing stool with mucus to severe complications such as malabsorption, bleeding, strictures, fistulas, and bowel obstruction. Involvement of the anal sphincter may result in fecal incontinence, while conditions like diabetes and peripheral arterial disease heighten the risk of chronic RP. Differentiating chronic RP from disease recurrence is crucial, especially in patients presenting with symptoms years after radiation therapy.

Treatment for mild to moderate cases involves anti-inflammatory agents such as short-chain fatty acid enema and sucralfate enema.[17] Short-chain fatty acids act by providing a source of energy for the colonic epithelial cells and reducing inflammation in the rectal mucosa. Sucralfate forms a protective barrier over ulcerated areas, preventing further injury and promoting healing. Hyperbaric oxygen therapy (HBOT) is another option, working by improving tissue oxygenation, potentially stimulating angiogenesis, and exerting antibacterial effects. Hyperbaric oxygen therapy (HBOT) entails inhaling pure oxygen within a pressurized chamber. This process facilitates the dissolution of oxygen in the blood plasma at elevated concentrations, thereby augmenting oxygen supply to tissues. This increased oxygen availability promotes tissue healing and may help alleviate symptoms of chronic RP.

In cases of severe and persistent symptoms, endoscopic interventions such as formalin application, Argon plasma coagulation or ND:YAG laser therapy may be necessary. Formalin application involves direct cauterization of ulcers and telangiectasias via rigid proctoscopy under sedation, to promote hemostasis. Argon plasma coagulation delivers a burst of ionized argon gas, generating heat to coagulate bleeding vessels and seal ulcerated areas. ND:YAG laser therapy achieves similar effects through selective photocoagulation of abnormal tissue.

Severe complications like perforation require urgent surgical intervention to prevent life-threatening outcomes.

7. *Painful gynecomastia:* Antiandrogen treatment used for prostrate cancer often leads to the development of gynecomastia and mastodynia, known as bicalutamide-induced breast events (BEs), due to an estrogen-androgen imbalance in breast tissue.[18] These adverse effects can be alleviated through pharmacological approaches like tamoxifen and anastrozole, which act on estrogen receptors and inhibit the aromatization of androgens, respectively. Additionally, low-dose radiotherapy (RT) of the breast tissue can induce hypoplasia or aplasia, reducing the number of ducts and preventing gynecomastia.

## Summary

The chapter highlights the significance of thorough pain assessment and tailored management in cancer pain. Understanding pain syndromes aids in prognosis, treatment decisions, and patient empowerment. A multidisciplinary approach, including pharmacological and non-pharmacological interventions, optimizes outcomes. In summary, individualized care plays a crucial role in easing distress and improving the well-being of patients amidst the challenges posed by cancer-related pain.

## References

1. Portenoy RK, Ahmed E. Cancer pain syndromes. Hematol Oncol Clin North Am. 2018;32(3):371–386. doi: 10.1016/j.hoc.2018.01.002. Epub 2018 Mar 22. PMID: 29729775.
2. Ps SK, Balan A, Sankar A, Bose T. Radiation induced oral mucositis. Indian J Palliat Care. 2009;15(2):95–102. doi: 10.4103/0973-1075.58452. PMID: 20668585; PMCID: PMC2902123.
3. Elad S, Cheng KKF, Lalla RV, Yarom N, Hong C, Logan RM, et al. Mucositis Guidelines Leadership Group of the Multinational Association of Supportive Care in Cancer and International Society of Oral Oncology (MASCC/ISOO). MASCC/ISOO clinical practice guidelines for the management of mucositis secondary to cancer therapy. Cancer. 2020 Oct 1;126(19):4423–4431. doi: 10.1002/cncr.33100. Epub 2020 Jul 28. Erratum in: Cancer. 2021;127(19):3700. PMID: 32786044; PMCID: PMC7540329.
4. Kennedy GD, Heise CP. Radiation colitis and proctitis. Clin Colon Rectal Surg. 2007;20(1):64–72. doi: 10.1055/s-2007-970202. PMID: 20011363; PMCID: PMC2780150.
5. Loprinzi CL, Lacchetti C, Bleeker J, Cavaletti G, Chauhan C, Hertz DL, et al. Prevention and management of chemotherapy-induced peripheral neuropathy in survivors of adult cancers: ASCO Guideline Update. Journal of Clinical Oncology. 2020;38(28):JCO.20.01399.
6. Younus J, Kligman L. Management of aromatase inhibitor-induced arthralgia. Curr Oncol. 2010;17(1):87–90. doi: 10.3747/co.v17i1.474. PMID: 20179809; PMCID: PMC2826784.

7. Wu Z, Guo W, Chen S, Zhuang W. Determinants of pain in advanced HCC patients recieving hepatic artery infusion chemotherapy. Invest New Drugs. 2021;39(2):394–9. doi: 10.1007/s10637-020-01009-x. Epub 2020 Oct 1. PMID: 33006020; PMCID: PMC7960585.
8. Jing D, Zhao Q, Zhao Y, Lu X, Feng Y, Zhao B, Zhao X. Management of pain in patients with bone metastases. Front Oncol. 2023;13:1156618. doi: 10.3389/fonc.2023.1156618. PMID: 37007073; PMCID: PMC10063159.
9. Jehn CF, Diel IJ, Overkamp F, Kurth A, Schaefer R, Miller K, et al. Management of metastatic bone disease algorithms for diagnostics and treatment. Anticancer Research [Internet]. 2016;36(6):2631–7. Available from: https://ar.iiarjournals.org/content/36/6/2631
10. Ortíz VMS, Ornelas GEA, Flores Cantisani JA, Torres JIR, Flores FC. Interventional techniques for head and neck cancer pain [Internet]. www.intechopen.com. IntechOpen; 2017. Available from: https://www.intechopen.com/chapters/56045
11. Jaeckle K. Available from: https://www.soc-neuro-onc.org/UploadedFiles/Levin/Levin_ch18_p413-422.pdf
12. Davis MP. Drug management of visceral pain: Concepts from basic research. Pain Research and Treatment. 2012;2012:1–18.
13. Mercadante S, Klepstad P, Kurita GP, Sjøgren P, Giarratano A. Sympathetic blocks for visceral cancer pain management: A systematic review and EAPC recommendations. Critical Reviews in Oncology/Hematology. 2015;96(3):577–83.
14. Hegarty D. Post thoracotomy pain syndrome: What pain management options do we have? J Surg Transplant Sci 2017;5(3):1059.
15. Kakati, Barnali; Nair, Nita; Chatterjee, Aparna. Post mastectomy pain syndrome at an Indian tertiary cancer centre and its impact on quality of life. Indian Journal of Cancer 2023;60(2):p 275–281. | DOI: 10.4103/ijc.ijc_861_21
16. Salati SA, Alsulaim L, Alharbi MH, Alharbi NH, Alsenaid TM, Alaodah SA, et al. Postmastectomy pain syndrome: A narrative review. Cureus. 2023;15(10): e47384. doi: 10.7759/cureus.47384. PMID: 38021812; PMCID: PMC10657609.
17. Dahiya DS, Kichloo A, Tuma F, Albosta M, Wani F. Radiation proctitis and management strategies. Clin Endosc. 2022;55(1):22–32. doi: 10.5946/ce.2020.288. Epub 2021 Nov 18. PMID: 34788934; PMCID: PMC8831406
18. Fagerlund A, Cormio L, Palangi L, Lewin R, Santanelli di Pompeo F, Elander A, Selvaggi G. Gynecomastia in patients with prostate cancer: A systematic review. PLoS One. 2015;10(8):e0136094. doi: 10.1371/journal.pone.0136094. PMID: 26308532; PMCID: PMC4550398.

Chapter 5

# Bone Pain

• Sukhada Savarkar

## INTRODUCTION

Cancer-induced bone pain (CIBP) is a common debilitating condition. It is linked to a reduced quality of life (QoL) and affects both the physical and mental well-being of individuals.

According to a WHO report[1] published in 1990, nearly 4 million people experience bone pain due to malignancy. With the current increasing global burden of cancer and improved survival due to technical and scientific advances; the incidence of CIBP is only expected to rise posing major challenge in cancer pain management. This chapter seeks to explore the epidemiology, mechanisms of CIBP and current treatment options for CIBP.

## EPIDEMIOLOGY OF CIBP

CIBP can be caused by bony metastasis or primary bone tumors. Incidence of primary bone tumors is relatively rare representing for only 0.2% of all cancers.[2] However bony involvement is seen in almost 60–84% of advanced metastatic cancers and nearly 70% of patients with bone metastasis experience CIBP.[3]

Skeleton is the third most common site of tumor metastasis after lungs and liver. Multiple myeloma and cancer of the breast, prostate, lungs, thyroid, kidneys, and ovaries are commonly associated with bone metastases. Up to 80% of all bone metastases are associated with cancer of the breast, lungs, and prostate.[4]

Breast cancer and prostate cancer contribute to approximately 65–75% of bone metastases in females and males respectively. Thyroid cancer, bladder cancer, renal cell carcinoma, and melanoma have relative incidences of bony metastases at 60%, 40%, 20–25%, and 14–45% respectively.[5] The most affected sites are the vertebrae (69%), followed by pelvic bones (41%), long bones (especially the proximal femur) (25%), and the skull (14%).

## CLINICAL FEATURES OF CIBP

In almost 20% patients, bone pain or a pathological bone fracture serves as the initial symptom of cancer. Pain may even precede radiological changes in bone in some cases.

Most of the patients with bone metastasis present with continuous pain that has a gradual onset and increases in intensity as the disease progresses over time.[3] Typically, it tends to be well localized to one or more specific areas. Pain is usually dull aching in nature with episodes of stabbing pain. Bony pain is usually associated with worsening of symptoms at night. It is crucial to understand that the intensity of pain is not always linked to the degree of bony metastases. It is difficult to predict the intensity of pain by tumor type or size. Patients with extensive bony lesions may experience only mild pain whereas a single lesion can be responsible for severe pain.

Bone metastases are often linked with incident pain, which is a form of breakthrough (episodic) pain. It can be defined as a transient flare of pain superimposed on an otherwise stable background pain which is being treated effectively with analgesics.[6] Bony metastases commonly cause movement related incident pain episodes. It may be induced by pain-inducing manoeuvres like body movement or weight-bearing. It is present in almost 75% of patients with bone metastases. Incident pain is usually acute, severe in intensity and difficult to treat due to its short lasting and unpredictable nature. It can significantly impact patients' daily lives and quality of life, presenting a major clinical challenge.

With progressive disease, the bone destruction becomes extensive and patients may experience pain due to pathological fractures, involvement, or compression of peripheral nerves, nerve roots, plexuses or spinal cord. Involvement of central or peripheral nervous system is responsible for neuropathic pain in these patients.

## MECHANISM OF CIBP

The pathophysiology underlying metastasis and CIBP is intricate and multifactorial, involving inflammatory, ischemic, neuropathic, compressive, or injurious mechanisms. Extensive research and experimental studies conducted over the past few decades have shed light on the nociceptive processes associated with bone metastases. This involves complex interactions among tumor cells, bone cells, activated inflammatory cells and bone-innervating neurons.

The initial step in bone metastasis involves the separation of cancer cells from the primary tumor into the systemic circulation. These tumor cells undergo a transition from epithelial to mesenchymal cells, facilitated by the loss of intercellular adhesion proteins on their surfaces, primarily mediated by matrix metalloproteinases (MMPs). Additionally, tumor cells produce vascular endothelial growth factor (VEGF) and chemokines from the CXCL family (e.g. CXCL12 and CCL2), which recruit leukocytes and endothelial cells into the tumor microenvironment, leading to the formation of an abnormal tumor vascular system distinguished by increased permeability and expression of cell adhesion molecules (CAMs). These factors collectively facilitate the penetration of tumor cells into the circulation.[7]

Upon entering the systemic circulation, tumor cells face the challenge of surviving in a new foreign environment. Normally, if the cancer cells lose intercellular connections, they undergo cell death. Inhibition of this physiologically programmed cell death occurs in cancer cells via the overexpression of tropomyosin receptor kinase B (TrkB) on the tumor cell membrane.[7]

The mechanism by which tumor cells enter bone tissue is not fully understood, but the CXCL12–CXC–chemokine receptor 4 chemokine system plays a crucial role in this process.[8] CXCL12 is involved in various cellular processes, including the upregulation of integrin $\alpha V\beta 3$ on tumor cell surfaces, which enhances the adherence of tumor cells to endothelial cells in the bone marrow.

Once in the bone tissue, metastatic tumor cells proliferate and cause progressive bone damage. Tumor cells, stromal cells, and inflammatory cells activated by tumor cells release various mediators that act on osteoblasts, osteoclasts, and bone-innervating nerve fibers. These mediators include endothelin, bradykinin, proteases, interleukin (IL) 6, hydrogen ions ($H^+$), colony-stimulating factors (CSFs), nerve growth factor (NGF), prostaglandin (PG) E2, serotonin, and tumor necrosis factor (TNF). Collectively, these mediators stimulate sensory nerve endings innervating the bone tissue, leading to nociception.

In a healthy bone, the density of sensory nerve supply varies across different compartments. The periosteum has the highest nerve density, followed by the bone marrow, while mineralized bone receives fewer nerve fibers, mainly consisting of thinly myelinated and unmyelinated A-δ or C-sensory nerve fibers.[9]

Numerous receptors and ion channels present on these sensory nerve endings play pivotal roles in detecting and transmitting noxious stimuli generated by tumor cells and associated cells (such as stromal and immune cells) through the release of various mediators as mentioned above. Endothelin receptor (ETAR), prostaglandin (PG) receptors, TrkA receptors, bradykinin receptors, cytokine receptors, chemokine receptors, TRPV1 (transient receptor potential channel, vanilloid subfamily member 1), acid-sensing ion channel 3 (ASIC3), and purinergic receptor (P2X3) are some of the key receptors involved in facilitating these processes.

Normally in a healthy bone; remodelling is a continuous process regulated by a delicate balance between bone-forming osteoblastic activity and bone resorption by osteoclasts. However, when cancer cells invade the bone, this balance is disrupted. Growth factors like IGF and TGF-beta, which are typically released into the bone marrow and utilized by osteoblasts to form new bone, instead facilitate the growth and survival of tumor cells. Cancer cells release endothelin, leading to osteoblast activation and proliferation, resulting in the formation of weak, fracture-prone new bone. Additionally, activated osteoblasts release RANKL (receptor activator of nuclear factor kappa ligand), promoting the proliferation and maturation of osteoclasts, which initiate bone resorption, leading to osteolysis and the release of growth factors that further promote tumor growth. This creates a vicious cycle between tumor cells, osteoblasts, and osteoclasts, exacerbating bone destruction while promoting tumor cell survival.

The tumor cells, thus damage the bone indirectly by primarily activating the RANKL/RANK system. The interaction between RANKL and RANK is crucial in the proliferation, differentiation, and maturation of osteoclasts, which actively resorb bone by creating a highly acidic resorption site, often referred to as a "bay" or "pit," between the osteoclast and the bone. This acidosis stimulates channels like TRPV1 or ASIC3, triggering cancer-induced bone pain (CIBP).[7] This disturbed homeostasis renders the bone more prone to skeletal-related events (SREs) like pathological fracture, spinal cord compression, need for surgery and hypercalcemia.

Depending on the radiological and histological appearance, bone metastases can be classified as osteolytic, osteosclerotic, or mixed. Breast cancer and multiple myeloma are typically associated with osteolytic lesions, whereas, osteoblastic lesions commonly occur in prostate cancer. Osteolytic lesions can be dangerous and are associated with the high-risk of fracture. Osteoblastic bone remodelling also increases the risk of pathological fractures but to a lesser extent. Eventually, irrespective of the type of metastasis (osteolytic, osteosclerotic, or mixed), continued destruction of the normal bone structure, compromised bone stability, and diminished mechanical resistance can result in pathological fractures across all types.

Tumor cells also stimulate abnormal proliferation of sensory and sympathetic nerve fibers, leading to the formation of a network of new nerve fibers with distinct morphology, organization, and density. Density of these fibers can be 10–70 times higher than the density of nerve fibers in normal bone. Studies have shown that NGF which is expressed abundantly in tumor cells and other inflammatory cells plays a significant role in creation of such neuroma like structures within tumor tissue.[10,11]

In normal bone, sensory and sympathetic nerve fibers are distinct from each other. Tumor cells stimulate sensory and sympathetic nerve fibers leading to neural reorganization and the formation of connections between these nerve fibers. As a result, nociception can also be produced by the activation of sympathetic fibers. This nerve sprouting and pathological nerve growth associated with bone metastasis contributes towards CIBP.[7,12]

## INVESTIGATIONS OF CIBP

Diagnosis of bone metastasis is generally easy even in patients with unknown primary tumor. Bone scans detect metastases with a high sensitivity. However, bone scans have a high false positive rate of around 40–50%. Therefore, any abnormality detected in bone scan needs to be confirmed by radiography.[3]

In comparison to bone scans, radiography is less sensitive but highly specific. It can detect lesions involving the bone marrow only when at least 50% of the bone in the X-ray's beam axis has been destroyed. However, it is more efficient at identifying lesions located in the bone cortex, even if they are relatively small. CT or MRI imaging can give additional information, especially for spine lesions, head neck tumors or intrathoracic tumors.

## TREATMENT OF CIBP

Effective pain management of CIBP is crucial as CIBP can have a significant negative impact on a patients' quality of life. Management of CIBP is often multimodal and involves a multidisciplinary approach (Fig. 5.1).

The aim of treatment is not only pain relief but also the prevention of SREs and improving quality of life. Hence a multimodal approach should be adopted for treatment of CIBP. Factors like life expectancy of the patients, stage of cancer, time take for pain relief by difference modalities must be included in a pain management plan.

### Pharmacological Options

#### *Surgery*

Surgery presents a valuable option for alleviating pain in patients with CIBP. Surgical interventions encompass a range of procedures, such as stabilizing or reconstructing an unstable spine or an impending fracture, decompression for vertebral bone metastases, reconstructing major joints, and fixing fractures in long bones. For patients with a favorable prognosis and bone metastases limited to a single site, surgical resection may be the preferred initial treatment. Even for patients with a limited life expectancy,

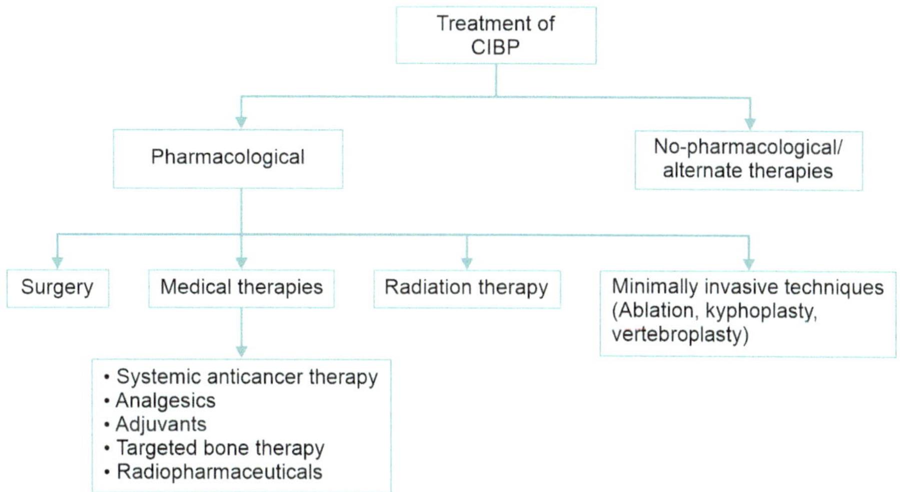


**Fig. 5.1:** Treatment options for cancer-induced bone pain (CIBP)

surgical interventions like fixation or decompression can provide significant pain relief and improve quality of life. Surgery offers a dual advantage of regaining mobility as well as pain relief. As per ESMO guidelines, surgery should be considered for patients with metastatic spinal cord compression, particularly those with spinal instability, unknown primary histology, recurrence post-radiotherapy, or a single compression site.[13]

### *Medical Therapies*

***Systemic anticancer therapy:*** Anticancer therapies, including hormonal therapy and chemotherapy, play an essential role in alleviating metastatic bone pain. In metastatic breast or prostate cancer, hormonal therapy alone can cause substantial pain relief aften as high as 60–80%. These therapies work by reducing the bulk of the tumor, thereby reducing the compressive, inflammatory, ischemic, and neuropathic component of CIBP. Early initiation of anticancer therapy is crucial for optimal pain management. However, it is important to note that the analgesic effects of systemic anticancer therapies may take 2–8 weeks to achieve pain relief. Therefore, it is essential to bridge this period with appropriate analgesic measures to ensure effective pain relief.

*Analgesics:* Aim of opioid and non-opioid analgesics is to reduce pain quickly. Given their fast onset of action compared to other modalities, analgesics should be started early.

***a. Non-opioid analgesics:*** *NSAIDs and paracetamol*–WHO recommends NSAIDs or Paracetamol alone or in combination with opioids for pain relief in cancer as first line agents depending on severity of pain. NSAIDs work by inhibiting COX enzymes and thereby reduce local inflammation and edema which makes them an attractive option for reducing bone pain. However, the evidence for its effectiveness in CIBP is limited.

In a Cochrane review by Derry and colleagues,[14] authors looked at safety and efficacy of NSAIDs in patients with cancer pain. They found that there is not strong evidence to say if NSAIDs, by themselves or with opioids, are helpful. They also noted that although some individuals with moderate or severe cancer pain might experience improvements within a short period, the evidence supporting this is limited. The main problem with using NSAIDs for a long time is that they can cause side effects like gastrointestinal irritation or bleeding, renal impairment, cardiovascular events, or bleeding disorders. For people at risk of renal impairment or gastrointestinal bleeding, paracetamol might be a safer choice and can be used instead. But there have not been any studies comparing the two directly in patients with cancer pain from bone metastases.

*b. Opioid analgesics:* CIBP generally responds well to opioid analgesics and form the mainstay of analgesic regimen in most patients. According to WHO guidelines, healthcare providers should consider any opioid for maintaining pain relief in adults and adolescents with cancer pain, based on their clinical evaluation and the severity of pain. Additionally, the selection of the opioid, its dose, and how it's administered should be tailored to the individual's specific pharmacokinetics, contraindications, and potential side effects, as outlined in the guidelines.[15]

A regular round the clock dosing should be prescribed as in most cases patients experience continuous pain. For breakthrough or incident pain, an immediate release formulation of opioid analgesic should be given. Management of incident pain can be difficult due to its sudden onset and short duration. Patients can be advised to take breakthrough opioids before starting an activity or movement which is responsible for sudden pain.

*Adjuvants:*

*a. Corticosteroids:* Steroid are frequently used as adjuvant analgesics in the management of CIBP due to their strong anti-inflammatory and anti-edema effect. Based on moderate-quality evidence, the WHO strongly advocates for the administration of corticosteroids in adults (including older persons) and adolescents with cancer pain if indicated. ESMO clinical guidelines for cancer pain recommend prompt use of steroids when the clinical and radiological diagnosis of metastatic spinal cord compression is confirmed.[13]

Despite its widespread use, there is limited data available on the effectiveness of corticosteroids in patients with CIBP. Generally, it is advised that corticosteroids be prescribed for the shortest duration possible, with individualized use. Clinicians should consider various factors such as the location and nature of pain, the risk of infection, diabetes mellitus, disease stage, and concurrent therapies when initiating steroid treatment.

*b. Anticonvulsants/antidepressants:* Anticonvulsants are being used increasingly in CIBP due to their effect on neuropathic pain. Few studies have demonstrated effectiveness of pregabalin in CIBP.[16,17] However, WHO makes no recommendation regarding the use of anticonvulsants/antidepressants for the treatment of cancer related neuropathic pain. Therefore, use of these agents should be individualized for every patient considering the side effect profile of these drugs.

*Targeted bone therapies:*

*a. Bisphosphonates (BPs):* Bisphosphonates exert a direct apoptotic effect on osteoclasts. These agents inhibit the differentiation and maturation of osteoclasts thereby preventing bone resorption, hypercalcemia, incidence of SREs. BPs reduce bone pain and requirement of analgesics. However, is it worth noting that their analgesic effects may take about a week to become apparent. Based on strong evidence from moderate-quality studies, the WHO recommends the use of bisphosphonates in adults for the prevention and treatment of bone pain.

Among the various bisphosphonates available, there is limited evidence demonstrating the superiority of one agent over another in terms of efficacy or duration of pain control.

Differences in nephrotoxic profiles often influence the choice of one agent over another. Generally, pamidronate and zoledronate are the most used agents for CIBP. However, it is important to acknowledge that bisphosphonates carry the risk of osteonecrosis of the jaw (ONJ), although the risk is less than 2% in the first year of therapy. Risk factors for ONJ include dentoalveolar surgery and poor dental hygiene. Therefore, a comprehensive dental evaluation and preventive measures are essential before initiating bisphosphonate therapy to minimize the risk of ONJ.[18]

*b. Denosumab:* Denosumab, a human monoclonal antibody, functions by binding to RANKL, thereby preventing its interaction with RANK. This interaction between RANKL and RANK is necessary for the differentiation and maturation of osteoclasts. Consequently, Denosumab reduces osteoclast activity, delays the onset of SREs, and enhances pain relief and quality of life in patients with bone metastasis.

According to ESMO guidelines,[13] Denosumab is suggested as an alternative to bisphosphonates for patients with bone metastases originating from solid tumors and myeloma. However, WHO has not issued a recommendation either for or against Denosumab in comparison to bisphosphonates for the prevention and treatment of bone pain.[15]

It is important to note that Denosumab carries a risk of ONJ. Although existing research indicates that Denosumab may decrease the occurrence of SREs and improve functional outcomes more effectively than bisphosphonates, it also raises the risk of osteonecrosis of the jaw without impacting bone pain or the time it takes to achieve pain relief. Further research is necessary to determine its suitability for routine use in CIBP management.

*c. Tanezumab:* Tanezumab is a humanized anti-NGF monoclonal antibody, which prevents NGF from binding to the TrkA receptor. Therefore, it inhibits the pathological sprouting and formation of new pathological nerve fiber networks mediated by NGF. While Tanezumab has been studied in patients with chronic musculoskeletal non-cancer pain, there is a scarcity of data regarding its effectiveness in alleviating cancer-induced pain. Only one study has compared tanezumab with a placebo in patients with painful bone metastases which did not demonstrate significant pain relief with Tanezumab.[19] Due to limited data, WHO guidelines neither recommend nor advise against its use.

*Radiopharmaceuticals:* In patients with diffuse metastatic osteoblastic or mixed lesions, radioisotope therapy may be offered when pain persists despite treatment with external beam radiation therapy.

Pain relief with radioisotopes usually starts 1–4 weeks after initiation. Bone marrow toxicity, effect on renal function, leukopenia, and thrombocytopenia are potential side effects of these agents and must be considered before starting the therapy.

Most studies on radioisotope therapy have focused on men with prostate cancer. Radium-223, for instance, has been assessed in patients with castration-resistant prostate cancer with bone metastases, demonstrating improvements in pain relief and a reduction in skeletal-related events (SREs).[20]

Currently, WHO guidelines make no recommendation for or against the use of radioisotopes.

### Radiation Therapy (RT)

Radiotherapy is effective in CIBP for reducing analgesic need, reducing risk of fracture, improving QoL. Based on high-quality evidence, both WHO and ESMO guidelines strongly recommend that a single-dose, low-fractionated RT should be used in adults with pain due to bone metastases if indicated and available. Typically, pain relief with radiotherapy starts within 1–2 weeks.

Research suggests that the efficacy of a single fraction (low-fractionated) of 8 Gy is comparable to longer treatment schedules, such as 5 fractions of 4 Gy (20 Gy). External beam radiotherapy (EBRT) is also considered a primary treatment option for most patients with metastatic spinal cord compression (mSCC).[13]

### Minimally Invasive Techniques

*Vertebroplasty/kyphoplasty:* Vertebroplasty and kyphoplasty are minimally invasive techniques used for treating painful metastatic vertebral compression fractures. Vertebroplasty was introduced in 1987 by a French group for treating hemangiomas. Later the technique was applied for treating painful metastatic, traumatic, or osteoporotic fractures.

It consists of injecting bone cement percutaneously into a vertebral body. Whereas, in kyphoplasty, a cavity is created in the vertebral body by a balloon before the cement injection.

Vertebroplasty or kyphoplasty can be recommended for patients with vertebral metastases who do not exhibit signs of metastatic spinal cord compression (mSCC) or spinal instability. Additionally, these procedures may be suitable for patients experiencing mechanical pain that does not respond to analgesics or for those with vertebral body collapse.

*Ablative therapies:* Radiofrequency ablation has shown to effectively local control of pain in around 64–77% of cases.[21] Ablative therapies can be combined with surgery as well as radiotherapy. They can be particularly useful in tumors which are in close proximity to vessels or spine.

## Non-pharmacological Treatment Options

Non-pharmacological or complementary and alternative medicine (CAM) therapies have experienced significant growth in their utilization for relieving cancer-induced pain and improving QoL. A diverse array of therapies are available, including cognitive behavioral therapies to acupuncture, acupressure, transcutaneous electrical nerve stimulation (TENS), yoga, hypnosis, guided imagery, biofeedback, aromatherapy, herbal remedies, massages, music therapy, and various other modalities. Research suggests that integrating these non-pharmacological therapies with conventional pharmacological methods can enhance the quality of life and pain relief for cancer patients.[22–24] However, despite their increasing usage among cancer patients, these therapies require further research and scrutiny within the scientific community to better understand their efficacy.

## Future Studies

Endothelin A (ET-A) receptor antagonists can have a potential for significant pain relief in patients with CIBP.[25] They show great promise especially in prostate cancer patients with bone metastasis.[26] Further research into it can possibly open a new avenue for pain relief in CIBP. Experimental research has demonstrated changes in sphingolipid metabolism within the spinal cord in rodent models of CIBP. The sphingosine 1-phosphate (S1P) receptor subtype 1 (S1PR1) is emerging as a potential novel target for therapeutic intervention in CIBP.[27] There is increasing interest in cannabinoids for reducing severe bone pain as well as inhibiting cancer growth, as evidenced by various animal studies. It has been suggested that the concurrent use of cannabis receptor agonists and opioids may reduce opioid dosage and associated morbidity. Therefore, cannabinoids can potentially serve as an effective adjunctive therapy in managing CIBP.[28,29]

## Conclusion

Bone metastases commonly occur as complications of cancer, with over 50% of affected patients experiencing moderate to severe pain. CIBP significantly impacts patients' daily functioning and mental well-being.

The mechanisms underlying bone pain are intricate and multifaceted. Tumor cells, bone matrix cells, and inflammatory cells produce mediators that activate nociceptors, damage nerve fibers, and secrete growth factors responsible for abnormal sensory and sympathetic nerve fiber growth and reorganization, leading to neuroma formation. These processes contribute to peripheral and central sensitization. Additionally, the interaction between metastatic cancer cells and osteoclasts forms a vicious circle, resulting in bone destruction, pathological fractures, and persistent pain.

Given the multifactorial nature of CIBP, tailored strategies targeting different disease stages and pain mechanisms are essential for optimal pain relief and quality of life. The therapeutic goal extends beyond pain management to include prevention of pain progression and skeletal-related events. Therefore, a multimodal approach combining pharmacological and non-pharmacological interventions, including anticancer treatment and symptomatic analgesia, is necessary. All interventions should be personalized to alleviate pain, enhance patients' QoL and functioning, and, where feasible, extend survival.

## References

1. Cancer pain relief and palliative care. Report of a WHO Expert Committee. World Health Organ Tech Rep Ser. 1990;804:1–75. PMID: 1702248.
2. Ramaswamy A, Rekhi B, Bakhshi S, Hingmire S, Agarwal M. Indian data on bone and soft tissue sarcomas: A summary of published study results. South Asian J Cancer. 2016 Jul-Sep;5(3):138–45. doi: 10.4103/2278-330X.187587. PMID: 27606300; PMCID: PMC4991135.
3. Bruera ED. Cancer pain: Assessment and management. Cambridge University Press (2011).
4. Smith HS. Painful bone metastases—Can we do better? Ann Palliat Med. 2012;1(1):81–2. doi: 10.3978/j.issn.2224-5820.2012.02.02. PMID: 25841433.
5. Coleman RE. Metastatic bone disease: clinical features, pathophysiology and treatment strategies. Cancer Treat Rev. 2001;27(3):165–76. doi: 10.1053/ctrv.2000.0210. PMID: 11417967.
6. Mercadante S. Malignant bone pain: pathophysiology and treatment. Pain. 1997;69(1-2):1–18. doi: 10.1016/s0304-3959(96)03267-8. PMID: 9060007.
7. Zaj czkowska R, Kocot-K pska M, Leppert W, Wordliczek J. Bone pain in cancer patients: mechanisms and current treatment. Int J Mol Sci. 2019 Nov 30;20(23):6047. doi: 10.3390/ijms20236047. PMID: 31801267; PMCID: PMC6928918.
8. Teicher BA, Fricker SP. CXCL12 (SDF-1)/CXCR4 pathway in cancer. Clin Cancer Res. 2010;16(11):2927–31. doi: 10.1158/1078-0432.CCR-09-2329. Epub 2010 May 18. PMID: 20484021.

9. Mantyh P. Bone cancer pain: causes, consequences, and therapeutic opportunities. Pain. 2013 Dec;154 (Suppl 1):S54–S62. doi: 10.1016/j.pain.2013.07.044. Epub 2013 Jul 31. PMID: 23916671.
10. Jimenez-Andrade JM, Bloom AP, Stake JI, Mantyh WG, Taylor RN, Freeman KT, et al. Pathological sprouting of adult nociceptors in chronic prostate cancer-induced bone pain. J Neurosci. 2010 Nov 3;30(44):14649–56. doi: 10.1523/JNEUROSCI.3300-10.2010. PMID: 21048122; PMCID: PMC3359142.
11. Bloom AP, Jimenez-Andrade JM, Taylor RN, Castañeda-Corral G, Kaczmarska MJ, Freeman KT. Breast cancer-induced bone remodeling, skeletal pain, and sprouting of sensory nerve fibers. J Pain. 2011 Jun;12(6):698–711. doi: 10.1016/j.jpain.2010.12.016. Epub 2011 Apr 15. PMID: 21497141; PMCID: PMC3111843.
12. Silverman DA, Martinez VK, Dougherty PM, Myers JN, Calin GA, Amit M. Cancer-associated neurogenesis and nerve-cancer cross-talk. Cancer Res. 2021 Mar 15;81(6):1431–1440. doi: 10.1158/0008-5472.CAN-20-2793. Epub 2020 Dec 17. PMID: 33334813; PMCID: PMC7969424.
13. Fallon M, Giusti R, Aielli F, Hoskin P, Rolke R, Sharma M, Ripamonti CI; ESMO Guidelines Committee. Management of cancer pain in adult patients: ESMO Clinical Practice Guidelines. Ann Oncol. 2018 Oct 1;29(Suppl 4):iv166-iv191. doi: 10.1093/annonc/mdy152. PMID: 30052758.
14. Derry S, Wiffen PJ, Moore RA, McNicol ED, Bell RF, Carr DB, McIntyre M, Wee B. Oral nonsteroidal anti-inflammatory drugs (NSAIDs) for cancer pain in adults. Cochrane Database Syst Rev. 2017 Jul 12;7(7):CD012638. doi: 10.1002/14651858.CD012638.pub2. PMID: 28700091; PMCID: PMC6369931.
15. WHO Guidelines for the Pharmacological and Radiotherapeutic Management of Cancer Pain in Adults and Adolescents. Geneva: World Health Organization; 2018. PMID: 30776210.
16. Gül K, Tepetam H, Gül HL. Duloxetine and pregabalin in neuropathic pain of lung cancer patients. Brain Behav. 2020;10(3):e01527. doi: 10.1002/brb3.1527. Epub 2020 Jan 22. PMID: 31967742; PMCID: PMC7066365.
17. Fallon MT. Neuropathic pain in cancer. Br J Anaesth. 2013 Jul;111(1):105–11. doi: 10.1093/bja/aet208. PMID: 23794652.
18. Kapoor R, Saxena AK, Vasudev P, Sundriyal D, Kumar A. Cancer induced bone pain: current management and future perspectives. Med Oncol. 2021;38(11):134. doi: 10.1007/s12032-021-01587-7. PMID: 34581894.
19. Sopata M, Katz N, Carey W, Smith MD, Keller D, Verburg KM, West CR, Wolfram G, Brown MT. Efficacy and safety of tanezumab in the treatment of pain from bone metastases. Pain. 2015 Sep;156(9):1703–1713. doi: 10.1097/j.pain.0000000000000211. PMID: 25919474.
20. Sartor O, Coleman R, Nilsson S, Heinrich D, Helle SI, O'Sullivan JM, et al. Effect of radium-223 dichloride on symptomatic skeletal events in patients with castration-resistant prostate cancer and bone metastases: results from a phase 3, double-blind, randomised trial. Lancet Oncol. 2014;15(7):738–46. doi: 10.1016/S1470-2045(14)70183-4. Epub 2014 May 13. PMID: 24836273.
21. Yevich S, Chen S, Metwalli Z, Kuban J, Lee S, Habibollahi P, et al. Radiofrequency ablation of spine metastases: A clinical and technical approach. Semin Musculoskelet Radiol. 2021 Dec;25(6):795–804. doi: 10.1055/s-0041-1740351. Epub 2021 Dec 22. PMID: 34937119.
22. Cepeda MS, Carr DB, Lau J, Alvarez H. Music for pain relief. Cochrane Database Syst Rev. 2006;(2):CD004843. doi: 10.1002/14651858.CD004843.pub2. Update in: Cochrane Database Syst Rev. 2013;10:CD004843. PMID: 16625614.
23. He Y, Guo X, May BH, Zhang AL, Liu Y, Lu C, Mao JJ, Xue CC, Zhang H. Clinical Evidence for Association of Acupuncture and Acupressure with Improved Cancer Pain: A Systematic Review and Meta-Analysis. JAMA Oncol. 2020;6(2):271–278. doi: 10.1001/jamaoncol.2019.5233. PMID: 31855257; PMCID: PMC6990758.
24. Singh P, Chaturvedi A. Complementary and alternative medicine in cancer pain management: a systematic review. Indian J Palliat Care. 2015;21(1):105–15. doi: 10.4103/0973-1075.150202. PMID: 25709198; PMCID: PMC4332115.
25. Khodorova A, Montmayeur JP, Strichartz G. Endothelin receptors and pain. J Pain. 2009;10(1):4–28. doi: 10.1016/j.jpain.2008.09.009. PMID: 19111868; PMCID: PMC2630124.
26. Aielli F, Ponzetti M, Rucci N. Bone metastasis pain, from the bench to the bedside. Int J Mol Sci. 2019 Jan 11;20(2):280. doi: 10.3390/ijms20020280. PMID: 30641973; PMCID: PMC6359191.

27. Grenald SA, Doyle TM, Zhang H, Slosky LM, Chen Z, Largent-Milnes TM, et al. Targeting the S1P/S1PR1 axis mitigates cancer-induced bone pain and neuroinflammation. Pain. 2017 Sep;158(9):1733–1742. doi: 10.1097/j.pain.0000000000000965. PMID: 28570482; PMCID: PMC5580091.

28. Lozano-Ondoua AN, Hanlon KE, Symons-Liguori AM, Largent-Milnes TM, Havelin JJ, Ferland HL 3rd. Disease modification of breast cancer-induced bone remodeling by cannabinoid 2 receptor agonists. J Bone Miner Res. 2013;28(1):92–107. doi: 10.1002/jbmr.1732. PMID: 22903605; PMCID: PMC4745976.

29. Mao Y, Huang Y, Zhang Y, Wang C, Wu H, Tian X, et al. Cannabinoid receptor 2 selective agonist JWH015 attenuates bone cancer pain through the amelioration of impaired autophagy flux induced by inflammatory mediators in the spinal cord. Mol Med Rep. 2019;20(6):5100–5110. doi: 10.3892/mmr.2019.10772. Epub 2019 Oct 25. PMID: 31661120; PMCID: PMC6854597.v

Chapter 6

# Chemotherapy Agents: Cause and Effect on Cancer Pain

• Manju Sengar • Venkatesh Kapu

## INTRODUCTION

Cancer affects a large number of people and is becoming more common as the population ages. Pain is a typical symptom of cancer diagnosis, and its prevalence increases throughout and after cancer therapy. Cancer pain syndromes are often classified as acute or chronic. Acute pain syndromes commonly follow diagnostic or therapeutic treatments, whereas chronic pain syndromes are typically directly connected to the tumor itself or to antineoplastic therapy.[1]

Majority of acute cancer pain syndromes are iatrogenic, related to a diagnostic test or treatment. Acute pain syndromes can be associated with all forms of antineoplastic therapy, including chemotherapy, targeted therapy, hormonal therapy, immunotherapy, and radiotherapy. Furthermore, chemotherapy infusion procedures may cause pain.

Acute pain syndromes related with chemotherapy infusion methods include venous spasm, intravenous infusion pain (e.g. oxaliplatin), phlebitis caused by drugs such as 5-fluorouracil, vinca alkaloids, vesicant extravasation, pain due to instillation of chemotherapy in the abdomen (intraperitoneal), intravesical and hepatic arteries.

Chemotherapy treats many type of cancers effectively however, similar to other antineoplastic treatments is also associated with side effects, one of which is pain. Chemotherapy induced pain includes:

- Oral mucositis
- Chemotherapy-induced peripheral neuropathy
- Chemotherapy-induced headaches
- Post chemotherapy acute limb ischemia
- Chemotherapy induced anginal pain
- Post chemotherapy gynecomastia
- Steroid-induced perineal burning and bone pains
- Flare syndrome
- Others

### Oral Mucositis

Oral mucositis is the most common acute painful disorder associated with antineoplastic therapy.[2] This complication can occur due to radiation therapy to the head and neck area as well as from several forms of systemic chemotherapy. Chemotherapy-associated mucositis can affect the mucosa of the entire gastrointestinal tract, but oral mucosal inflammation (stomatitis) is the most common cause of pain. Oral mucositis usually manifests clinically within the first week after chemotherapy administration. The frequency of chemotherapy-induced oral mucositis varies depending on the medication schedule and dosage, the usage of concurrent therapies (particularly radiation therapy), the tolerance of the individual patient, genetic variations in drug metabolizing pathways, immune signaling, cell injury/repair mechanisms, and potentially tobacco use and smoking history. The frequency and severity are both drug and dose dependent. The three most commonly used cytotoxic agents associated with oral mucositis are doxorubicin, fluorouracil (FU), and methotrexate. Oral mucositis affects on an average 20 to 40 percent of patients receiving conventional-dose cytotoxic chemotherapy. The frequency is higher (up to 80 percent) in those undergoing hematopoietic cell transplantation (HCT), particularly myeloablative allogeneic HCT. At three weeks post-transplant, half of the patients still experience significant pain that requires opioid use. Oral mucositis has been observed in 30 to 40 percent of patients undergoing therapy with molecularly targeted agents (vascular endothelial growth factor receptors) like sunitinib, sorafenib, lenvatinib, and regorafenib; 25 percent of patients treated with palbociclib, an inhibitor of cyclin-dependent kinase 4/6; 20 percent of patients treated with poly (ADP-ribose) polymerase (PARP) inhibitors, such as Olaparib and niraparib; and 10 to 45 percent of patients treated with agents that target the epidermal growth factor receptor (EGFR), such as cetuximab, erlotinib, dacomitinib, and mobocertinib; majority of cases are moderate to mild. Moreover, oral mucosal lesions have been observed in as many as 73% of patients receiving treatment with the mTOR inhibitors temsirolimus and everolimus. These lesions include both discrete aphthous-like ulcerations with an underlying inflammatory mechanism and typical ulcerations caused by loss of mucosal integrity. Immune checkpoint inhibitor use can cause mucosal toxicities such as stomatitis, periodontal disease, oral lichen planus, xerostomia, and, in rare cases, salivary gland-related Sjögren's disease and mucous membrane pemphigoid-like lesions.

Both the drug and the dose affect the frequency and severity. The three most often cytotoxic drugs associated with oral mucositis are methotrexate, fluorouracil (FU) and doxorubicin. The National Cancer Institute Common Terminology Criteria for Adverse Events (NCI CTCAE) criteria is typically used to grade the severity of mucositis (Table 6.1), taking into account the intensity of pain and the presence or absence of life-threatening complications.

### *Management*

***Prophylactic oral care:*** A thorough oral examination must be performed prior to the start of systemic anticancer treatment for the majority of patients as part of their preventive oral care. The European Society of Medical Oncology (ESMO) and the Multinational Association of Supportive Care in Cancer (MASCC)/International Society of Oral Oncology (ISOO)[3] have updated their joint guidelines, which align with this recommendation.[4] Dental caries treatment, scaling and root planning, and endodontic therapy, if necessary, should all be part of pretherapy oral hygiene protocols. When odontogenic pathology is severe, tooth extraction is recommended.

### *Preventive Treatments that may be Beneficial*

***Oral cryotherapy:*** Patients who are undergoing chemotherapy with bolus FU may benefit from oral cryotherapy, which involves swishing ice chips around the mouth for 30 minutes. This therapy has been shown to be beneficial and cost effective.

**Table 6.1: NCI CTCAE v 5.0 adverse events**

| Adverse event | Grade 1 | Grade 2 | Grade 3 | Grade 4 | Grade 5 |
|---|---|---|---|---|---|
| Mucositis oral[$] | Asymptomatic or mild symptoms; intervention not indicated | Moderate pain or ulcer that does not interfere with oral intake; modified diet indicated | Severe pain, interfering with oral intake | Life-threatening consequences; urgent intervention indicated | Death |
| Palmar-plantar erythrodysesthesia syndrome[#] | Minimal skin changes or dermatitis (e.g. erythema, edema, or hyperkeratosis) without pain | Skin changes (e.g. peeling, blisters, bleeding, fissures, edema, or hyperkeratosis) with pain; limiting instrumental ADL | Severe skin changes (e.g. peeling, blisters, bleeding, fissures, edema, or hyperkeratosis) with pain; limiting self-care ADL | | |

[$]Mucositis oral is characterized by ulceration or inflammation of the oral mucosa.

[#]A disorder characterized by redness, marked discomfort, swelling, and tingling in the palms of the hands or the soles of the feet. Also known as Hand-Foot syndrome.

(NCI CTCAE: National Cancer Institute Common Terminology Criteria for Adverse Events)

*Palifermin:* In accordance with updated guidelines from MASCC/ISOO and other expert groups, patients undergoing autologous hematopoietic stem cell transplantation with a preparative regimen involving total body radiation could well be prevented from oral mucositis by using Palifermin, a recombinant keratinocyte growth factor, which stimulates proliferation and differentiation of epithelial cells, including those of the digestive tract.

*Photobiomodulation (low level laser therapy):* According to updated guidelines from the MASCC/ISOO, photobiomodulation, may be beneficial in preventing oral mucositis in patients undergoing HCT conditioned with high-dose chemotherapy, either with or without total body irradiation.

*Chlorhexidine:* It's unclear if using mouthwash containing chlorhexidine is beneficial. In order to prevent recurrences in subsequent cycles, patients who experienced severe mucositis in previous cycles must reduce their dosage.

*Treatment of established mucositis:* The mainstay of treatment for mucositis caused by traditional cytotoxic chemotherapy is symptom management. It combines topical mucosal protectants, systemic or topical analgesia, and oral hygiene (including rinses with saline and/or sodium bicarbonate).

*Routine oral care:* Routine mouth care for patients with established mucositis should be done every four hours. This includes taking out dentures, cleaning the mouth gently, and rinsing it with a weak solution of baking soda and salt (one teaspoon baking soda and half a teaspoon salt in a quart of water). The MASCC/ISOO expert panel determined that these inert, mild oral rinses that increase clearance may be helpful in maintaining oral hygiene and enhancing patient comfort, despite the paucity of data regarding saline or bicarbonate rinses for the prevention or treatment of oral mucosal mucositis. Although a soft toothbrush or foam swab can effectively clean teeth, patients suffering from moderate to severe stomatitis may find them excessively painful.

Foods that don't require much chewing should be the only foods consumed during severe mucositis; foods that are acidic, salty, or dry should be avoided.

*Analgesia:* Mucositis-related pain has been treated with topical and systemic approaches, such as topical lidocaine solutions, which reduce pain but need to be applied four to six times a day. Topical lidocaine is commonly paired with agents for cleaning and/or coating; this combination is commonly called "miracle mouthwash." These mixtures are compounded differently by individual pharmacies, most of which do not have a set formula, and there is no standard formulation. These mouthwashes typically contain a topical anesthetic (like lidocaine), antacids and/or mucosal protective agents (like magnesium-aluminum), and astringent/anticholinergic agents (like sodium bicarbonate, diphenhydramine).

Notably, a systematic review of the treatment of oral mucositis came to the conclusion that there was no evidence to support the use of mouthwashes with mixed medications to treat mucositis caused by radiation or chemotherapy.[5] Adverse effects from lidocaine and diphenhydramine may occur in patients. Regarding mixed-medication mouthwash use, the Mucositis Study Group of the MASCC/ISOO guidelines for 2020 make no recommendations. Alternatively, regular and regular use of a soft toothbrush and a homemade salt-and-soda mouthwash (one teaspoon each of salt and sodium bicarbonate in a liter of water) can be employed for oral hygiene.

Even in the absence of significant systemic absorption, topical application of morphine sulphate (0.2%, 2 mg/mL in water, 15 mL swish for two minutes and expectorate) may reduce the duration and intensity of mouth pain. A specific recommendation for other groups could not be made, but the updated 2020 MASCC/ISOO guidelines suggested that this approach be restricted to patients receiving chemoradiotherapy for head and neck cancer. Parenteral or systemic oral opioids may be necessary if the pain is severe enough. For patients who are unable to swallow, morphine is advised as the first-choice opioid for patient-controlled analgesia. If the patient is able to swallow, oral administration is advised. Transdermal fentanyl is an additional option for patients who are incapable of swallowing. Patient-controlled analgesia with morphine and suitable locks to enable timely delivery of analgesics is especially advised for severe mucositis in the context of high dose chemotherapy. For adequate analgesia, narcotics are usually administered at a basal rate as well as in intermittent bolus doses. In order to maintain adequate nutrition and continue analgesics until recovery, patients with severe mucositis may benefit from total parenteral nutrition.

### Chemotherapy-induced Neuropathy

Multiple chemotherapy drugs have neurotoxic effects. Patients undergoing chemotherapy may experience acute neuropathic pain that manifests as polyneuropathy or, less frequently, as mononeuropathy.[6] The first cases of polyneuropathy associated with chemotherapy were reported in patients receiving vincristine, a vinca alkaloid. In addition the following medications have a high rate of polyneuropathy: bortezomib, cisplatin, oxaliplatin, thalidomide, and paclitaxel. Acute paresthesias and dysesthesias can be caused by any of these medications. While oxaliplatin-induced pharyngo laryngeal spasm is one example of an acute presentation, neuropathy-related pain in patients receiving these medications typically starts slowly. Neuropathic pain induced by chemotherapy typically gets better over time when the treatment is discontinued or the dosage is lowered. Neuropathic pain can occasionally turn chronic.

*Anti-microtubule drugs* such as paclitaxel and docetaxel are used to treat a wide range of tumors. Although docetaxel appears to be less neurotoxic than paclitaxel (overall incidence of any grade neuropathy: 15 percent versus 60%), both are linked to a primarily sensory neuropathy. Furthermore, paclitaxel more frequently causes severe (grade 3 or 4) sensory neuropathy than docetaxel. Severe arthralgias and myalgias with numbness and tingling are the hallmarks of taxane-associated acute pain syndrome, which usually starts one to two days after treatment and lasts for a median of four to five days.

*Vincristine:* Vincristine is used against a variety of cancers. An axonal neuropathy caused by disruption of the microtubules within axons and interference with axonal transport is the dose-limiting toxicity. Both sensory and motor fibers can be affected by neuropathy, but small sensory fibers are more commonly affected. Nearly every patient on vincristine has some degree of neuropathy. Paresthesias in the fingertips and feet, with or without pain, cramping in the muscles, and/or mild distal weakness, are typically the initial symptoms. Likewise, medications such as thalidomide, eribulin, and ixabepilone also result in excruciating neuropathy symptoms.

*Bortezomib:* One of the main nonhematologic toxicities of bortezomib is peripheral nerve damage. When it manifests, the excruciating sensory neuropathy can impair one's quality of life and ability to carry out everyday tasks. It may also necessitate changing one's dosage or stopping treatment altogether.

*Retinoic acid:* Acute promyelocytic leukemia is treated with all-trans retinoic acid, which in rare cases can result in multiple mononeuropathies and pseudotumor cerebri. On the other hand, fatigue and headaches are common during treatment.

Using antidepressants like duloxetine can help reduce the symptoms of chemotherapy-induced peripheral neuropathy (CIPN), including pain. Other adjuvant analgesics (such as tricyclic antidepressants, anticonvulsants), opioids, physical modalities like cutaneous electrical stimulation, and/or interventional procedures may be indicated for symptomatic patients with chronic neuropathy who do not respond to duloxetine. Acupuncture is advised by the National Comprehensive Cancer Network (NCCN) for patients whose supportive medications are not working.[7] Acupuncture also produced improvements in overall and CIPN-specific quality-of-life and clinically significant reductions in pain interference and intensity.

### Chemotherapy-induced Headaches

Chemotherapy-induced headaches are rather common following treatment with all trans retinoic acid (ATRA) for leukemia, or with intrathecal methotrexate for lymphoma, leptomeningeal carcinomatosis, and leukemia. Nuchal rigidity, fever, lethargy, irritability, and vomiting are possible side effects that could or might not occur with repeated administration of the medication. These side effects could last for several days or longer.

### Post Chemotherapy Acute Limb Ischemia

Acute limb ischemia following chemotherapy, also known as Raynaud's phenomenon, was reported in testicular cancer survivors receiving bleomycin, vinblastine, and cisplatin therapy. This condition is caused by a decreased blood supply to the fingers and toes.

### Fluoropyrimidine-induced Angina

The drugs capecitabine and fluorouracil (FU) lead to increased risk of cardiac ischemic episodes, which are thought to be caused by coronary vasospasm.

### Post Chemotherapy Gynecomastia

A common side effect of treatment for testicular cancer is usually painful and only lasts a brief time.

### Steroid-induced Perineal Burning

Dexamethasone at moderate to high intravenous doses (ranging from 12 mg to 200 mg) was used to treat and prevent nausea and vomiting related to chemotherapy. Within seconds of the intravenous injection, the pain begins abruptly, generally lasts for only 20 to 30 seconds, and was frequently described as itching, burning, and squeezing.[8] The brief duration of pain may indicate the amount of time needed for the compound to be hydrolyzed into phosphate ions and dexamethasone, although the pathogenesis of this event remains unexplained.

Moreover, perianal pain is frequently observed in patients with febrile neutropenia who need IV antibiotics, topical and systemic analgesics, good hygiene, and supportive care medications.

### Flare Syndrome

Increased bone pain is a characteristic of advanced prostate cancer following the start of LHRH (lutenizing hormone releasing hormone) agonist alone. This pain can occasionally be linked to an increased risk of cord compression, bladder outlet obstruction, and hypercoagulability. Injection site pain can also occur due to LHRH antagonists like degarelix and agonists like leuprolide. Diffuse musculoskeletal pain, skin erythema, altered liver function and hypercalcemia are indicative of advanced breast cancer. It may occur following the first dose of tamoxifen or other agonists of the estrogen receptor. Severe pain can also be experienced at the injection site from injections like fulvestrant, which is used in patients with breast cancer.

### Others

Myalgias, or joint pain, which may be accompanied by fever and extreme fatigue, are linked to interferons. These symptoms usually appear soon after the treatment and become less severe with subsequent doses.

Bone pain is a common side effect of using growth factors like filgrastim and pegfilgrastim. Moreover, using all transretinoic acid (ATRA) has been linked to diffuse bone pain.

Due to deep intramuscular injection, L-asparginase may produce pain at the injection site. It may also cause abdominal pain from pancreatitis or a severe headache from sagittal venous thrombosis.

Palmar-plantar erythrodysesthesia syndrome, also known as hand-foot syndrome, acute erythema, or toxic erythema of the palms and soles, is a painful skin condition that has been linked to a number of medications, including high-dose methotrexate, liposomal doxorubicin, continuous fluorouracil, capecitabine, paclitaxel, tyrosine kinase inhibitors (sorafenib and sunitinib), mTOR inhibitors (everolimus). As the rash worsens, blisters and desquamation may appear.

Treatment includes preventative measures suchas topical emollients. If palmar-plantar erythrodysesthesia is diagnosed, it is recommended to carefully monitor the worsening of the severity and, in severe cases, to stop drug treatment till further improvement. Once improved, the treatment is restarted either with lower doses or the drug is changed. Santosh, et al. recent study demonstrated that topical diclofenac 1% is linked to a significant decrease in hand-foot syndrome events, capecitabine dose reductions, and an improvement in quality of life at 12 weeks.

## CHRONIC PAIN SYNDROMES RELATED TO CHEMOTHERAPY

### Chemotherapy-related Neuropathy

While most patients with cytotoxic therapy experience temporary relief from their painful peripheral neuropathy, some may experience chronic pain that lasts for long time. Similar to other axonopathies, the pain initially affects the feet and distal legs before moving on to the hands and arms. The type of chemotherapy the patient received, as well as the dosage, have a significant impact on the level of pain and the existence and severity of neurological deficits. The platinum compounds cisplatin and oxaliplatin are the most frequently linked to different types of neurotoxicity among the widely used anticancer medications. A common side effect of cisplatin therapy is symmetrical, primarily sensory peripheral neuropathy, which usually manifests in most patients only after a cumulative dose of 300 $mg/m^2$ is reached.[9] Once established, there is no effective therapy available; instead, care is limited to treating symptoms. The majority of patients gradually get better, but recovery is frequently not complete. When carboplatin is administered at conventional dosages, peripheral neuropathy and central nervous system toxicity are rare. However, when high-dose carboplatin is used in conjunction with hematopoietic cell transplantation, severe neuropathy can develop. Although other factors, such as diabetes or the severity of acute neuropathy, may also play a role, cumulative dose is the main factor that determines the incidence and severity. After treatment is stopped, oxaliplatin neurotoxicity usually gets better. On the other hand, it might worsen for several months after treatment is stopped (a condition known as "coasting"). About 80% of patients have neuropathy that is at least partially reversible.

### Bone Complications and Glucocorticoids

Avascular necrosis of the femoral or humeral head, characterized by excruciating arthropathy, is often the consequence of long-term glucocorticoid usage. It may take several months following the initial report of pain for radiologic changes to become apparent on an MRI or CT scan. In addition, steroids hasten the onset of osteoporosis, which increases the risk of vertebral compression fractures linked to either acute or chronic back pain.

### Drug-related Osteonecrosis

Patients with metastatic bone disease who are treated with potent bisphosphonates or denosumab to prevent bone-related events may experience a rare but potentially serious side effect known as drug-related osteonecrosis of the jaw.

## ROLE OF CHEMOTHERAPY IN PALLIATION OF CANCER PAIN

Chemotherapy administered in a non-curative context with the goals of optimizing symptom control, enhancing quality of life (QoL), and, ideally, extending survival is referred to as palliative chemotherapy. Palliative chemotherapy is frequently given in addition to curative care and at any point during the course of treatment, despite the common misconception that it is a last resort.

### Conditions in which Palliative Chemotherapy is used to Relieve Pain

Palliative chemotherapy can be used for a variety of cancers.[10] The type of cancer determines the drug is to be used in the chemotherapy. There are some types of cancer in which palliative chemotherapy has shown certain significant benefits.

In malignant spinal cord compression, immediate corticosteroids and Radiotherapy, while chemotherapy in highly chemo-sensitive tumors like lymphoma, plasma cell tumors help in relieving symptoms. Similarly, initiation of hormonal therapy like Degarelix which is a LHRH antagonist in prostate cancer in addition to radiotherapy can help in pain relief.

Nerve root compressions associated with huge nodal mass or tumors causing significant pain can be relieved with immediate chemotherapy based on histology.

Raised intracranial pressure with severe headaches due to disease involvement can be relieved with corticosteroids and intrathecal chemotherapy regimens such as methotrexate, cytarabine, pemetrexed, etc. based on the type of cancer.

*Pancreatic cancer:* Palliative chemotherapy with either taxanes or fluoropyrimidine analogue based regimens can reduce pain, physical function and improve life expectancy of a pancreatic cancer patient. It also slows down appetite loss and onset of other symptoms.

*Non-small cell lung cancer:* Palliative chemotherapy can help with cough, dyspnea, and pain associated with non-small cell lung cancer.

*Breast cancer:* Palliative chemotherapy enhances quality of life and reduces fatigue.

*Cervical cancer* patients experience severe pain due to obstruction of ureters, compression of nerves due to nodes and also patients with penile carcinoma experience severe pain in penile region and also leads to nerve root compression due to heavy nodal mass.

Similarly, in *head and neck cancers*, patients experience severe pain impairing their nutrition and QoL

Evidence supports the role of chemotherapy in preserving or enhancing a patient's quality of life and managing bothersome symptoms. Palliative chemotherapy, which is based on the histology of the tumor, has an established role and successfully accomplishes these goals for certain patients with a variety of metastatic solid tumors.[11]

## Conclusion

Multifactorial factors can contribute to pain in cancer patients. Early detection of adverse events and prompt intervention can lead to better outcomes because pain syndromes associated with chemotherapy can cause a variety of complications that impair quality of life.

## References


1. Chronic cancer pain syndromes. In: Oxford Textbook of Palliative Medicine, 6th ed, Cherny NI, Fallon MT, Kaasa S, et al (Eds), Oxford University Press, Oxford 2021.
2. Elad S, Yarom N, Zadik Y, Kuten-Shorrer M, Sonis ST. The broadening scope of oral mucositis and oral ulcerative mucosal toxicities of anticancer therapies. CA Cancer J Clin. 2022;72(1):57–77. doi:10.3322/caac.21704
3. Elad S, Cheng KKF, Lalla RV, et al. MASCC/ISOO clinical practice guidelines for the management of mucositis secondary to cancer therapy [published correction appears in Cancer. 2021 Oct 1;127(19):3700]. Cancer. 2020;126(19):4423–4431. doi:10.1002/cncr.33100
4. Peterson DE, Boers-Doets CB, Bensadoun RJ, Herrstedt J. ESMO Guidelines Committee. Management of oral and gastrointestinal mucosal injury: ESMO Clinical Practice Guidelines for diagnosis, treatment, and follow-up. Ann Oncol. 2015;26 Suppl 5:v139–v151. doi:10.1093/annonc/mdv202
5. McGuire DB, Fulton JS, Park J, et al. Systematic review of basic oral care for the management of oral mucositis in cancer patients. Support Care Cancer. 2013;21(11):3165–3177. doi:10.1007/s00520-013-1942-0
6. Burgess J, Ferdousi M, Gosal D, et al. Chemotherapy-Induced Peripheral Neuropathy: Epidemiology, Pathomechanisms and Treatment. Oncol Ther. 2021;9(2):385–450. doi:10.1007/s40487-021-00168-y
7. Swarm RA, Paice JA, Anghelescu DL, et al. Adult Cancer Pain, Version 3.2019, NCCN Clinical Practice Guidelines in Oncology. J Natl Compr Canc Netw. 2019;17(8):977–1007. doi:10.6004/jnccn.2019.0038
8. Neff SP, Stapelberg F, Warmington A. Excruciating perineal pain after intravenous dexamethasone. Anaesth Intensive Care. 2002;30(3):370–371. doi:10.1177/0310057X0203000319
9. Krarup-Hansen A, Helweg-Larsen S, Schmalbruch H, Rørth M, Krarup C. Neuronal involvement in cisplatin neuropathy: prospective clinical and neurophysiological studies. Brain. 2007;130(Pt 4):1076–1088. doi:10.1093/brain/awl356
10. Neugut AI, Prigerson HG. Curative, Life-Extending, and Palliative Chemotherapy: New Outcomes Need New Names. Oncologist. 2017 Aug;22(8):883–885. doi: 10.1634/theoncologist.2017-0041. Epub 2017 May 26. PMID: 28550031; PMCID: PMC5553954.
11. Roeland EJ and LeBlanc TW. "Palliative chemotherapy: oxymoron or misunderstanding?." BMC palliative care vol. 15 33. 21 Mar. 2016, doi:10.1186/s12904-016-0109-4.

# Section II

# Cancer Pain Management

Chapter 7

# WHO Ladder and Role of Opioids in Treatment of Cancer Pain

• Ashwini Rane

Pain is one of the common presenting symptom of cancer. Around 30–40% patients suffer pain even at diagnosis.[1] Pathophysiology of cancer pain is complex, caused either by direct tissue injury, metastatic disease, and/or cancer-related inflammatory processes.[2] Though the cancer pain may be controlled in patients after receiving curative treatment, it could persist in some as well as remain poorly controlled especially in patients with advanced disease.[1]

In addition, there are concerns about opioid overprescribing, dependence, and addiction. To ensure appropriate use, healthcare providers should possess a thorough understanding of optimal dosing, potential side effects, and effective management strategies for these side effects.

This chapter outlines principles of WHO ladder, its validity and drawback in cancer pain management and proposed changes in ladder. Additionally, the chapter provides brief details about opioids which helps to take informed decisions regarding opioids for cancer pain management, prioritizing patient safety.

## WHO LADDER OF CANCER PAIN

In 1986, World Health Organization published the guideline for cancer pain management.[3] The group of experts involved, provided a unique step ladder, which is acclaimed as the 'WHO Ladder (Fig. 7.1). The WHO analgesic ladder, provides a framework for prescription of analgesia based on pain intensity, is relatively straightforward and has since been the globally applicable approach to cancer pain management. It has proved highly valuable, especially in resource-limited settings with limited access to pain specialists. WHO ladder recommends use of analgesics based on the pain intensity. Pain intensity divided into mild, moderate and severe. The first step (mild pain) involves prescribing simple non-opioid analgesics, the second step (moderate pain) involves addition of weak opioids, while strong opioids are employed in the third step of the ladder instead of the weak opioids. Adjuvants also known as co-analgesics are a group of drugs which were developed for a different indication other than pain, but may be used to improve analgesia in certain conditions. The classes of the drugs that come under this term include, corticosteroids, anticonvulsants (Pregabalin, Gabapentin), antidepressants (Amitriptyline, Nortriptyline), bisphosphonates. Adjuvants can be added at all the three steps, if there is additional component to the nociceptive pain that are poorly managed by non-opioids and opioids (ex-neuropathic pain, post radiotherapy and chemotherapy inflammation)[4]

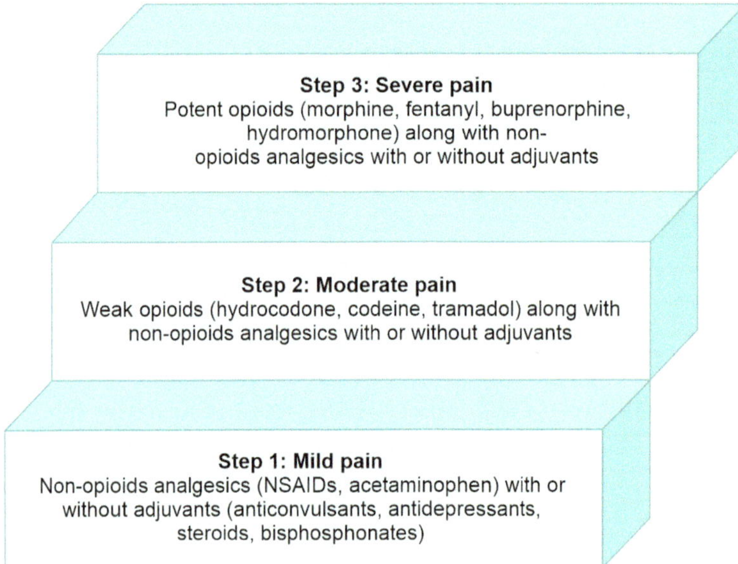


**Fig. 7.1:** The WHO ladder

*Recommendations for the analgesics were:*

- *By the mouth/oral medication*: Easily available pharmacological approach
- *By the clock/regular or fixed intervals:* Medication should be prescribed to be taken on the round the clock basis
- Dose has to be adjusted according to the individual patient
- *By the ladder:* Treatment started according to pain intensity

Since the introduction of the WHO ladder, several studies have been published about the efficacy of the ladder in management of the pain.[5,6] Although it has shown satisfactory pain relief in 70–80% patients.[7] Ladder approach is not without its own drawbacks.

## Drawbacks of the Ladder

- Focused only on adult cancer pain management, does not apply to pediatric patients.
- Ladder involves only pharmacological management of pain. Interventional pain procedures are not included in the guidelines.
- Non-opioids at the base of the ladder, perceived as a simple treatment without much side effects and patients tend to continue these medications for a prolonged period of time, however, prolonged treatment with NSAIDs is associated with serious side effects.[8]
- Cannot be used as a guide for acute pain in cancer patient or for pain in immediate postoperative period after cancer surgery.[9]
- The ladder is not as effective in the management of pure neuropathic pain. Pure neuropathic pain occurs due to injury to somatosensory nervous system patho-physiology of neuropathic pain is complex, use of the opioids in neuropathic pain is controversial.[10] Two practice guidelines recommend to use tricyclic antidepressants and anticonvulsants as a 1st line of management.[4,11]

WHO's three-step analgesic ladder, originally intended for cancer pain and emphasizing a medication-centric approach, could contribute to opioid misuse and exacerbate the opioid crisis.[9]

On the basis of updated literature, WHO introduced new guidelines in 2018 for management cancer pain.

### Features in 2018 Guidelines

- Originally devised for adults with cancer pain, it has now been adapted for use in children.
- Recommended addition of radiopharmaceutical drugs and radiotherapeutic management.[12]
- Provides for dose titration and description of opioids.[12]

With newer updates in the literature, various new techniques for pain managements few changes in the ladder are proposed/suggested such as the recommendation of low doses of strong opioids have also been recommended for use at the step II of the ladder,[14] removal of step II,[13] interventional pain procedures (nerve blocks, epidural analgesia, intrathecal medications, ablative procedures, neurosurgical procedure) to be added as a fourth step[8,15,16] for improved pain management.

## OPIOIDS

Opium is a mixture of alkaloids derived from seeds of papaver somniferum. Opiate is a naturally occurring alkaloid (morphine and codeine).[17]

Opioids are naturally occurring, semisynthetic or synthetic compounds that bind specifically to opioid receptors and share the properties of one or more of the naturally occurring endogenous opioids.

Despite growing concerns and alternative medications, opioids retain their value in managing severe pain.

### Classification of Opioids[18–20]

Morphine is prototypical opioid for clinical use. Various semisynthetic opioids are derived from morphine by changes in chemical composition (diamorphine, dihydrocodeine, buprenorphine, nalbuphine and oxycodone). Later synthetic opioids were developed (pethidine, fentanyl, methadone, alfentanil, remifentanil).

The International Union of Pharmacology in 2000 changed the nomenclature of opioids to what is the current classification as mentioned, opioids acting on μ (mu) opioid receptor (MOP), κ (kappa) opioid (KOP), δ (delta) opioid receptor (DOP), NOP (nociceptin orphanin FQ peptide receptor). These are G protein couple receptors located at cortex, medulla, hippocampus, amygdala, dorsal horn, periaqueductal gray matter.

Depending upon the action on opioid receptors, opioids can be divided into (Table 7.1)

- *Pure agonist:* Drug produces maximal response at the receptor
- *Partial agonist:* Produces partial response irrespective of amount of drug
- *Antagonist:* Does not produce any response at the receptor site.

Table 7.1: Opioid analgesics

| Pure agonist | Agonist-antagonist | Partial agonist | Antagonist |
|---|---|---|---|
| Morphine | Pentazocine | Buprenorphine | Naloxone |
| Fentanyl | Nalbuphine | | Naltrexone |
| Codeine | Nalorphine | | Nalmefine |
| Oxycodone | | | |
| Methadone | | | |
| Meperidine | | | |
| Hydrophone | | | |

## Mechanism of Action of Opioids[21,22]

Binding of an opioid agonist to the transmembrane part of opioid receptor, leads to conformational changes in the α subunit of the receptor. This leads to a cascade of events and overall effect is in form of $Ca^{++}$ ion channel closure and $K^+$ channel opening. Thus, causing neuronal hyperpolarization and reducing the neurotransmitter release. The nociceptive action of opioids is directly mediated by reduced afferent transmission of signals at the level of ascending pain pathway, spinal cord (substantia gelatinosa), periaqueductal gray (PAG), locus coeruleus (LC) and rostroventral medulla (RVM) and indirectly by activating the descending inhibitory pain pathway.

## Commonly used Opioids

### *Morphine*

It is a preferred opioid of choice in cancer pain management.[29] It is metabolised in the liver by glucuronidation to M3G (morphine-3-glucuronide) (55–80%) and M6G (morphine-6-glucuronide) (10–15%), latter contributing to the analgesic and other effects of morphine due to its potent action on mu-receptors. Significance of M3G metabolite is unclear. Both metabolites are excreted by kidneys and thus cumulate in renal failure with side effects. Hence morphine is not advised in those with renal impairment.[22,30,31]

### *Oxycodone*

It is a semisynthetic compound derived from codeine with strong μ-receptor agonist and mild κ and δ receptors agonist action. It is metabolised in liver into noroxycodone and oxymorphone respectively, latter being more potent than the original drug.[30] It is available as injectable and oral formulations. It is as effective as other opioids.[32] It is not available in India.

### *Hydrocodone*

A synthetic opioid derivative of codeine. Similar to oxycodone, hydrocodone is metabolised in liver.[30] Availability is restricted to some countries, including India.

### *Hydromorphone*

A semisynthetic opioid with a pharmacological profile similar to morphine. It is available as oral and injectable formulation. It is metabolised in liver mainly to hydromorphone-3-glucuronide (H3G). It does not have analgesic effect but is a potent neuro-excitatory molecule. Renal impairment does result in an increased risk of side-effects, however, there are no absolute contraindications to use of hydromorphone.[30]

*Fentanyl*

Fentanyl is a synthetic, lipid-soluble drug which is almost 100 times more potent than morphine. It is a strong μ-receptor agonist. Due to its lipid soluble nature, fentanyl gets sequestrated in body lipids and central nervous system, thus causing less constipation and peripheral effects as compared to morphine. Fentanyl is metabolised in number of inactive metabolites in liver by cytochrome P450 enzyme system. Its metabolism is decreased in severe liver failure. Some evidence suggests accumulation of parental compound in chronic renal failure.[33] However, the metabolites of fentanyl are inactive and, therefore, is relatively safe in patients with chronic kidney disease. There are limited clinical trials for transdermal patches in dialysis dependent patients, case reports have shown successful pain management with transdermal patches in dialysis dependent patient.[34,35]

*Buprenorphine*

It is a synthetic compound, with partial agonist action on μ and OPRL-1 receptors and antagonist action on κ and δ receptors.[22] The main analgesic effect of buprenorphine is attributed to its effect on μ-receptors. It causes less respiratory depression as compared to the other opioids.[36] Buprenorphine is excreted by hepatic metabolism, it should be used with reduced initial doses and increased interval in doses in hepatic dysfunction.[37] It can be safely used in patient with renal impairment.[38]

*Methadone*

Methadone is a synthetic opioid, μ and δ opioid receptor agonist. It is a lipophilic drug, with a large volume of distribution and 60–90% protein binding. It is metabolized in the liver and has a biphasic elimination pattern with a high individual variability in plasma half-life ranging from 8–120 hours.[39] Due to this methadone may tend to accumulate in body and there is uncertain correlation between plasma levels and analgesic effect of methadone.

*Side effects:* QT prolongation, respiratory depression, variable plasma half-life, variable conversion ratios with morphine, potential drug interactions. It is advisable that methadone should be used by a pain management expert, as the doses need to titrated carefully with optimal monitoring of risks and benefits.[30]

*Codeine*

Codeine is a weak opioid used for pain management. It is metabolized to codeine-6-glucuronide (80%) by conjugation in liver and morphine (10–20%) by demethylation. Codeine has poor evidence for use as a single agent or in combination with other drugs for use in cancer pain management. It is contraindicated in children below 12 years of age and should be used with caution in adolescents (12–18 years).[30]

*Tramadol*

It is a synthetic centrally acting analgesic with agonist effect on mu-opioid receptors and serotonin as well as norepinephrine reuptake inhibitor. It is a prodrug and gets metabolized in liver to desmethyltramadol which is a potent active molecule. It is useful in management of nociceptive as well as neuropathic pain due to a different mechanism of action. It should be used cautiously in patients with risk of developing seizures as it reduces the seizure-threshold.[22,31]

*Tapentadol*

It is a synthetic, centrally acting, strong μ-opioid receptor agonist, with inhibitory action on noradrenaline reuptake. It is available only as an oral formulation and undergoes extensive hepatic metabolism mainly by glucuronidation. Less side effects as compared to other opioids.[22]

## OPIOID RECEPTOR ANTAGONISTS

### Centrally Acting Opioid Antagonists

*Naloxone*

A competitive antagonist.[40] Available in parenteral formulations. FDA approved for opioid emergencies such as (overdose or opioid induced respiratory depression.) The CDC Guideline recommends prescription of naloxone in patients with a history of substance use disorder, high-risk and/or history of overdose, higher opioid dose (>50 morphine milligram equivalent daily dosing).[41]

*Naltrexone*

Available in oral and parenteral formulations. FDA approved for opioid and alcohol use disorder for maintenance treatment.

Opioids commonly used in cancer pain management along with the various preparations and routes of administration are given in Table 7.2.

## OPIOID AVAILABILITY IN INDIA

India has limited opioids legally available for medical use.[42] These include morphine, methadone, fentanyl, tramadol, and meperidine. Popular opioids in other parts of the world, such as hydrocodone and oxycodone, though legal in India are unavailable.

### Opioid Formulations (Table 7.2)

Various formulations of opioids are available world-wide and include tablets/syrup/intravenous form of morphine, transdermal/intravenous/oral transmucosal preparation of fentanyl, transdermal/sublingual tablet of buprenorphine and syrup of methadone. Various newer formulations of the opioids have been introduced to improve pain management and reduce opioid use disorder. Morphine oral formulations such as Embeda (morphine extended release tablet with naltrexone sequestered tablet) and MorphaBond ER (morphine extended release tablet) have approved by FDA as a opioid deterrent formulations.[43] Sublingual tablet, nasal sprays of fentanyl for breakthrough pain.[44] Subcutaneous dept formulations and long acting implant of the buprenorphine is FDA approved in opioid use disorder.[45] However, most of these are unavailable in India. In India, in addition to the intravenous preparations, morphine is available in tablet forms both the quick release and controlled release preparations, fentanyl in transdermal patch and oral transmucosal preparation, buprenorphine in a sublingual tablet and as

**Table 7.2: Commonly used opioids in cancer pain management**

| Opioid | Route of administration | Dose | |
|---|---|---|---|
| *Strong opioids* | | | |
| **1. Morphine**<br>*Formulations*<br>• Oral-immediate-release tablets, modified-release tablets and capsules, liquid<br>• Rectal-suppository<br>• Parenteral-intravenous (IV) and subcutaneous (SC) solutions | PO | Opioid tolerant: 10 mg q4 hr[23]<br>Opioid naïve or frail: 5 mg q4 hr mild-mod renal failure: 5–10 mg q6h–q8 hr[24,25] | Potency ratio of oral morphine to SC or IV morphine is 2:1 or 3:1 with individual variability[26] |
| | IV | 1 mg IV bolus repeat every 5–10 min till adequate pain relief is achieved[23,24] | In severe pain (pain score >8) |
| **2. Fentanyl**<br>*Formulations*<br>• Oral-lozenges<br>• Parenteral<br>• Local-TD (transdermal) | TD | 12, 25, 50 µg/hr patches should be changes every 72 hours. | • TD should be started in patients after achieving adequate pain relief with oral or parenteral route.[25]<br>• Equianalgesic dose should be calculated<br>• Breakthrough pain relief medications should be prescribed<br>• Transmucosal, nasal, buccal formulations to be used only for breakthrough pain |
| | IV/SC/IM | 10–50 µg by PCA/ Syringe pump[23] | |
| **3. Methadone**<br>*Formulation*<br>• Oral<br>• Parenteral<br>• Transmucosal | Oral | Opioid naïve<br>2.5–5 mg BD<br>Elderly: 1–2 mg | Clinicians with limited experience should consult a pain specialist before starting or rotation to methadone.[27] |
| **4. Oxycodone**<br>*Formulations*<br>• Oral- (IR and MR*)<br>• Parenteral | Oral | 5 mg q4 hr[24] | Can combine with acetaminophen |
| **5. Buprenorphine**<br>*Formulations*<br>• Local: TD<br>• Oral: SL (sublingual) | TD | 5, 10, 15, 20 µg/hr every 7days[23] | |
| | SL | 200, 400 µg<br><br>2, 8 mg tablets (NCG)[23] | |

*(Contd..)*

**Table 7.2: Commonly used opioids in cancer pain management** (*Contd...*)

| Opioid | Route of administration | Dose | |
|---|---|---|---|
| *Weak opioids* | | | |
| **1. Tapentadol** Oral | Oral | IR-50 mg q3 hr, q4 hr Titrated as 100 mg q4 hr and 150 mg q6 hr TDS (Max <600 mg/day) ER: 50–150 mg BD[23] | • Mild liver impairment IR 50 mg TDS (max <200 mg/day) • Should be avoided in severe renal and hepatic impairment |
| **2. Tramadol** (IV, Tablet-IR and ER both oral and rectal formulations) | Oral | IR- 50 mg QID (max 600 mg/day)[23] ER-single dose 100–300 mg In renal impairment 50 mg BD max 200 mg/day | • It should be avoided in hepatic impairment • The drug-drug interactions with antidepressants, antimigraine • Drugs, antiarrhythmics, antipsychotics, anticonvulsants, antiparkinsonian agents, and ondansetron. • It precipitates seizure may also cause tramadol related deaths[28] |
| **3. Codeine** *Formulation*: Oral | PO | 30 mg QID [23] (ref NCG) | • Always available in combination with Paracetamol • Should be avoided in <18 years |

*IR: immediate release, MR: modified release

a transdermal patch, methadone in syrup formulation. Codeine, tramadol, tapentadol all available as tablets of various strengths and in combination with paracetamol.

## Intrathecal Drug Delivery Systems (IDD)

These are novel devices which deliver the drug into the subarachnoid space where it acts directly at the dorsal horn of the spinal cord. Small doses of the drug results in rapid and adequate analgesia without crossing the blood–brain barrier with less systemic side effects as compared to other routes of administration.[46] The device consists of a pump which is surgically placed in the subcutaneous space and the catheter which is subcutaneously tunnelled after inserting into the intrathecal space.[47] Fentanyl, morphine and sufentanil are the commonly used intrathecal opioids.[48] These pumps can deliver the drug at a fixed or a variable rate with the option of intermittent boluses or patient controlled analgesia (PCA).[46] Intrathecal analgesia is preferred when other options for pain management have either exhausted and pain is intractable or intolerable side effects provided the patient has an expected 3 months survival. However, it is associated with complications such as local site infection, meningioma, granuloma, CSF leak at the insertion site, drug related complications (respiratory depression, somnolence, urinary retention, hyperalgesia, tolerance, withdrawal).[49]

## OPIOID TITRATION

Before starting the analgesics, the goal of treatment such as adequate analgesia (a 30–50% reduction in pain intensity), optimum activity, minimal side effects should be discussed with the patient and caregiver, details of the medications with common side effects should be explained.[12, 24]

Opioids are started for moderate to severe pain. Starting dose depends upon whether the patient is opioid naïve or opioid tolerant, and other comorbidities affecting drug pharmacokinetics and dynamics.

Patients are considered opioid naïve[50,51] if they have never taken opioid analgesics in the past.

Opioid tolerant[50] are patients on oral morphine 60 mg/24 hours or 30 mg daily oxycodone or fentanyl patch 25 μg/hr on the round the clock basis for a week or longer.

Low dose pure μ agonists can be used. Oral mode of drug delivery is preferred during titration. Immediate release (IR) or short acting formulations are preferred at titration. The extended release (ER) formulations are preferred once the patient is already on a stable dose of opioids. However, one randomized trial has shown no difference between IR and ER formulations.[52] Morphine is the most common opioid used for titration, the lowest tolerable IR dose should be started (refer to Table 7.2) with aim to titrate up by 30–50% of daily dose till adequate pain relief (30–50% reduction in pain intensity) is achieved.

Patient should be re-evaluated frequently after starting the treatment to ensure adequate analgesia without side effects. Patients may have breakthrough pain (BTP) episodes during a 24-hour period on a otherwise stable back ground pain. Small BTP doses of opioids should be made available for use during such episodes (breakthrough Pain has been discussed in detail in Chapter 8). An adjuvant can be considered if necessary to further improve analgesia.

Chemotherapy, radiation and surgery, all are known to reduce tumor load and thereby result in some amount of pain relief. Opioids however, should not be stopped abruptly to prevent any withdrawal symptoms or worsening of pain, but should be de-escalated slowly or tapered off. Opioid dose reduction should be considered if pain relief is satisfactory without any breakthrough pain episodes, completion of acute event, completion of treatment of the cancer or side effects of opioids are unmanageable.

Taper or reduce the dose of the opioid by 10–20% of the starting dose. Further reductions are done slowly with constant re-evaluation of pain relief.[12] In case of dose reduction for unmanageable side effects such as sedation, a 25–50% dose reduction should be done.[24] Patients should be monitored frequently for increase in pain intensity or withdrawal symptoms.

Longer the opioid use, longer will be the duration of tapering. Usual tapering involves 10–20% every 4 weeks. Opioid tapering should be done on individual basis, should be started after discussing with the patient, the risks and benefits. Tapering can be done as rapid reduction (by 10% per week) or slow reduction (by 10% per month) or slower till 30% of total dose is reached and then reduced by 10% of the remaining per week).[53]

## OPIOID SIDE EFFECTS

### 1. Gastrointestinal

Nausea, vomiting, early satiety, bloating, constipation, abdominal pain are common problems with opioid treatment. Most of these adverse effects get relieved with pharmacological tolerance over time, except constipation which requires active management.

#### *i. Opioid Induced Constipation (OIC)*

Patients should be regularly administered a laxative when an opioid is prescribed and they should be routinely evaluated for. The prevalence of constipation when on opioids is as high as 60–90%. Other contributory factors should be ruled out.

*Prevention of OIC* **(Fig. 7.2)**

- Prophylactic laxatives should be started at a lower dose and then titrated according to clinical efficacy (dose).
- Identify and correction of other metabolic disorders (hypercalcemia, hypothyroid).
- Lifestyle modification as increase water intake, increase the amount of fibre in the diet, increase mobility, encourage squatting position for defecation.

*Treatment of OIC:* Various studies have failed to show any difference between better efficacy of laxatives in OIC patients.[55] Transdermal fentanyl patch causes less constipation than oral morphine.[56] Peripherally acting μ-receptor antagonists (naltrexone, naldemedine, naloxegol, and naloxone) have been suggested for the refractory constipation.[57]

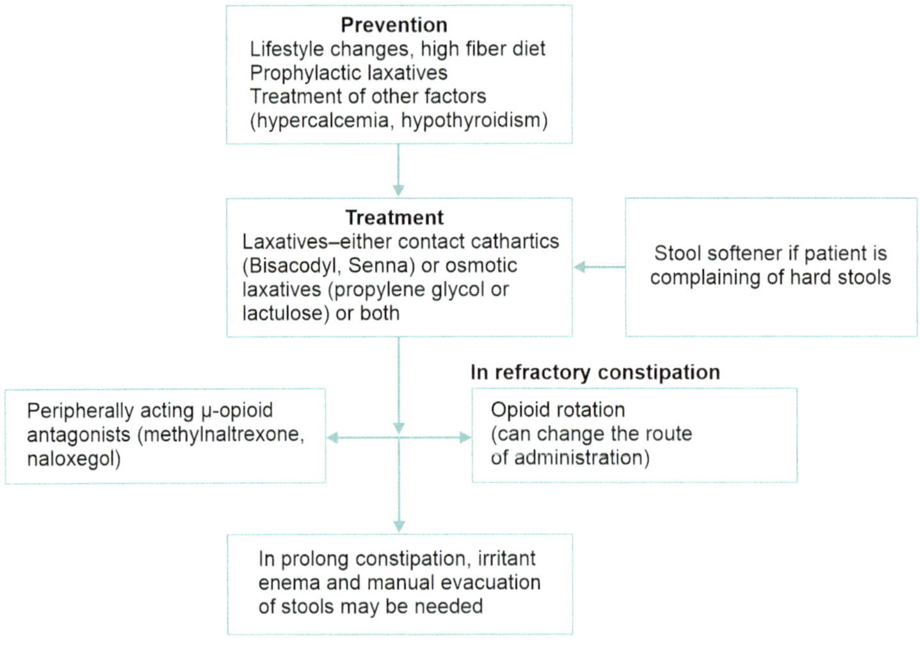


**Fig. 7.2:** Management of opioid induced constipation (OIC)

*ii. Nausea and Vomiting*

It is commonly seen with early part of opioid treatment and decreases after 3–4 days of start of the therapy. Dopamine antagonist, such as prochlorperazine or metoclopramide, or a serotonin receptor antagonist, such as ondansetron are effective. Treatment strategy is formulated with proper assessment of the patient. Changing route of administration may be helpful in refractory cases.[38] Based on association of nausea and vomiting after food ingestion then metoclopramide is useful, if its associated with epigastric pain then PPI (proton pump inhibitor) and $H_2$ receptor blockers (ranitidine) is useful, if it is occurs with movement the anticholinergic or antihistaminics are useful.

Narcotic bowel syndrome is rare but usually under diagnosed condition. It occurs due to with chronic use or increasing the dose of opioids. Diagnosis is generally by excluding other causes. Treatment generally includes rotation of opioids or decreasing the dose of opioid or replaced with of the other non-opioid analgesics.[58]

## 2. Neurological Side Effects

*i. Sedation and Confusion*

Sedation is commonly seen in the initial phase of the treatment. Other contributing factors for sedation are concomitant use of other CNS depressing drugs, fatigue due to disease, metabolic disorders, renal and hepatic impairment, sepsis, etc. Validated tools such as the Epworth Sleepiness Scale (ESS) and Stanford Sleepiness Scale are available for quantifying sedation.[30] If sedation causes impairment of daily routine activities, dose of the opioid can be decreased and adjuvant analgesic, interventional pain procedures can be helpful. Psychostimulants (methylphenidate, dextroamphetamine, modafinil, donepezil) may be used where the pain relief is adequate with prescribed dose of opioid, but patient complains of sedation or sleepiness.[59] However, psychostimulants are associated with certain side effects such as hallucination, delirium, psychosis.

*ii. Cognitive Failure*

Cognitive changes are usually seen in initial phase of the start of the treatment usually subsides within a week of the opioid therapy.

Risk factors for delirium and cognitive failure:

- Advanced disease (more common with lung cancer, time since diagnosis <15 days)
- Elderly population
- Higher dose of opioid (oral morphine >400 mg)
- On other psychoactive medications.

Pathophysiology is poorly understood. Infection, metabolic abnormality (hypercalcemia, hyponatremia, paraneoplastic syndrome), infection, renal and hepatic impairment and dehydration are the contributory factors. In general, patients should be advised to refrain from driving, operating machines, and performing tasks that require significant concentration and psychomotor skills for a period of 3–4 days after start of opioid therapy as well as after significant increases (30–50%) in their daily dose of opioid.[30]

*iii. Delirium*

Opioid can cause onset or worsen the delirium, treatment include ruling out and treatment of underlying cause, careful dose reduction by (25–50% can be considered) or opioid rotation and/or addition of other analgesics.

*iv. Hallucination*

Usually infrequent and difficult to diagnose. Mood change can be an only organic sign to suspect hallucinations. It associated with advanced disease and chronic opioid use.[60]

*v. Myoclonus*

Most commonly seen with high dose of morphine, hydromorphone, meperidine, fentanyl and its derivatives and diamorphine.[30] No specific evidence-based treatment available, can consider low dose clonazepam or lorazepam. Opioid rotation or reduction of the dose can be considered.

### 3. Respiratory Depression

Central action of the opioid is responsible for this side effect especially when started in larger doses in relatively opioid naïve patients. Patients usually develop tolerance to the respiratory depression with continue stable therapy. Simultaneous administration of CNS depressing drugs (benzodiazepine, gabapentin, pregabalin),[61] opioid rotation with improper dose equivalent ratios, liver and renal impairment usually put the patient at risk.[30]

It is treated with IV naloxone 0.04 to 0.08 mg slow IV every min till the opioid effect is reversed. Other adjuvant drugs or non-opioids are used for analgesia. Patient should be monitored for recurrence of respiratory depression as it may recur after antagonist gets metabolised (half-life: 30 min).[62]

### 4. Pruritus

Pruritus is known to occur in 2 to 10 percent of patients receiving chronic opioids.[63] Pathophysiology of opioid induced pruritus is poorly understood. There have been evidences that morphine causes histamine release from mast cells but other opioids have failed to do so. Recent evidences suggested that pruritis is a result of direct action on mu-opioid receptors.[64] It is treated only in severe cases, with antihistaminics (diphenhydramine, cetirizine). If the pruritus persists then rotation of opioid is considered.[46] Change of morphine to hydromorphone has been shown effective.[30]

### 5. Urinary Retention

Although it is more frequently seen in opioid use in neuraxial blockade in acute pain management, rarely it is seen with enteral use of opioid. It causes sphincter muscle to contract, detrusor muscle relaxation. Rarely does the patient require catheterization. Low dose opioid antagonist, opioid rotation may help.

### 6. Opioid Induced Hyperalgesia

Opioid induced hyperalgesia (OIH) is a paradoxical response seen in patients who have been exposed to opioids, wherein they demonstrate an excessively increased sensitivity to a noxious stimulus. It is seen especially in the patients who have been exposed to opioids for a short duration. May present with hyperalgesia (increased response to a painful stimulus) and allodynia (pain following an otherwise non-painful stimulus). The precise mechanism is as yet unknown, though many have been proposed and NMDA receptor activation may have some major role. Detailed hypothesis of OIH has been discussed in detail in Chapter 19.

To come to a diagnosis of OIH, one has to differentiate it from the other possible reasons for increasing pain and need for increasing doses of opioids such as:[65]

- Opioid tolerance
- Opioid withdrawal
- Opioid use disorder

Pain of OIH however, worsens despite an increase in opioid dose, as opposed to the other conditions, where the pain actually improves with increase in opioid dose.

*Treatment of OIH*

Reduce the opioid dose gradually or change to another alternative opioid or opioid rotation

- Prescribe a non-opioid analgesic for opioid sparing action such as antidepressants, anticonvulsants and NSAIDs
- Consider addition of a NMDA receptor antagonist, for example, ketamine which could help block the over sensitized pain receptors in those with hyperalgesia
- Consider non-pharmacological interventions, for example, physical therapies, psychological therapies, or interventional therapies including spinal cord stimulators.

## OPIOID TOLERANCE

Described as a decrease in analgesic efficacy of the opioid over time that compels the need to increase the dose of opioid. It is suspected when the rapid dose escalation is required to obtain the desired relief.

## OPIOID DEPENDENCE

It is defined as a disorder of regulation of opioid use resulting in a physical and psychological dependence on the opioid chiefly due to repeated and prolonged use of the opioid. Dependence makes it difficult for the person to stop taking the opioid when it is no longer needed. Prescription of any opioid may lead to substance disorder. Certain studies have claimed that weak opioids are more addictive than strong opioid.[66] Opioid dependence results in a strong internal urge for opioid consumption, characterised by over usage, higher prioritization of opioids over alternative activities and continued usage despite adverse consequences.

## OPIOID ADDICTION

It is characterized by inability to consistently abstain, impairment in behavioral control, craving, diminished recognition of significant problems with one's behaviors and interpersonal relationships, and a dysfunctional emotional response.[67]

To prevent the above, opioid stewardship, defined as 'coordinated interventions designed to improve, monitor, and evaluate the use of opioids to support and protect human health has been introduced in clinical practice.[68] The healthcare provider should plan the opioid titration and de-escalation for individual patients. Patients should be educated about the abuse potential of the drug. Patients should be explained about the proper storage and disposal opioids.[9]

## OPIOID ROTATION

Opioid rotation is switching from one opioid to another or to another route of administration to improve pain relief or reduce unwanted side effects.

### Opioid Rotation is Indicated[27]

- Refractory pain despite escalating opioid dose
- Excessive side effects
- Other route of administration of opioid is warranted (vomiting, sepsis)
- Cost and other logistic issues of the previous opioid treatment

Opioid rotation is complex due to interindividual variability in response to the opioids, cross tolerance, dose conversion challenges and hence requires an individualized approach. Knowledge about the potency of the opioid and equianalgesic dose helps in opioid rotation. The equianalgesic dose as well as the clinical factors and patient factors should be accounted for.[69] Table 7.3 shows a compiled equianalgesic dose conversions of the commonly used opioids in India.[29] These relative potency ratios should be used as an approximate guide for opioid rotation. Calculated dose should be reduced to 25–50%. Patient should be evaluated regularly for titration of the dose or side effects while undergoing an opioid rotation. Switching of opioid to oral methadone is effective.[70] Methadone is also useful in patients, if they develop nausea, vomiting, myoclonus with first line opioid. However due to interindividual variability in the pharmacokinetics of methadone, the process could be more challenging.

### NDPS Act and Regulations for Opioid Use

The Narcotic Drugs and Psychotropic Substances (NDPS) Act, 1985,[71] regulates the production, possession, use and distribution of narcotic drugs and psychotropic substances in India.

**Table 7.3: Equianalgesic doses of opioids**

| Opioid | Dose of equivalent to morphine per oral (PO) | Conversion factor |
|---|---|---|
| Morphine | 30 mg | 1 |
| Codeine | 200 mg | 0.15 |
| Fentanyl TD (µg/hr) | 12.5 | 2.4 |
| Methadone<br>1–20 mg/d<br>21–40 mg/d<br>41–60 mg/d<br>>61–80 mg/d | <br>7.5 mg<br>3.75 mg<br>3 mg<br>2.5 mg | <br>4<br>8<br>10<br>12 |

*Regulations*

- The NDPS Act classifies various drugs into different schedules based on their potential for abuse and dependence. Opioids are placed in schedules I, II, and III, with varying degrees of strictness associated with each schedule.
- Only registered medical practitioners can prescribe opioids as per NDPS Act. They must also undergo specific training in pain management and palliative care to be eligible for prescribing certain opioids.
- Medical practitioners are required to maintain detailed records of opioid prescriptions, including patient details, diagnosis, and quantity dispensed.

  After 1985 several amendments were made to the NDPS.[72]

*In 2014–2014 amendment:* Aim was to facilitate the use of opioids for medical purposes.

*2021 amendment:* This amendment further streamlined the process for availing essential narcotic drugs for specific medical conditions.

## Conclusion

Pain is the persistent symptom, which is present at all stages of the of cancer management. Despite various recent guidelines, cancer pain remains poorly managed in advanced disease. Lack of knowledge, financial restrictions, limited availability of the drugs hinders effective management of the pain. WHO ladder provides the analgesic path with an aim to provide effective strategy to manage cancer pain. The three step ladder emphasises on starting non-opioid drugs and then escalating to opioids according to pain severity. Although opioids remain essential for management of the cancer pain, they are associated with unavoidable side effects and opioid use disorders. With proper knowledge of pharmacodynamics and pharmacokinetics will help in opioid selection and titration. Individualized assessment and titration of pain medication are crucial for achieving satisfactory pain control and improving quality of life.

## References

1. Snijders RAH, Brom L, Theunissen M, van den Beuken-van Everdingen MHJ. Update on Prevalence of Pain in Patients with Cancer 2022: A Systematic Literature Review and Meta-Analysis. Cancers (Basel). 2023 Jan;15[3].
2. Portenoy RK. Treatment of cancer pain. Lancet (London, England). 2011 Jun;377[9784]:2236–47.
3. Ventafridda V, Saita L, Ripamonti C, De Conno F. WHO guidelines for the use of analgesics in cancer pain. Int J Tissue React. 1985;7[1]:93–6.
4. Dworkin RH, O'Connor AB, Backonja M, Farrar JT, Finnerup NB, Jensen TS, et al. Pharmacologic management of neuropathic pain: evidence-based recommendations. Pain. 2007 Dec;132[3]:237–51.
5. Jadad AR, Browman GP. The WHO analgesic ladder for cancer pain management: stepping up the quality of its evaluation. Jama. 1995;274[23]:1870–3.
6. Eisenberg E. Time to modify the WHO analgesic ladder? Pain Clin Updat. 2005;13[5]:1–4.
7. Orhan ME, Bilgin F, Ergin A, Dere K, Güzeldemir ME. [Pain treatment practice according to the WHO analgesic ladder in cancer patients: eight years experience of a single center]. Agri Agri Dernegi'nin Yayin organidir = J Turkish Soc Algol. 2008 Oct;20[4]:37–43.
8. Szeto C-C, Sugano K, Wang J-G, Fujimoto K, Whittle S, Modi GK, et al. Non-steroidal anti-inflammatory drug (NSAID) therapy in patients with hypertension, cardiovascular, renal or gastrointestinal comorbidities: joint APAGE/APLAR/APSDE/APSH/APSN/PoA recommendations. Gut. 2020 Apr;69[4]:617–29.

9. Crush J, Levy N, Knaggs RD, Lobo DN. Misappropriation of the 1986 WHO analgesic ladder: the pitfalls of labelling opioids as weak or strong. Vol. 129, British Journal of Anaesthesia. Elsevier; 2022. p. 137–42.
10. McNicol ED, Midbari A, Eisenberg E. Opioids for neuropathic pain. Cochrane database Syst Rev. 2013 Aug;2013[8]:CD006146.
11. Moulin DE, Clark AJ, Gilron I, Ware MA, Watson CPN, Sessle BJ, et al. Pharmacological management of chronic neuropathic pain—consensus statement and guidelines from the Canadian Pain Society. Pain Res Manag. 2007;12[1]:13–21.
12. Organization WH. WHO guidelines for the pharmacological and radiotherapeutic management of cancer pain in adults and adolescents. 2018.
13. Vadalouca A, Moka E, Argyra E, Sikioti P, Siafaka I. Opioid rotation in patients with cancer: a review of the current literature. J Opioid Manag. 2008;4[4]:213–50.
14. Fallon M, Dierberger K, Leng M, Hall PS, Allende S, Sabar R, et al. An international, open-label, randomised trial comparing a two-step approach versus the standard three-step approach of the WHO analgesic ladder in patients with cancer. Ann Oncol Off J Eur Soc Med Oncol. 2022 Dec;33[12]:1296–303.
15. Napoli R Di, Esposito G, Cascella M. Intrathecal Catheter. StatPearls.
16. Cascella M, Muzio MR, Viscardi D, Cuomo A. Features and Role of Minimally Invasive Palliative Procedures for Pain Management in Malignant Pelvic Diseases: A Review. Am J Hosp Palliat Care. 2017 Jul;34[6]:524–31.
17. Williams J. Basic Opioid Pharmacology. Rev pain. 2008 Mar;1[2]:2–5.
18. Dhawan BN, Cesselin F, Raghubir R, Reisine T, Bradley PB, Portoghese PS, et al. International Union of Pharmacology. XII. Classification of opioid receptors. Pharmacol Rev. 1996 Dec;48[4]:567–92.
19. Pathan H, Williams J. Basic opioid pharmacology: an update. Br J pain. 2012 Feb;6[1]:11–6.
20. Trivedi M, Shaikh S, Gwinnutt C. Pharmacology of opioids II. Anaesthesia, UK. 2007;
21. Freye E, Levy JV. Mechanism of Action of Opioids and Clinical Effects. Opioids in Medicine: A Comprehensive Review on the Mode of Action and the Use of Analgesics in Different Clinical Pain States. 2008. p. 85–187.
22. Azzam AAH, McDonald J, Lambert DG. Hot topics in opioid pharmacology: mixed and biased opioids. Br J Anaesth. 2019;122[6]:e136–45.
23. Approach to managing cancer pain. National cancer grid, 2021.
24. Swarm RA, Paice JA, Anghelescu DL, Are M, Bruce JY, Buga S, et al. Adult cancer pain, version 3.2019, NCCN clinical practice guidelines in oncology. J Natl Compr Cancer Netw. 2019;17[8]:977–1007.
25. Fallon M, Giusti R, Aielli F, Hoskin P, Rolke R, Sharma M, et al. Management of cancer pain in adult patients: ESMO Clinical Practice Guidelines. Ann Oncol. 2018;29:iv166–91.
26. Lasheen W, Walsh D, Mahmoud F, Sarhill N, Rivera N, Davis M, et al. The intravenous to oral relative milligram potency ratio of morphine during chronic dosing in cancer pain. Palliat Med. 2010;24[1]:9–16.
27. Paice JA, Bohlke K, Barton D, Craig DS, El-Jawahri A, Hershman DL, et al. Use of opioids for adults with pain from cancer or cancer treatment: ASCO guideline. J Clin Oncol. 2023;41[4]:914–30.
28. Gibbison B, Bailey CR, Klein AA. Tramadol—the Marmite (TM) drug. Vol. 70, Anaesthesia. England; 2015. p. 125–30.
29. Thota RS, Ramanjulu R, Ahmed A, Jain P, Salins N, Bhatnagar S, et al. Indian Society for Study of Pain, Cancer Pain Special Interest Group Guidelines on Pharmacological Management of Cancer Pain (Part II). Indian J Palliat Care. 2020;26[2]:180–90.
30. Eduardo B, Portenoy R. cancer pain: assesment and managment. seccond. UK: cambridge university; 2009. 230–254 p.
31. Gupta R. Pain management: essential topics for examinations. Springer; 2014.

32. Schmidt-Hansen M, Bennett MI, Arnold S, Bromham N, Hilgart JS. Efficacy, tolerability and acceptability of oxycodone for cancer-related pain in adults: an updated Cochrane systematic review. BMJ Support Palliat Care. 2018;8[2]:117–28.
33. Dean M. Opioids in renal failure and dialysis patients. J Pain Symptom Manage. 2004 Nov;28[5]:497–504.
34. Han J, Saraf SL, Gordeuk VR, Gowhari M. Safety of chronic transdermal fentanyl use in patients receiving hemodialysis. Am J Heal Pharm [Internet]. 2016 Jul 1;73[13]:947–8. Available from: https://doi.org/10.2146/ajhp150748
35. Coluzzi F, Caputi FF, Billeci D, Pastore AL, Candeletti S, Rocco M, et al. Safe Use of Opioids in Chronic Kidney Disease and Hemodialysis Patients: Tips and Tricks for Non-Pain Specialists. Ther Clin Risk Manag. 2020;16:821–37.
36. Yassen A, Olofsen E, Romberg R, Sarton E, Teppema L, Danhof M, et al. Mechanism-based PK/PD modeling of the respiratory depressant effect of buprenorphine and fentanyl in healthy volunteers. Clin Pharmacol Ther. 2007 Jan;81[1]:50–8.
37. Wilcock A, Charlesworth S, Prentice W, Selby P, McKenna M, Cripps S, et al. Prescribing in Chronic Severe Hepatic Impairment. J Pain Symptom Manage. 2019 Sep;58[3]:515–37.
38. Böger RH. Renal impairment: a challenge for opioid treatment? The role of buprenorphine. Palliat Med. 2006;20 Suppl 1:s17-23.
39. Bryson J, Tamber A, Seccareccia D, Zimmermann C. Methadone for treatment of cancer pain. Curr Oncol Rep. 2006 Jul;8[4]:282–8.
40. Waldhoer M, Bartlett SE, Whistler JL. Opioid receptors. Annu Rev Biochem. 2004;73:953–90.
41. Dowell D, Haegerich TM, Chou R. CDC Guideline for Prescribing Opioids for Chronic Pain--United States, 2016. JAMA. 2016 Apr;315[15]:1624–45.
42. Viswanath V, Palat G, Chary S, Broderick A. Challenges of Using Methadone in the Indian Pain and Palliative Care Practice. Indian J Palliat Care. 2018 Jan;24[Suppl 1]:S30–5.
43. Litman RS, Pagán OH, Cicero TJ. Abuse-deterrent Opioid Formulations. Anesthesiology [Internet]. 2018 May 1;128[5]:1015–26. Available from: https://doi.org/10.1097/ALN.0000000000002031
44. Christrup LL, Lundorff L, Werner M. Novel formulations and routes of administration for opioids in the treatment of breakthrough pain. Clin Pract. 2009;6[5]:695.
45. Rosenthal RN. Novel Formulations of Buprenorphine for Treatment of Opioid Use Disorder. Focus (Am Psychiatr Publ). 2019 Apr;17[2]:104–9.
46. Cohen SP, Dragovich A. Intrathecal analgesia. Anesthesiol Clin. 2007 Dec;25[4]:863–82, viii.
47. Smith HS, Deer TR, Staats PS, Singh V, Sehgal N, Cordner H. Intrathecal drug delivery. Pain Physician. 2008 Mar;11[2 Suppl]:S89–104.
48. Deer TR, Prager J, Levy R, Rathmell J, Buchser E, Burton A, et al. Polyanalgesic Consensus Conference 2012: recommendations for the management of pain by intrathecal (intraspinal) drug delivery: report of an interdisciplinary expert panel. Neuromodulation. 2012;15[5]:436.
49. Bhatia G, Lau ME, Koury KM, Gulur P. Intrathecal Drug Delivery (ITDD) systems for cancer pain. F1000Research. 2013;2:96.
50. Califf DD. Dr. Robert M Califf, MD Commissioner of Food and Drugs US Food and Drug Administration 10903 New Hampshire Avenue Silver Spring, MD 20993. 2022;
51. Lee C, Ye M, Weaver O, Jess E, Gilani F, Samanani S, et al. Defining opioid naïve and implications for monitoring opioid use: A population based study in Alberta, Canada. Pharmacoepidemiol Drug Saf. 2023;
52. Caraceni A, Hanks G, Kaasa S, Bennett MI, Brunelli C, Cherny N, et al. Use of opioid analgesics in the treatment of cancer pain: evidence-based recommendations from the EAPC. Lancet Oncol. 2012;13[2]:e58–68.
53. Dowell D, Compton WM, Giroir BP. Patient-centered reduction or discontinuation of long-term opioid analgesics: the HHS guide for clinicians. Jama. 2019;322[19]:1855–6.

54. Sande TA, Laird BJA, Fallon MT. The use of opioids in cancer patients with renal impairment-a systematic review. Support care cancer Off J Multinatl Assoc Support Care Cancer. 2017 Feb;25[2]:661–75.
55. Candy B, Jones L, Goodman ML, Drake R, Tookman A. Laxatives or methylnaltrexone for the management of constipation in palliative care patients. Cochrane database Syst Rev. 2011 Jan;[1]:CD003448.
56. Ghoshal A. Fentanyl, morphine, and opioid-induced constipation in patients with cancer-related pain. Indian J Palliat Care. 2020;26[4]:535.
57. Lang-Illievich K, Bornemann-Cimenti H. Opioid-induced constipation: a narrative review of therapeutic options in clinical management. Korean J Pain. 2019 Apr;32[2]:69–78.
58. Farmer AD, Gallagher J, Bruckner-Holt C, Aziz Q. Narcotic bowel syndrome. Lancet Gastroenterol Hepatol. 2017 May;2[5]:361–8.
59. Stone P, Minton O. European Palliative Care Research collaborative pain guidelines. Central side-effects management: what is the evidence to support best practice in the management of sedation, cognitive impairment and myoclonus? Palliat Med. 2011 Jul;25[5]:431–41.
60. Sivanesan E, Gitlin MC, Candiotti KA. Opioid-induced Hallucinations: A Review of the Literature, Pathophysiology, Diagnosis, and Treatment. Anesth Analg. 2016 Oct;123[4]:836–43.
61. Macleod J, Steer C, Tilling K, Cornish R, Marsden J, Millar T, et al. Prescription of benzodiazepines, z-drugs, and gabapentinoids and mortality risk in people receiving opioid agonist treatment: Observational study based on the UK Clinical Practice Research Datalink and Office for National Statistics death records. PLoS Med. 2019 Nov;16[11]:e1002965.
62. van Lemmen M, Florian J, Li Z, van Velzen M, van Dorp E, Niesters M, et al. Opioid overdose: limitations in naloxone reversal of respiratory depression and prevention of cardiac arrest. Anesthesiology. 2023;139[3]:342–53.
63. American Academy of Hospice and Palliative Medicine [Internet]. Available from: www.aahpm.org/certification/index.html
64. Okutani H, Lo Vecchio S, Arendt-Nielsen L. Mechanisms and treatment of opioid-induced pruritus: Peripheral and central pathways. Eur J Pain. 2024;28[2]:214–30.
65. Velayudhan A, Bellingham G, Morley-Forster P. Opioid-induced hyperalgesia. Contin Educ Anaesthesia, Crit Care Pain. 2014;14[3]:125–9.
66. Rivas SR, Tessner AC, Goldwyn EE. Calculating prescription rates and addiction probabilities for the four most commonly prescribed opioids and evaluating their impact on addiction using compartment modelling. Math Med Biol. 2021 Jun;38[2]:202–17.
67. Services USD of H and H. Pain management best practices inter-agency task force report: updates, gaps, inconsistencies, and recommendations. Washington, DC US Dep Heal Hum Serv. 2019;
68. Levy N, Lord LJ, Lobo DN. UK recommendations on opioid stewardship. Vol. 372, bmj. British Medical Journal Publishing Group; 2021.
69. Mercadante S, Bruera E. Opioid switching in cancer pain: From the beginning to nowadays. Crit Rev Oncol Hematol. 2016 Mar;99:241–8.
70. Good P, Afsharimani B, Movva R, Haywood A, Khan S, Hardy J. Therapeutic challenges in cancer pain management: a systematic review of methadone. J Pain Palliat Care Pharmacother. 2014 Sep;28[3]:197–205.
71. Narcotic Drugs and Psychotropic Substances Act,1985. India; 1985.
72. Parmar A, Narasimha VL, Nath S. National Drug Laws, Policies, and Programs in India: A Narrative Review. Indian J Psychol Med. 2023;02537176231170534.

Chapter 8

# Non-opioids in Cancer Pain

• Veer Thakkar

## INTRODUCTION

Cancer pain is multifactorial with complex etiologies including injury to soft tissues, mechanical distortion (tumor expansion in viscera, bone/fascia), tissue lysis (tumor erosion of bone or skin), release of neuro-hormones that activate small afferents; and nerve injury secondary to tumor compression, activation of immune processes, or iatrogenic injuries such as nerve sectioning for tumor excision.

Though opioids are the gold standard for treatment of moderate to severe cancer pain, the World Health Organization (WHO) ladder has since its inception in 1986, recommended the use of simple analgesics for treating mild cancer pain. Simple analgesics include paracetamol and non-steroidal anti-inflammatory drugs (NSAIDs) which are non-opioid analgesics. Since then, the list of non-opioids has increased beyond paracetamol and NSAIDs to encompass a spectrum of other drugs popularly referred to as adjuvant analgesics or co-analgesics. In this chapter we shall outline these drugs and their current role in managing cancer pain.

Non-opioid analgesics include:

1. NSAIDs
2. Corticosteroids
3. Antidepressants
4. Anticonvulsants
5. Topical agents
6. Ketamine
7. Cannabinoids

## PARACETAMOL AND NSAIDs

### Acetaminophen

Although acetaminophen has been historically classified as an NSAIDs, multiple investigations have failed to demonstrate the anti-inflammatory actions of acetaminophen. It exerts its pharmacological effects largely at the central nervous system (CNS) level and not as a peripheral Cyclooxygenase (COX) inhibitor. It readily crosses the blood–brain barrier and is homogenously distributed throughout the CNS. It is here that acetaminophen produces the selective inhibition of the COX pathway. Thus it is devoid of the adverse effects seen with the use of other NSAIDs such as gastric ulcerations and platelet dysfunction. Within the CNS, the action of acetaminophen is explained by the 'peroxide theory'. It does not directly bind to the active site of the COX enzyme, rather it reduces the active form of the enzyme, rendering it catalytically deficient. This mechanism of inhibition is seen only in tissues where the peroxides are low in concentration, such as the brain. It also explains why acetaminophen is ineffective at sites where the peroxide levels are high, such as in inflamed tissues.

Analgesic effects of acetaminophen are attributed to two distinct mechanisms. The first one involves the modulation of the endogenous cannabinoid system. Acetaminophen is transformed to N-arachidinoyl-phenolamine (AM404) in the brain, spinal cord and dorsal root ganglia. This conversion occurs in two steps, initially by de-acetylation to p-aminophenol and subsequently is conjugated with arachidonic acid by fatty acid amide hydrolase to AM404. Because of structural similarity between AM404 and N-arachidonoylethanolamine (AEA), which is an endogenous cannabinoid neurotransmitter, the former acts as a weak agonist at the cannabinoid receptors type 1 and 2 (CB1 and CB2). AM404 also doubles up as an inhibitor of the anandamide membrane transporter (AMT), leading to increased levels of endogenous cannabinoids.[1,2] In addition, it also potently activates the vanilloid subtype 1 receptors (TRPV1). Both the vanilloid and cannabinoid mechanisms are present in the thermoregulatory and pain center in the brain.[2-4]

## Role of Acetaminophen in Cancer Pain Management

Acetaminophen has been effectively used as a single agent in mild pain. It is also part of many fixed drug combinations with opioids (codeine, tramadol, hydrocodone or oxycodone). When used with opioids, it has an opioid sparing effect. These combinations may be initiated in patients with moderate pain.

For moderate to severe pain, the addition of acetaminophen to a strong opioid has limited evidence.[5–14] However, most randomized controlled trials that suggest limited benefit of acetaminophen were underpowered. In 2017, a Cochrane review of three double-blind randomized controlled trials compared acetaminophen alone with a placebo, or acetaminophen in combination with an opioid comparing with the same dose of opioid alone for at least five days duration; concluding that risk of bias was high in all of the three studies, and that there is no high-quality evidence to support or refute the use of acetaminophen in patients with any severity of cancer pain.[8] However, a network meta-analysis in 2019, of therapeutics for cancer pain concluded that the top-ranking drug classes for global efficacy included nonopioid analgesics such as acetaminophen, NSAIDs and opioids.[5]

Acetaminophen is administered via intravenous, oral or rectal routes. The onset of action of intravenous acetaminophen is 5 to 10 minutes, while that of oral and rectal varies from as low as 10 minutes to more than 60 minutes. The dose for a 50 kg adult is 650 mg every four hours or 1000 mg every 6 hours, the total daily dose not exceeding 4 g. The dose should be reduced in patients with low body weight, hepatic insufficiency, chronic alcoholism, malnutrition or dehydration. Patients with renal impairment may get the usual dose but the time interval between two doses should not be less than 6 hours.

Although the side effect profile of acetaminophen is exceedingly good, the therapeutic index is relatively narrow and the main toxicity being liver injury. Hepatotoxicity secondary to acetaminophen overdose is a serious concern and can be life threatening.

Acetaminophen induced hepatic injury has been generally attributed to doses of more than 4 g/day.[15–17]

## NSAIDs

NSAIDs have a potent inhibitory effect on cancer pain secondary to tissue invasion. Thus reflecting the role of prostaglandins in mediating pain secondary to the lytic process of tumor invasion. These drugs are the first line of implementation in the WHO's step-ladder approach to the management of cancer pain.

In contrast to opioids, NSAIDs relieve pain without interacting with opioid receptors, decrease elevated body temperature, possess anti-inflammatory and anti-platelet activities. They do not cause sedation and are non-addictive. Pharmacologically they are weakly acidic (ionization constants varying from 3.0 to 5.0); have varying degrees of lipid solubility and are almost completely absorbed orally; highly bound to albumin, have small volume of distribution and are metabolized by the liver. The various classes of NSAIDs have been included in Table 8.1. Their use as a single agent in treatment of mild cancer pain has been well established.[5] Additionally, when used in conjunction with opioids, they have additive analgesic effects, thus reducing the total opioid requirement. This also helps to lessen the opioid-related side effects.

The anti-inflammatory action of NSAIDs lies in their ability to inhibit the activity of the COX enzyme. This leads to decreased production of the pro-inflammatory prostaglandins. COX enzyme catalyzes the first step in the synthesis of prostaglandins, during inflammation, from arachnoid acid. The subsequently formed prostanoids include PGH2, PGE2, PGD2, PGI2 and TXA2 (Fig. 8.1).

The COX enzyme exists in two isoforms: COX-1 and COX-2. The former is more of a house-keeping enzyme, present in nearly all cell types and plays an important role in tissue homeostasis (cyto-protection of the stomach lining, platelet aggregation). COX-2 activity is normally absent from cells but is inducible by mediators involved in acute and chronic inflammatory processes. Thus COX-1 is physiological whereas COX-2 is usually, but not always, pathological. All non-selective NSAIDs inhibit the activity of both these enzymes at therapeutic doses. Most of the side effects of these drugs like

**Table 8.1: Classification of NSAIDs**

| Class | Examples |
|---|---|
| A. Nonselective COX inhibitors | |
| 1. Salicylates | Aspirin |
| 2. Propionic acid derivatives | Ibuprofen, naproxen, ketoprofen, flurbiprofen |
| 3. Aryl-acetic acid derivatives | Diclofenac, aceclofenac |
| 4. Oxicam derivatives | Piroxicam, tenoxicam |
| 5. Pyrrolo-pyrrole derivatives | Ketorolac |
| 6. Indole derivative | Indomethacin |
| B. Preferential COX-2 inhibitors | Meloxicam, nimesulide |
| C. Selective COX-2 inhibitors | Celecoxib, etoricoxib |
| D. Analgesic-antipyretics with poor anti-inflammatory action | Paracetamol (acetaminophen) |

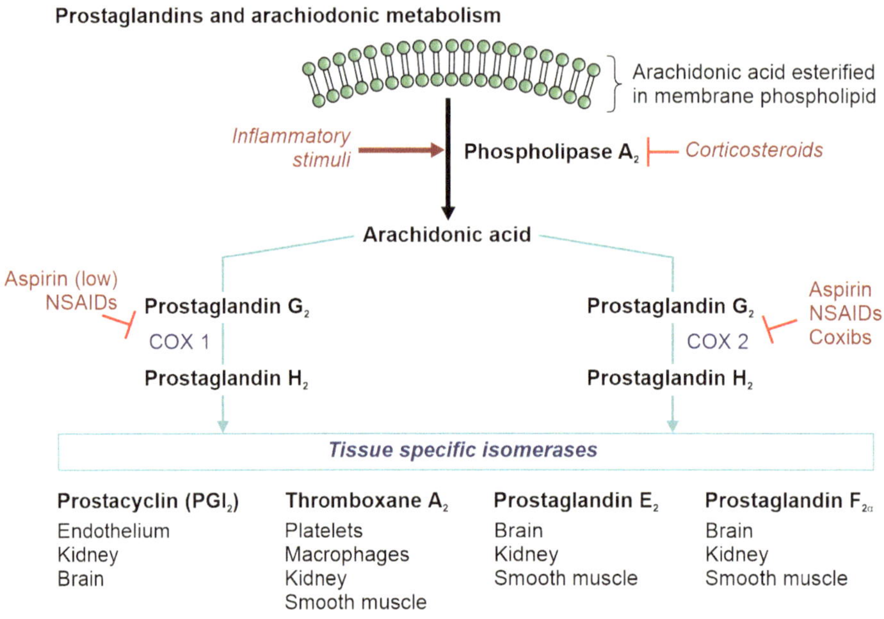


**Fig. 8.1:** Cyclooxygenase pathway

gastrointestinal (GI) ulcerations and GI bleeds, platelet dysfunction, etc. are due to the suppression of COX-1 derived prostanoids. Also inhibition of COX-1 is responsible for hypersensitivity to aspirin and other NSAIDs in chronic asthmatics and patients with chronic urticarial-angioedema.

## Role of NSAIDs in Cancer Pain Management

NSAIDs are effective in treating cancer pain when used alone or in combination with an opioid.[13,18,19] Evidence regarding the efficacy of NSAIDs as an additive analgesic with an opioid is slightly more than the combination of acetaminophen with an opioid.[8,13,18]

In 2017, Cochrane review was conducted that included eleven randomized trials comparing different NSAIDs or a step three opioid with or without an NSAID. There were no trials comparing an NSAID with a placebo. Initially moderate to severe pain was reduced to no less than mild pain after one or two weeks in four studies. The authors noted that all the studies were at high-risk of bias for lack of blinding, incomplete data or small sample size. Thus, the authors concluded that there were no high-quality trials to support or refute the benefit of NSAIDs, alone or in combination with opioids for any severity of cancer pain.[8] The lack of high-quality evidence with respect to the analgesic efficacy of NSAIDs in cancer pain was reiterated in a 2019 systematic review.[18] On the other hand, a 2019 network meta-analysis concluded that NSAIDs, like acetaminophen and opioids were one of the top-ranking drug classes for the global efficacy for chronic cancer pain therapeutics.[5]

A systematic review conducted in 2021, evaluated the opioid sparing effects of one NSAIDs (ketorolac) in patients with chronic cancer pain, including nine studies. The data was insufficient to draw conclusions but one study found a significant degree of morphine sparing.[19] Clinically, NSAIDs may be particularly useful in treating patients having bone pain or pain that is grossly due to inflamed lesions. They are relatively less effective in treating neuropathic pain.

The major adverse effects of NSAIDs include cardiovascular toxicity, gastrointestinal toxicity, bleeding, nephrotoxicity and hepatotoxicity.

The risk of major cardiovascular events such as myocardial infarction, stroke and death is same with all nonselective NSAIDs at high doses. The prothrombotic effects of nonselective NSAIDs are seen at the initiation of therapy but the risk of adverse cardiovascular events is cumulative over time.

NSAIDs produce gastrointestinal toxicities in the form of both dyspepsia and peptic ulcer disease. Although the risk seems to be low with selective COX-2 inhibitors than with nonselective agents such as ibuprofen and naproxen.[20,21]

Most NSAIDs interfere with platelet aggregation, except nonacetylated salicylates and selective COX-2 inhibitors. Aspirin irreversibly inhibits platelet aggregation for the life time of the platelets (five to seven days), the antiplatelet action of other NSAIDs usually lasts for two days.

Reversible renal insufficiency occurs due to renal vasoconstriction, acute intestinal nephritis and acute tubular necrosis in patients with low renal perfusion. But prolonged use of NSAIDs may cause chronic nephropathy, which may be irreversible.

Hepatotoxicity is seen with NSAIDs even at usual doses. However, the elevation is liver enzymes is usually mild and reverts back to normal on discontinuation of the offending agent.

## ADJUVANT ANALGESICS

Adjuvant analgesics are a heterogeneous group of drugs which are usually indicated for purposes other than pain relief. But over the past few decades they have been used as analgesics in patients who are on opioid therapy.[22] The number and types of these 'adjuvants' used in clinical practice for the management of cancer pain has increased dramatically (Table 8.2).

The decision to initiate adjuvant analgesic therapy is based on clinical judgement and there is no published data on the timing of starting these drugs. These drugs are often considered for patients with chronic cancer pain who are poorly responsive to opioids, in other words in such cases where titrating the optimum dose of opioids is difficult, to achieve analgesia and manage the side effects related to opioids. There are two approaches followed for starting these drugs. In the first approach, where a patient may benefit from the non-analgesic effect of an adjuvant drug (e.g. mood enhancement from an antidepressant or reduction in skeletal related events by using a bisphosphonate), early administration of these drugs before the full dose of opioids has been ascertained may be beneficial. On the other hand, a second approach to starting an adjuvant advocates delaying these drugs till efforts have been made to optimize the opioid therapy. Starting an adjuvant in tandem with an opioid may have better outcomes associated with an opioid sparing effect. While the delayed approach ensures that the drug is indeed needed, reducing the risk of additive toxicity by sequencing drug titration efforts, and decreases the confusion with regards to the offending agent in case an adverse drug reaction occurs. This delayed approach of initiation of a co-analgesic has limited support in a systematic review.[23]

**Table 8.2: Adjuvant analgesics in cancer pain treatment**

| Group of drugs | Class | Subclass | Drugs |
|---|---|---|---|
| Multipurpose analgesics | Corticosteroids | | Dexamethasone, prednisolone, methylprednisolone |
| | Anti-depressants | Tricyclic | Amitriptyline, nortriptyline, desipramine |
| | | Serotonin norepinephrine reuptake inhibitors (SNRIs) | Duloxetine |
| | | Selective serotonin reuptake inhibitors (SSRIs) | Paroxetine, citalopram |
| | | Others | Bupropion |
| | Alpha-2 adrenergic agonists | | Tizanidine, clonidine |
| | Cannabinoids | | Dronabinol, nabilone, nabiximols |
| | Topical analgesics | | Local anesthetics (lignocaine), capsaicin, TCA, NSAIDs |
| Drugs for neuropathic pain | Anti-convulsant | | Gabapentin, pregabalin, valproate, phenytoin, carbamazepine, oxcarbazepine, topiramate, lamotrigine |
| | Sodium channel blockers | Sodium channel modulator | Lacosamide |
| | | Sodium channel blocker | Mexiletine, intravenous lignocaine |
| | NMDA receptor antagonists | | Ketamine, memantine, dextromethorphan, amantadine |
| | GABA agonists | GABAa agonists | Clonazepam |
| | | GABAb agonists | Baclofen |
| Drugs for bone pain | Osteoclast inhibitors | Bisphosphonates | Pamidronate, zolendronate, ibandronate |
| | | | Calcitonin |
| | | RANKL inhibitor | Denosumab |
| | Radiopharmaceuticals | | Strontium-89, samarium-153, radium-223 |
| Drugs for bowel obstruction | Anticholinergic agents | | Scopolamine, atropine, glycopyrrolate |
| | Somatostatin analog | | Octreotide |

## 1. Corticosteroids

Steroids have been used to decrease cancer related pain since a long time. They have shown to improve appetite, nausea, pain, and overall quality of life.[24] Despite being used as a co-analgesic in cancer related pain, the mechanism by which steroids impart analgesia is unknown and may be multifactorial. They reduce peritumoral edema, alleviating pain by decreasing the mass effect and reducing the stretch on pain-sensitive structures. Anti-inflammatory properties inhibit the release of compounds that sensitize the primary afferent nerves, and directly inhibit the abnormal discharges produced by the injured nerves leading to decrease in neuropathic pain. Additionally, pain may be reduced secondary to the potentially mood elevation effects of steroids.

Evidence regarding the clinical benefits of steroids in the treatment of cancer-related pain is sparse. The number of trails aimed at assessing the analgesic properties of steroids in cancer patients have been small and have produced mixed results.[25–27] A Cochrane review conducted in 2015, reviewed 6 randomized trials and found that steroid therapy resulted in modest decrease in pain compared to control treatments (placebo or standard therapy) at one week. The authors concluded that additional trials were needed to evaluate the efficacy of steroid therapy for management of cancer related pain in adults.[28]

Notwithstanding the lack of evidence, there is enough clinical experience suggesting the usefulness of steroids in treating pain arising due to a variety of cancers. Neuropathic and bone pain, pain associated with stretch of the organ capsule or duct obstruction, pain related to lymphedema and headaches secondary to raised intracranial pressures are few of the conditions where steroids have proven to be effective in mitigating the pain.

A risk-to-benefit analysis should be done before considering steroids for pain management due to their potential toxicities. These include increased risk of myopathy, infections, diabetes, hypertension, cushingoid habitus, and skin breakdown. When patients are put on long-term steroid therapy, serious side effects like gastrointestinal bleeding and neuropsychiatric syndromes (ranging from mild dysphoria to severe anxiety or depression, or psychosis) should also be kept in mind.

In the setting of advanced illness where opioid regimes are not yielding satisfactory results and the prognosis is of a very short duration (days to weeks), a low dose steroid is added to tackle pain and other symptoms such as nausea, fatigue, or dysphoria. This treatment is usually continued until the patient dies. On the other hand, where steroids need to be started in patients with a longer life expectancy to treat neuropathic pain, the risks of prolonged steroid therapy are usually too substantial to consider open-end therapy. In such cases a short course of steroids (steroid pulse), tapered over a course of two weeks may be started until other drugs (like pregabalin), started for neuropathic pain have reached therapeutic levels.

Dexamethasone is the most commonly used steroid for cancer related pain, presumably due to its long half-life and relatively low mineralocorticoid effects reflecting a better safety profile. Although to date there is no evidence to suggest that this drug is better than other alternatives like prednisolone or methylprednisolone for treating cancer pain.

A high dose steroid therapy was recommended for some conditions. A loading dose of dexamethasone as high as 96 mg followed by rapid tapering beginning at 24 mg four times a day was advocated for 'pain crisis' associated with epidural spinal cord compression (ESCC). The dose is titrated over two weeks, usually till radiotherapy has shrunk the tumor. Although better pain relief was the rationale of administering steroids at such high doses, no high-quality comparative studies justified the use of this regime. In one study of patients with ESCC, this high dose regime did have better pain relief and preserved ambulation after six months, it was associated with substantial (11%) risk of side effects including gastrointestinal bleeds and psychosis.[29] Considering the risk of permanent neurological damage, this high dose regime is followed by some clinicians, in the absence of quality evidence. The other alternative to this is starting a loading dose of dexamethasone at 10–20 mg followed by a dose of 16 mg/day in divided doses. This is followed by the dose down-titration to the lowest dose that maintains pain relief while other analgesics are added. The decision to start either depends solely on the clinical judgement of the treating physician.

## 2. Antidepressants

The analgesic effects of antidepressants have been recognized since the 1960s. Antidepressants have been used in cancer patients suffering from a depressed mood and are poorly responsive to opioids. These drugs have been studied in populations with chronic pain for a variety of conditions and meta-analyses have shown that they are effective as multipurpose analgesics in conditions including low back pain, various types of neuropathic pain and fibromyalgia.[22,30–33] Although there is limited evidence to support their use in cancer patients, tricyclic antidepressants have been studied extensively and have proven their efficacy in neuropathic pain.[34] The analgesic effect of antidepressants is mainly related to the enhanced availability of monoamines at the synapses within the neural pathways that are part of a descending pain modulating system. Inhibition of norepinephrine reuptake is thought to be the most important mode of action, but serotonergic and dopaminergic effects may also play a part in analgesia.[35]

Although antidepressants comprise several subclasses and many drugs, analgesic efficacy has been best established for tricyclic antidepressants (TCAs)[36,37] and selective-norepinephrine reuptake inhibitors (SNRIs).[38–42] Better side effect profile of SNRIs, among patients with serious medical illnesses including cancer, makes them the first line analgesic antidepressants as opposed to TCAs in cancer patients.

The SNRIs include duloxetine, milnacipran, venlafaxine and desvenlafaxine. Amongst these, duloxetine has the best analgesic properties.[40–43] A five-week randomized trial in cancer patients with chemotherapy-induced peripheral neuropathy (CIPN) secondary to taxanes or platinum agents found that duloxetine acted as an analgesic at a dose of 30 to 60 mg.[43] There are no trials comparing the analgesic efficacy of drugs within the SNRI group. The side effects of SNRIs include nausea, sexual dysfunction and somnolence or mental clouding.

The TCAs include tertiary amine compounds like amitriptyline, and secondary amine compounds such as nortriptyline and desipramine. The secondary amine compounds, which are more selective at the norepinephrine reuptake sites have a more favorable side effect profile as compared to amitriptyline. Thus, when an antidepressant is to be started in a medically ill patient, nortriptyline or desipramine is preferred. All the TCAs are contraindicated in patients with serious heart disease, severe prostatic hypertrophy and narrow-angle glaucoma.

The initial toxicity profile of antidepressants has to be kept in mind while initiating these drugs, especially TCAs. Starting with low dose, gradual increments are made until benefit occurs, side effect supervene or the conventional maximum dosage is reached. SNRIs are usually titrated in one or two doses, but for TCAs, it may take several steps to achieve the desired analgesic effects. For antidepressants, the analgesic dose range is much lower than the antidepressant dose range and analgesia, usually, but not always appears at lower doses than mood elevation. When TCAs are used in high doses, their plasma concentration and electrocardiogram should be monitored. These drugs can prolong the QTc interval and may precipitate cardiac arrhythmias, and should be used with caution in patients who are on other drugs which affect the QTc interval. Duloxetine is usually started at a dose of 20–30 mg/day, which is gradually increased over a week to 60 mg/day. A higher dose of 120 mg/day may be considered thereafter. The starting dose of nortriptyline is 10–25 mg/day at night. This dose is increased up to 50–150 mg/day till desired analgesic effect is achieved or intolerable side effects occur. Plasma concentration should be monitored in patients receiving doses more than 100 mg/day.

Antidepressants should not be discontinued suddenly. They should preferably be tapered before stopping if they have been administered for several weeks, particularly at high doses. The antidepressant discontinuation syndrome may mimic flu-like symptoms and psychiatric phenomenon.

### 3. Anticonvulsants

These are a group of drugs which work in various clinical scenarios and have various mechanisms of action. Two anticonvulsants, the gabapentinoids, namely gabapentin and pregabalin have been approved for use in patients with neuropathic pain without accompanying morbid depression. They are used as a first-line treatment for neuropathic cancer pain, other than CIPN.[44]

The gabapentinoids act by binding to the alpha-2-delta protein, which a subunit of a system that modulates the flux through the N-type, voltage gated calcium channels. This reduces the influx of calcium ions and decreases the likeliness of depolarization. They are not metabolised in the liver and have a few drug interactions. But they do enhance the central depressive action of other centrally acting drugs including opioids. Thus they should be added with caution in cancer patients who are already on opioids or other central nervous system depressants.[45–46] Both these drugs are excreted through the kidneys, this makes it necessary to decrease the dose in renal impairment patients. The common side effects include mental clouding, dizziness and somnolence. Weight gain and edema are less common side effects.

Although gabapentin and pregabalin have been studied extensively for other types of neuropathic pain including post-herpetic neuralgias and painful diabetic neuropathies, evidence to support their efficacy in cancer related neuropathic pain is limited. Three small randomized placebo-controlled trials tested the addition of gabapentin and pregabalin in patients with cancer-related neuropathic pain, who were already on opioid therapy. All three studies concluded that addition of gabapentinoids significantly improved the neuropathic pain and dysesthesias.[47–49] On the other hand, a placebo-controlled randomised trial on the use of gabapentin for CIPN failed to show any benefit. Pregabalin alone (without opioids) was studied for the treatment of radiotherapy related neuropathic pain in head and neck cancer survivors. These patients had a significant decrease in their pain intensities. Pregabalin also improved their mood states and quality of life, and the number of rescue pain medication was also low.[50]

A systematic review conducted to determine the efficacy of adjuvant analgesic drugs (antidepressants and anticonvulsants) alongside standard opioid therapy for pain related directly to cancer, concluded that adjuvants improved pain control within 4–8 days when added to an opioid for cancer pain. But reduction of pain intensity greater than 1 point on a 0-10 numerical scale is unlikely. This was especially true in patients with non-cancer neuropathic pain.[51]

On the other hand, another systematic review was conducted to evaluate the beneficial and adverse effects of various pharmacological agents used for the treatment of neuropathic cancer pain. The authors concluded that the absolute benefit of all agents (antidepressants and anticonvulsants) greatly outweighed the risks for harm. But all the studies included in the review had low methodologic quality, precluding conclusions about the relative effect sizes of different medication groups.[52]

The major difference that differentiates the gabapentinoids is the pharmacokinetics. The absorption of gabapentin in facilitated by a transporter in the small bowel and the CNS. This transporter is saturable at higher doses, such as 1800 mg/day. At these doses the kinetics become nonlinear as less absorption occurs with each dose increment. Thus gabapentin has a pharmacokinetic ceiling along with a pharmacodynamic ceiling, which is seen with other adjuvant analgesics as well. Pharmacodynamics ceiling is when responders reach a maximum response level and further dose escalation does not increase the benefit effect.

Pregabalin is usually initiated at the dose of 50 to 75 mg a day. The dose is further escalated to 150 to 300 mg twice daily in two to three steps over one or two weeks. The starting dose is decreased to 25 mg per day in frail cancer patients with slower titration. The starting dose of gabapentin is often 300 mg per day. This dose is slowly increased over a few days to almost double, while monitoring analgesia and side effects. If pain relief is inadequate and in the absence of pharmacodynamic ceiling and side effects the dose can be escalated to as high as 3600 mg per day, given in two to three divided doses.[53]

## 4. Topical Agents

Many topical agents have been used for various pain syndromes and may be considered for multimodal analgesia. The advantage of topical agents is that they can be applied directly at the site of pain and they lack the relative systemic toxicities that are especially relevant in clinically ill patients. Although neuropathic pain is the main indication where these agents are used they may have a broader application. Local anesthetics, capsaicin, NSAIDs and TCAs have been used as topical agents with varying degrees of pain relief.

### *a. Local Anesthetics*

Lignocaine is the most commonly used local anesthetic for topical application. 5% lignocaine patches are applied for treatment of focal or regional pain of all types. Creams and gels containing lignocaine may also be used but they need to be applied two to four times a day.

Although a 2014 systematic review concluded that topical lidocaine has limited evidence to support its use for neuropathic pain, individual studies and clinical experience suggest that it can be effective in certain situations.[54] The currently approved formulations use a 12-hour regime. Multiple patches are often used together. There is limited evidence to indicate high level of safety with four patches applied for 24 hours a day for up to 72 hours.[55] The most commonly reported side effect of lignocaine patches is skin irritation, although this may be attributed to the vehicle rather than to lignocaine. There is only a remote chance of systemic toxicity for absorption of lignocaine, but the risk may be higher in patients with renal or hepatic dysfunction.[56,57]

Eutectic mixture of local anesthetic (EMLA), which is a combination of lignocaine and prilocaine is capable of penetrating intact skin and produces dense local cutaneous anesthesia. EMLA may be applied in cancer patients undergoing painful procedures like lumbar puncture, biopsies or subcutaneous ports being accessed through a needle.

#### *b. Capsaicin*

Capsaicin is a naturally occurring constituent of chili peppers. It depletes substance P from the terminals of afferent C fibers. Topical application of capsaicin low-dose transdermal patches (0.025 to 0.1%), have shown benefit in controlled trials in patients with cancer-related neuropathic pain. Application site burning sensation, often transient, is the most common side effect and the reason for discontinuation of treatment. The patch is applied two to three times a day for at least a week to determine clinical benefit.

#### *c. Anti-inflammatory Drugs*

There is no data to support the use of NSAIDs as a patch or gel for local application in cancer pain. Nonetheless, efficacy and safety evidence is sufficient to warrant a trial in patients with a small area of local or locoregional pain of any cause. Diclofenac is the most commonly used drug as a topical agent.

### 5. Ketamine

Ketamine is often used in palliative medicine to treat refractory pain, in end of life care.[58] Even though there is limited data to support its use, ketamine may be used in the earlier course of illness especially in treatment refractory neuropathic pain.

Ketamine acts as a N-methyl-D-aspartate (NMDA) receptor antagonist. NMDA is responsible for sensitization of central neurons and the functioning of opioid receptors.

Ketamine is used as a brief infusion in sub-anesthetic doses for treatment of severe pain.[58] Prolonged infusions and oral ketamine have been used to treat refractory pain associated with advanced disease.[59] A 2017 Cochrane review of three trails concluded that the evidence was insufficient to assess the benefits and harms of ketamine as an adjuvant to opioids for relief of refractory cancer pain.[60,61] Nevertheless, use of parenteral ketamine for chronic pain is supported in consensus guideline from the American Society of Regional Anesthesia and Pain Medicine, the American Academy of Pain Medicine and the American Society of Anesthesiologists.[62] Psychotomimetic effects are the most problematic side effects of ketamine. These include symptoms of dissociation, hallucinations, and delirium. These can be reduced by co-administration of a benzodiazepine, lorazepam, or a neuroleptic, haloperidol.[62]

## 6. Cannabis and Cannabinoids

The term 'cannabinoids' refer to the compounds derived from cannabis plant which contains more than sixty cannabinoids. Some of these compounds have pharmacological effects which mimic the effects of endogenous cannabinoids by interacting with receptors in the CNS and other tissues. The primary psychoactive ingredient is tetrahydrocannabinol (THC). A trial of non-inhaled cannabinoid should be given to patients with cancer related pain not responding adequately to conventional opioids and adjuvant therapies. However, these agents appear to have limited analgesic efficacy and relatively high side effect liability and also the social stigmata of being considered as a drug of abuse. Although the evidence is limited and at times conflicting, clinical trials have suggested analgesic efficacy of cannabinoid drugs and also inhaled cannabis.[63–66] Few studies have been conducted on cancer patients.[64, 67–69] These studies indicate that cannabinoids may be used as multipurpose analgesics for patients with refractory pain secondary to advanced disease.

## 7. Other Agents

### *a. Baclofen*

Baclofen acts as a GABA receptor modulator. It reduces the release of excitatory neurotransmitters by binding to the GABAb presynaptic receptors in the brainstem, dorsal horn of the spinal cord and other CNS sites. It is especially effective in the treatment of spasticity and trigeminal neuralgia. Based on clinical experience baclofen has been used in various types of neuropathic pain including cancer pain.[70] It is started at a dose of 5 mg twice a day and gradually increased up to 200 mg per day.

### *b. Drugs for Bowel Obstruction*

Cancer patients with malignant bowel obstruction (MBO) who are not candidates for surgical interventions are treated with opioids (for adequate pain control), anticholinergic agents and octreotide (to decrease intraluminal secretions and peristaltic movements) and/or corticosteroids (to lessen the peritumoral edema).

The evidence on the use of somatostatin analogs like octreotide in patients with advanced cancers and MBO to relieve distressing gastrointestinal symptoms is quiet conflicting. Octreotide inhibits gastric, pancreatic and intestinal secretions, reduces gastrointestinal motility and may relieve pain and other distressing symptoms of bowel obstruction. A systematic review noted that at least four small randomized trials of high or unclear risk of bias concluded that octreotide was superior to an anticholinergic agent given alone for the symptomatic management of MBO.[71] On the other hand, two adequately powered multi-centric randomized trials with low-risk of bias reported no significant difference between a long-acting somatostatin analog and a placebo.[72,73] The usual starting dose of octreotide is 100 μg two to three times a day and is administered subcutaneously.

Anticholinergic agents like scopolamine (hyoscine) may be added to patients with MBO who have a high level of obstruction or to limit the colicky abdominal pain, along with octreotide.

## Summary

Management of cancer pain requires a holistic approach. In addition to the cancer related pain, cancer patients often suffer from other illnesses such as clinical depression, which may perpetuate pain or may aggregate it. Opioid analgesics may play the central role in the treatment of cancer pain, but the role of adjuvant analgesics or the co-analgesics cannot be undermined in the multimodal approach to cancer pain management. However, these agents should be used with caution keeping in mind their long-term side effects. The dosages of the commonly used co-analgesics have been summarized in Tables 8.3 and 8.4.

**Table 8.3: Non-opioids in cancer pain**

| **Drug** | **Usual analgesic dose** | **Maximum dose per day** | **Remarks** |
|---|---|---|---|
| *NSAIDs* | | | |
| Diclofenac | 50 mg q8 hr to q12 h | 150 mg | Bone pain |
| Ibuprofen | 400 mg q4–6 h or 600 mg to 800 mg q 6–8 h | 3200 mg (acute)<br>2400 mg (chronic) | |
| Aspirin | 325 to 1000 mg q4–6 h | 4000 mg | Irreversibly inhibits platelet function |
| Celecoxib | 200 mg once daily or 100 mg q12 hr | 400 mg | Less risk of GI toxicity relative to nonselective NSAIDs<br>CVS and kidney risks are dose related and may be similar to nonselective NSAIDs |
| Etoricoxib | 30 to 60 mg once daily | 60 mg (chronic)<br>120 mg (acute pain up to 8 days) | May be associated with severe dose related CVS effects |
| *Non-NSAID analgesic* | | | |
| Acetaminophen (paracetamol) | 325 to 650 mg q 4–6 h or 1000 mg q 6 h (up to 3 times a day) | 3000 mg<br>4000 mg in selected medically supervised patients<br>Avoid or use a lower dose (max 2000 mg/day) in patients at risk of hepatotoxicity (old age, regular alcohol use, malnourished) | Doses <2000 mg/day do not appear to increase risk of GI complications<br>Does not alter platelet function<br>Can cause hepatotoxicity in chronic or acute overdose |

**Table 8.4: Co-analgesics used in cancer pain**

| Class | Drug | Dosage | Remarks |
|---|---|---|---|
| Corticosteroids | Dexamethasone | 1 to 2 mg twice daily | Neuropathic, bone, visceral pain, brain edema, spinal cord compression |
| | Prednisolone | 5 to 10 mg twice daily | |
| Antidepressants | Duloxetine | 20 to 30 mg daily max 60 to 120 mg daily | Neuropathic pain |
| | Nortriptyline | 10 to 20 mg at bedtime max 50 to 150 mg at bedtime | |
| Anti-convulsant | Gabapentin | 100 to 300 mg twice daily max 300 to 1200 mg thrice daily | Neuropathic pain |
| | Pregabalin | 50 to 75 mg twice daily max 150 to 300 mg twice daily | |
| GABAb agonists | Baclofen | 5 mg twice a day max 200 mg per day | Spasticity |
| Drugs for bowel obstruction | Octreotide (somatostatin analogue) | 0.1 to 0.3 mg q12 h, subcutaneously | Anti-secretory |

## References


1. De Petrocellis PL, Bisogno T, Davis JB, Pertwee RG, Di Marzo V. Overlap between the ligand recognition properties of the anandamide transporter and the VR1 vanilloid receptor: inhibitors of anandamide uptake with negligible capsaicin-like activity. FEBS Lett. 2000; 483:52–56.
2. Szallasi A, Di Marzo V. New perspectives on enigmatic vanilloid receptors. Trends Neurosci. 2000; 23:491–97.
3. Karai L, Brown DC, Mannes AJ, Connelly ST, Brown J, Gandal M, Wellisch OM, Neubert JK, Olah Z, Iadarola MJ. Deletion of vanilloid receptor 1-expressing primary afferent neurons for pain control. J Clin Invest. 2004; 113:1344–52.
4. Piomelli D, Giuffrida A, Calignano A, Rodriguez de Fonseca F. The endocannabinoid system as a target for therapeutic drugs. Trends Pharmacol Sci. 2000; 21:218–24.
5. Huang R, Jiang L, Cao Y, et al. Comparative Efficacy of Therapeutics for Chronic Cancer Pain: A Bayesian Network Meta-Analysis. J Clin Oncol 2019; 37:1742
6. Curatolo M, Sveticic G. Drug combinations in pain treatment: a review of the publishedevidence and a method for finding the optimal combination. Best Pract Res ClinAnaesthesiol 2002; 16:507.
7. Sima L, Fang WX, Wu XM, Li F. Efficacy of oxycodone/paracetamol for patients with bone-cancer pain: a multicenter, randomized, double-blinded, placebo-controlled trial. J ClinPharm Ther 2012; 37:27.
8. Wiffen PJ, Derry S, Moore RA, et al. Oral paracetamol (acetaminophen) for cancer pain.Cochrane Database Syst Rev 2017; 7:CD012637.
9. Axelsson B, Borup S. Is there an additive analgesic effect of paracetamol at step 3? Adouble-blind randomized controlled study. Palliat Med 2003; 17:724.
10. Stockler M, Vardy J, Pillai A, Warr D. Acetaminophen (paracetamol) improves pain andwell-being in people with advanced cancer already receiving a strong opioid regimen: arandomized, double-blind, placebo-controlled cross-over trial. J Clin Oncol 2004; 22:3389.
11. Israel FJ, Parker G, Charles M, Reymond L. Lack of benefit from paracetamol(acetaminophen) for palliative cancer patients requiring high-dose strong opioids: arandomized, double-blind, placebo-controlled, crossover trial. J Pain Symptom Manage 2010; 39:548.

12. Cubero DI, del Giglio A. Early switching from morphine to methadone is not improved by acetaminophen in the analgesia of oncologic patients: a prospective, randomized, double-blind, placebo-controlled study. Support Care Cancer 2010; 18:235.
13. Nabal M, Librada S, Redondo MJ, et al. The role of paracetamol and nonsteroidal anti-inflammatory drugs in addition to WHO Step III opioids in the control of pain inadvanced cancer. A systematic review of the literature. Palliat Med 2012; 26:305.
14. Straube C, Derry S, Jackson KC, et al. Codeine, alone and with paracetamol (acetaminophen), for cancer pain. Cochrane Database Syst Rev 2014; :CD006601.
15. Dart RC, Bailey E. Does therapeutic use of acetaminophen cause acute liver failure?Pharmacotherapy 2007; 27:1219.
16. Larson AM. Acetaminophen hepatotoxicity. Clin Liver Dis 2007; 11:525.
17. Whitcomb DC. Acetaminophen poisoning and liver function. N Engl J Med 1994;331:1311.
18. Magee DJ, Jhanji S, Poulogiannis G, et al. Nonsteroidal anti-inflammatory drugs and painin cancer patients: a systematic review and reappraisal of the evidence. Br J Anaesth2019; 123:e412.
19. Butcher B, Hutchings E, Fazekas B, et al. Opioid-sparing effects of ketorolac in palliativecare patients receiving opioids for chronic cancer-related pain: A systematic literaturereview. Palliat Med 2022; 36:71.
20. Coxib and traditional NSAID Trialists' (CNT) Collaboration, Bhala N, Emberson J, et al.Vascular and upper gastrointestinal effects of non-steroidal anti-inflammatory drugs:meta-analyses of individual participant data from randomised trials. Lancet 2013;382:769.
21. Chan FKL, Ching JYL, Tse YK, et al. Gastrointestinal safety of celecoxib versus naproxen inpatients with cardiothrombotic diseases and arthritis after upper gastrointestinal bleeding (CONCERN): an industry-independent, double-blind, double-dummy, randomised trial. Lancet 2017; 389:2375.
22. Portenoy RK. A Practical Approach to Using Adjuvant Analgesics in Older Adults. J AmGeriatr Soc 2020; 68:691.
23. Kane CM, Mulvey MR, Wright S, et al. Opioids combined with antidepressants orantiepileptic drugs for cancer pain: Systematic review and meta-analysis. Palliat Med2018; 32:276.
24. Mercadante SL, Berchovich M, Casuccio A, et al. A prospective randomized study of corticosteroids as adjuvant drugs to opioids in advanced cancer patients. Am J Hosp Palliat Care 24:13–19, 2007.
25. Bruera E, Moyano JR, Sala R, et al. Dexamethasone in addition to metoclopramide forchronic nausea in patients with advanced cancer: a randomized controlled trial. J Pain Symptom Manage 2004; 28:381.
26. Paulsen O, Klepstad P, Rosland JH, et al. Efficacy of methylprednisolone on pain, fatigue,and appetite loss in patients with advanced cancer using opioids: a randomized, placebo-controlled, double-blind trial. J Clin Oncol 2014; 32:3221.
27. Yennurajalingam S, Frisbee-Hume S, Palmer JL, et al. Reduction of cancer-related fatiguewith dexamethasone: a double-blind, randomized, placebo-controlled trial in patients with advanced cancer. J Clin Oncol 2013; 31:3076.
28. Haywood A, Good P, Khan S, et al. Corticosteroids for the management of cancer-related pain in adults. Cochrane Database Syst Rev 2015; :CD010756.
29. Sørensen S, Helweg-Larsen S, Mouridsen H. Effect of high dose dexamethasone in carcinomatous metastatic spinal cord compression treated with radiotherapy: a randomised trial. EurJ Cancer 1994; 30A:22–7.
30. Urits I, Peck J, Orhurhu MS, et al. Off-label Antidepressant Use for Treatment and Management of Chronic Pain: Evolving Understanding and Comprehensive Review. CurrPain Headache Rep 2019; 23:66.
31. Griebeler ML, Morey-Vargas OL, Brito JP, et al. Pharmacologic interventions for painfuldiabetic neuropathy: An umbrella systematic review and comparative effectivenessnetwork meta-analysis. Ann Intern Med 2014; 161:639.
32. Mease PJ, Dundon K, Sarzi-Puttini P. Pharmacotherapy of fibromyalgia. Best Pract ResClin Rheumatol 2011; 25:285.

33. Ferreira GE, McLachlan AJ, Lin CC, et al. Efficacy and safety of antidepressants for thetreatment of back pain and osteoarthritis: systematic review and meta-analysis. BMJ2021; 372:m4825.
34. Dworkin RH, O'Connor AB, Backonja M, et al. Pharmacologic management of neuropathic pain: evidence-based recommendations. Pain 2007; 132:237–51.
35. Woolf CJ, American College of Physicians, American Physiological Society. Pain: moving from symptom control toward mechanism-specific pharmacologic management. AnnIntern Med 2004; 140:441.
36. Sindrup SH, Gram LF, Skjold T, et al. Concentration-response relationship in imipramine treatment of diabetic neuropathy symptoms. Clin Pharmacol Ther 1990; 47:509.
37. Max MB, Lynch SA, Muir J, et al. Effects of desipramine, amitriptyline, and fluoxetine onpain in diabetic neuropathy. N Engl J Med 1992; 326:1250.
38. Sindrup SH, Bach FW, Madsen C, et al. Venlafaxine versus imipramine in painful polyneuropathy: a randomized, controlled trial. Neurology 2003; 60:1284.
39. Rowbotham MC, Goli V, Kunz NR, Lei D. Venlafaxine extended release in the treatment of painful diabetic neuropathy: a double-blind, placebo-controlled study. Pain 2004; 110:697
40. Arnold LM, Rosen A, Pritchett YL, et al. A randomized, double-blind, placebo-controlled trial of duloxetine in the treatment of women with fibromyalgia with or without major depressive disorder. Pain 2005; 119:5.
41. Wernicke JF, Pritchett YL, D'Souza DN, et al. A randomized controlled trial of duloxetine in diabetic peripheral neuropathic pain. Neurology 2006; 67:1411.
42. Matsuoka H, Iwase S, Miyaji T, et al. Additive Duloxetine for Cancer-Related Neuropathic Pain Nonresponsive or Intolerant to Opioid-Pregabalin Therapy: A Randomized Controlled Trial (JORTC-PAL08). J Pain Symptom Manage 2019; 58:645.
43. Smith EM, Pang H, Cirrincione C, et al. Effect of duloxetine on pain, function, and quality of life among patients with chemotherapy-induced painful peripheral neuropathy: a randomized clinical trial. JAMA 2013; 309:1359.
44. Shkodra M, Caraceni A. Treatment of Neuropathic Pain Directly Due to Cancer: An Update. Cancers. 2022; 14(8):1992. https://doi.org/10.3390/cancers14081992
45. Gomes T, Greaves S, van den Brink W, et al. Pregabalin and the Risk for Opioid-Related Death: A Nested Case-Control Study. Ann Intern Med 2018; 169:732.
46. Gomes T, Juurlink DN, Antoniou T, et al. Gabapentin, opioids, and the risk of opioid-related death: A population-based nested case-control study. PLoS Med 2017;14:e1002396.
47. Caraceni A, Zecca E, Bonezzi C, et al. Gabapentin for neuropathic cancer pain: a randomized controlled trial from the Gabapentin Cancer Pain Study Group. J Clin Oncol2004; 22:2909
48. Mishra S, Bhatnagar S, Goyal GN, et al. A comparative efficacy of amitriptyline,gabapentin, and pregabalin in neuropathic cancer pain: a prospective randomized double-blind placebo-controlled study. Am J Hosp Palliat Care 2012; 29:177.
49. Keskinbora K, Pekel AF, Aydinli I. Gabapentin and an opioid combination versus opioid alone for the management of neuropathic cancer pain: a randomized open trial. J Pain Symptom Manage 2007; 34:183.
50. Jiang J, Li Y, Shen Q, et al. Effect of Pregabalin on Radiotherapy-Related Neuropathic Pain in Patients With Head and Neck Cancer: A Randomized Controlled Trial. J Clin Oncol 2019; 37:135.
51. Bennett MI. Effectiveness of antiepileptic or antidepressant drugs when added to opioids for cancer pain: systematic review. Palliat Med 2011; 25:553.
52. Jongen JL, Huijsman ML, Jessurun J, et al. The evidence for pharmacologic treatment of neuropathic cancer pain: beneficial and adverse effects. J Pain Symptom Manage 2013;46:581.
53. Bruera E and Portenoy RK (2010). Cancer pain: Assessment and management. Cambridge: Cambridge University Press.
54. Derry S, Wiffen PJ, Moore RA, Quinlan J. Topical lidocaine for neuropathic pain in adults. Cochrane Database Syst Rev 2014; :CD010958.

55. Gammaitoni AR, Alvarez NA, Galer BS. Pharmacokinetics and safety of continuously applied lidocaine patches 5%. Am J Health Syst Pharm 2002; 59:2215.
56. Gabra BH, Abidi MH, Al-Khadimi Z, et al. Systemic absorption of topical lidocaine in abone marrow transplant recipient with hepatic sinusoidal obstruction syndrome. Am J Health Syst Pharm 2011; 68:135.
57. De Martin S, Orlando R, Bertoli M, et al. Differential effect of chronic renal failure on the pharmacokinetics of lidocaine in patients receiving and not receiving hemodialysis. Clin Pharmacol Ther 2006; 80:597.
58. Jackson K, Ashby M, Howell D, et al. The effectiveness and adverse effects profile of "burst" ketamine in refractory cancer pain: The VCOG PM 1-00 study. J Palliat Care 2010;26:176.
59. Mercadante S, Arcuri E, Tirelli W, Casuccio A. Analgesic effect of intravenous ketamine in cancer patients on morphine therapy: a randomized, controlled, double-blind, crossover, double-dose study. J Pain Symptom Manage 2000; 20:246
60. Bell RF, Eccleston C, Kalso EA. Ketamine as an adjuvant to opioids for cancer pain. Cochrane Database Syst Rev 2017; 6:CD003351.
61. Cohen SP, Bhatia A, Buvanendran A, et al. Consensus Guidelines on the Use of Intravenous Ketamine Infusions for Chronic Pain From the American Society of Regional Anesthesia and Pain Medicine, the American Academy of Pain Medicine, and the American Society of Anesthesiologists. Reg Anesth Pain Med 2018; 43:521.
62. Krystal JH, D'Souza DC, Karper LP, et al. Interactive effects of subanesthetic ketamineand haloperidol in healthy humans. Psychopharmacology (Berl) 1999; 145:193.
63. Skrabek RQ, Galimova L, Ethans K, Perry D. Nabilone for the treatment of pain in fibromyalgia. J Pain 2008; 9:164.
64. Johnson JR, Burnell-Nugent M, Lossignol D, et al. Multicenter, double-blind, randomized, placebo-controlled, parallel-group study of the efficacy, safety, and tolerability of THC:CBD extract and THC extract in patients with intractable cancer-related pain. J Pain Symptom Manage 2010; 39:167.
65. Wilsey B, Marcotte T, Tsodikov A, et al. A randomized, placebo-controlled, crossover trial of cannabis cigarettes in neuropathic pain. J Pain 2008; 9:506.
66. Wilsey B, Marcotte T, Deutsch R, et al. Low-dose vaporized cannabis significantly improves neuropathic pain. J Pain 2013; 14:136.
67. Bowles DW, O'Bryant CL, Camidge DR, Jimeno A. The intersection between cannabis andcancer in the United States. Crit Rev Oncol Hematol 2012; 83:1.
68. Portenoy RK, Ganae-Motan ED, Allende S, et al. Nabiximols for opioid-treated cancer patients with poorly-controlled chronic pain: a randomized, placebo-controlled, graded-dose trial. J Pain 2012; 13:438.
69. Lichtman AH, Lux EA, McQuade R, et al. Results of a Double-Blind, Randomized, Placebo-Controlled Study of Nabiximols Oromucosal Spray as an Adjunctive Therapy in Advanced Cancer Patients with Chronic Uncontrolled Pain. J Pain Symptom Manage 2018; 55:179.
70. Yomiya K, Matsuo N, Tomiyasu S, et al. Baclofen as an adjuvant analgesic for cancer pain. Am J Hosp Palliat Care 2009; 26:112.
71. Obita GP, Boland EG, Currow DC, et al. Somatostatin Analogues Compared With Placebo and Other Pharmacologic Agents in the Management of Symptoms of Inoperable Malignant Bowel Obstruction: A Systematic Review. J Pain Symptom Manage 2016; 52:901.
72. Currow DC, Quinn S, Agar M, et al. Double-blind, placebo-controlled, randomized trial of octreotide in malignant bowel obstruction. J Pain Symptom Manage 2015; 49:814.
73. Khoo D, Hall E, Motson R, et al. Palliation of malignant intestinal obstruction using octreotide. Eur J Cancer 1994; 30A:28.

Chapter 9

# Understanding Breakthrough Pain and its Management

• Anjana Wajekar

## INTRODUCTION

Cancer-related pain is pain due to cancer itself, its metastasis or cancer related therapies (surgery, chemotherapy or radiation). The International Classification of Diseases ICD-11, published in 2019, included chronic cancer related pain for the first time as a separate entity.[1] It is a combination of mixed nociceptive and neuropathic pain. Cancer-related pain is multi-morphic and often presents with fluctuations in pain intensity. The characteristics of cancer pain comprises a continuous background pain juxtaposed with intermittent episodic pain. ICD-11 has not included the term 'breakthrough pain' in their list but have used the term intermittent episodic pain which encompasses all significant pain flares.[1] Breakthrough pain (BTP) is defined as the transitory increase in pain intensity from a baseline pain of mild-moderate intensity in patients on regularly administered analgesic treatment.[2–5] High prevalence of BTP among cancer patients is a predictor of worsening severity of pain, pain-associated distress, functional impairment, and poorer quality of life. Literature mentions a 40–80% prevalence of BTP in cancer patients.[3,4,6–8] BTP is commonly prevalent not only adults but also in children, although it is frequently underdiagnosed. A small cross-sectional study has reported episodes of BTP in 60% of children with controlled background pain of varied origins.[9] Studies have reported a significant negative impact of BTP on patient reported outcomes on quality-of-life indicators.[7]

## CLASSIFICATION/TYPES OF BTP

Breakthrough pain can be triggered by an event (incident) or spontaneous.[7] BTP triggered by an event can be further categorized as predictable, e.g. pain caused due to weight-bearing or an activity (movement, swallowing, coughing, defaecation, repeated dressing changes or bladder spasm after voiding), or unpredictable but still triggered by an event. Incident pain is the most frequent subtype of BTP, precipitated by movement and associated with bony metastasis or fractures.[3,7] Background pain may be absent or mild-moderate at rest but may exacerbate on movement. The onset is typically sudden, reaching maximum intensity within a few minutes. This leads to patient anticipating pain and thus restricting his or her movements, depending on the site of bony involvement. This type of pain significantly impacts the patients' mood, anxiety, functional autonomy and quality of life. Treatment of incident pain can be a challenge as freedom from pain on movement only is difficult to achieve.

Spontaneous or idiopathic pain is not associated with an identifiable cause or a precipitating event and occurs without any warning, e.g. biliary colic, stabbing pain associated with nerve injury.[3,7] It is a sudden sharp pain which peaks within minutes. It is more frequently associated with neuropathic pain and pain control may take a long time.

Some practitioners prescribe to a third group of end-of-dose failure, which does not fit into the definition of BTP but never the less exists and can be controlled with modifications to the basal analgesic regimen.[10] This kind of pain manifests as an exaggeration of the background pain, corresponding to the time of wearing off of the last analgesic dose. Episodic pain related to clinical procedures (injections or needle biopsies) is regarded as acute pain and not included within the nomenclature of chronic pain.

## CHARACTERISTICS

BTP occurs in patients suffering from cancers of soft tissue, bone, viscera and nervous system. About 50% of cancer patients may experience two or more types of BTP and the cause is a predictable event in one-third of them.[7,11] BTP characteristics show both inter-patient and intra-patient variabilities. It is usually rapid in onset, moderate to severe intensity, lasting a short duration. Studies report that the maximum time to peak intensity is 10 minutes in 66% of the patients with mean duration lasting up to 45 minutes. Mean pain intensity is also found to be around numeric rating scale (NRS) 7 when the underlying background pain is around 3–4.[11] A BTP with a neuropathic mechanism is associated with more severe pain and require a longer duration for optimal pain control.[11] Two commonest BTP are the movement associated bony pain due to metastasis and swallowing associated oropharyngeal pain due to mucositis.[10]

## ASSESSMENT

It is of prime importance to differentiate breakthrough pain from persistent pain. Initial and ongoing evaluation of both the background pain intensity as well as the worst pain intensity are paramount. These patients should undergo a detailed, structured pain assessment which includes the frequency, duration, intensity and precipitating factors of each BTP episode, along with previous and current pain treatments for baseline (persistent) pain and their effectiveness. Pain assessment should also mention the pathophysiological mechanisms of the pain syndrome. Utilizing the ICD-11 taxonomy of cancer pain—bone pain, neuropathic pain and visceral pain, for BTP facilitates tailored treatment which helps achieve optimal pain control. The brief pain inventory is a simple tool for evaluating both the background pain and BTP and its relation to the function and quality of life. It includes several questions on pain intensity which allows the patient to differentiate between average pain as well as the worst pain in last 24 hours, possibly as an indicator of BTP. A few other patient-reported questionnaires include the McGill Pain Questionnaire, Alberta Breakthrough Pain Assessment Tool and breakthrough pain assessment tool (BAT) but they have not yet found widespread acceptance.[2,12–14]

Understanding the patient's perspective in pain assessment is also of paramount importance. The patient should be trained to maintain a pain diary with daily records of the pain intensity, site, medications used and duration of relief. Visual analogue scales, numerical rating scales (0–10), and verbal rating scales, are the traditional pain assessment measures, suitable for this purpose. These scores should be charted frequently, through the whole spectrum from the onset until the episode ends either spontaneously or after a specific treatment, and when the pain recurs. The duration between the onset of the episode and the administration of drugs, and the onset of its effect should be recorded. Onset of pain, peak intensity, location, quality, predictability, precipitating factors, and those factors that provide relief or prevent it, should also be recorded for every episode of BTP. Spontaneous BTP is more challenging to predict. The origin and presentation of this type of pain can be either neuropathic, with short pain episodes, or visceral, such as a colic. It may be quite distressing and difficult to manage. Maintenance of a pain diary by patients can help in diagnosing such pain.

A pilot study has reported that patients use qualitatively similar pain descriptors for both background pain and BTP, the higher intensity of BTP being reflected in the more intense terms.[14] Another study has reported that BTP is commonly a brief exacerbation on a relatively well controlled background pain and is located at the same site.[15]

## MANAGEMENT

Both prevention and treatment are a part of BTP management. A different therapeutic approach is indicated depending upon the subtype of BTP. For example, neuropathic pain necessitates pre-emptive therapy whereas others may be treated only when required. The same patient may experience different types of BTP over the course of their cancer detection and varied management strategies.

## NON-PHARMACOLOGICAL

Patient or caregivers can help alleviate the BTP episodes by use of various non-pharmacological methods such as change in position, use of heat or cold compress, massage, meditation, mindfulness and other distraction therapy modalities.[6] These can also be useful, allowing time for the onset of the rescue medication administered. Use of orthotic devices for upper limb bony lesions or surgical stabilisation can help improve the quality of patients' life.

## OPTIMIZATION OF BASAL TREATMENT

Various opioid and non-opioid medications are generally used for the around-the-clock (ATC) medications. Oral opioids such as morphine are routinely used for baseline control of analgesia in moderate to severe pain. Transdermal fentanyl or buprenorphine is useful in cases of patients who cannot swallow, suffer constipation and have poor compliance. Optimisation of basal analgesia along with careful titration to prevent adverse events must be done. Either the interval between dosages can be decreased or their dose can be increased, depending on the drug and patient profile. It is recommended to optimise the basal regimen with an extended-release formulation if four or more rescue doses are needed.[3,16] In some cases, it is difficult to manage sudden pain such as BTP occurring during coughing, change in position or in cases where intense BTP last for mere seconds or minutes. Sometimes patients with incident pain may be on acceptable basal regimen, but remain confined to bed with restricted mobility in an effort to prevent BTP. Opioid switching to improve response during escalation to maximum tolerated dose is one of the methods to optimise the basal regimen. This may necessitate the use of adjuvant drugs such as anti-emetics and laxatives pre-emptively to limit the opioid side effects. Non-steroidal anti-inflammatory drugs (NSAIDs) have an adjuvant role in improving basal analgesia and also help in preventing or mitigating the effect of BTP.[6] Literature is scarce on the presence of BTP in patients with neuropathic pain. Regular use of adjuvants like anti-convulsants and anti-depressants may have some benefit in limiting the BTP. Additionally, use of topical drugs like capsaicin and eutectic mixture of local anesthetic (EMLA) may have some benefit by preventing transmission at local level in neuropathic pain. Similarly, ketamine can be an excellent option for central desensitization in patients with neuropathic pain. Severe incident pain may be an indication to consider intrathecal local anesthetics and opioids. The ideal combination of various opioids and non-opioid medications to arrive at an optimum basal regimen with the added aim of reducing the frequency and intensity of BTP episodes needs to be individualized to the probable pathophysiological mechanisms of pain. The use of single fraction external beam radiotherapy (EBRT) and bisphosphonates has direct implications in treatment of bony pain both for background pain and indirectly reducing the BTP episodes.

## MANAGEMENT OF BTP EPISODES

Opioids are the cornerstone of cancer pain management. The mainstay of treatment for episodic or breakthrough pain is the administeration of additional oral opioids as a rescue to the continuous basal regimen. Current recommendations favor the use of an oral short acting opioid such as morphine in a dose proportional to the total daily opioid dose.[16,17] The WHO guidelines for management of cancer pain in adults and adolescents recommend immediate release morphine dose equivalent to 50–100% of the routine 4 hourly dose for severe BTP.[18] Oral oxycodone or hydromorphone are other alternatives. However, these preparations are unavailable in India. Oral medications have a slow peak action time of up to 1 hr, making its use ideal in patients with predictable BTP, e.g. an additional oral dose 30 minutes prior to intended physical activity or dressing change is an option.[3] Presence of mucositis or xerostomia may necessitate use of other routes. Also, in cases of unpredictable events, severe cancer pain or a BTP necessitating immediate relief, parental opioids have been proven to be highly efficacious and safe. Subcutaneous morphine for at home injections have been found to be safe whereas intravenous morphine (1.5 mg every 10 minutes) is reserved for administration in a hospital setup.[16] Parenteral opioids such as morphine or fentanyl, may also be administered for longer duration with use of patient-controlled analgesia devices.

## NON-INVASIVE FAST DELIVERY SYSTEMS

Transmucosal delivery of lipophilic substances such as fentanyl, have gained popularity for fast onset and quick relief of BTP. Fentanyl is a lipophilic, synthetic opioid which is hundred times more potent than morphine. Transmucosal drug delivery system, for fentanyl include atomization devices, nasal sprays, sublingual tablets, buccal soluble films, lozenges, effervescent tablets, etc.[16,17] Of these only oral transmucosal fentanyl citrate (OTFC) or lozenges are available in India. These routes have the advantages of bypassing the first-pass effect of liver, thus improving the bioavailability in the blood, leading to rapid pain relief. But there are no double blind randomised controlled trial

**Table 9.1 Transmucosal fentanyl deliver systems[10]**

| S.No. | Formulation | Onset (minutes) | Duration of action (minutes) |
|---|---|---|---|
| 1 | Lozenge | 15–30 | 40 |
| 2 | Buccal tablet | 15 | 45 |
| 3 | Sublingual tablet | 10–15 | 40 |
| 4 | Buccal soluble film | 15 | 60 |
| 5 | Intranasal spray | 5–10 | 20 |
| 6 | Fentanyl pectin nasal spray | 5–10 | 20 |

comparing the various formulations or any evidence of the superiority of any one formulation over other. The potency and rapid onset with fast relief also raise concerns for misuse, abuse and overdosage of these formulations. Current recommendations favour the use of transmucosal fentanyl use only if the total daily morphine dose exceeds 60 mg or its equivalent.[3,10] Both fentanyl buccal tablet and sublingual tablets are tolerated well and have been found to be safe up to 12 months.[10] All other formulations have only been assessed for safety and tolerability outcomes for periods ranging from 12 to 16 weeks. It is recommended to start with the smallest dose of these fast delivery fentanyl, and repeated if there is unsatisfactory pain relief after 15–30 minutes depending on the formulation. These medications should be restricted to a maximum of two doses per BTP episode and a maximum of four BTP episodes treated per day.[16]

Ketamine through sublingual routes and intranasal sprays (10 mg per spray at 90 second interval to a maximum of 5 sprays in adults) have also been reported to be effective for BTP treatment.[19]

### Other Approaches

Local application of benzocaine gel 15 minutes prior, can alleviate oral ulcer pain prior to chewing food. Anti-tussives should be prescribed for patients with BTP associated with coughing.

## TREATMENT CHALLENGES IN DIFFERENT LOCATIONS

The prevalence of BTP in outpatient departments is around 40% whereas in palliative care units as high as 80%.[7] Also, with long-term usage of baseline opioids with periodically increasing dosage, patients become tolerant over time. Use of oral morphine for at home relief is the first line recommendation.[10,16] The use of non-invasive fast drug delivery systems is suitable for BTP on outpatient basis depending upon their availability and rigorous prescriber and patient education. In some countries with pain-nurse driven at-home care, patient or their relatives are educated regarding subcutaneous use of morphine and sometimes even nurse administered intravenous morphine.[17] Patients in palliative wards or during hospital admission, can be prescribed parental opioids and non-opioids under the monitoring by a dedicated pain service team. Patients in palliative intensive care units may also be prescribed intrathecal opioids and local anesthetics for BTP relief.

## FUTURE DEVELOPMENTS

Most of the available data on BTP are primarily sourced from cross-sectional studies. Due to the dynamic nature of cancer and its treatment strategies, the nature and intensity of BTP can vary over long-term. More longitudinal studies are required for mapping of BTP and individualizing the treatment plans. Patient education to improve the compliance, prevent anxiety related to excess use of pain killers and the management of adverse effects need to be focused upon. Similarly, education for medical professionals in the field of cancer management should also be stressed upon. Newer drug delivery systems for fast relief with limited side effect profile are in various stages of research whose results may very well completely alter the management of BTP. With improvements in the life expectancy of patients with cancer, the long-term safety profile of these newer delivery systems also need to be evaluated.

### Summary

Cancer-related pain is multifaceted and often presents with inter-patient and intra-patient fluctuations in pain intensity. Every patient is different and strategies to manage pain also needs to be individualized. Breakthrough pain is a transient and exacerbating pain on a background of chronic controlled pain. A trifecta of in-depth evaluation, categorization and optimal management strategy can significantly help control pain and thereby lead to an improvement in patient related outcome measures. Maintenance of a pain diary by the patient is paramount. The need for regular pharmacological treatment of BTP episodes, more than four times a day, necessitates titration of basal regimen. After optimization of basal analgesia, use of oral morphine for at home relief is a first line recommendation. The use of non-invasive fast drug delivery systems, although revolutionary in BTP treatment, is limited by their availability, limited literature on safety and tolerability profile and potential for misuse or abuse. A holistic approach inclusive of non-pharmacological approaches, forms the foundation of optimum BTP management.

### References

1. Bennett MI, Kaasa S, Barke A, et al. The IASP classification of chronic pain for ICD-11: Chronic cancer-related pain. Pain 2019; 160: 38–44.
2. Løhre ET, Hjermstad MJ, Brunelli C, et al. Pain Intensity Factors Changing Breakthrough Pain Prevalence in Patients with Advanced Cancer: A Secondary Analysis of a Cross-Sectional Observational International Study. Pain Ther. 2018 Dec;7(2):193–203.
3. Fallon M, Giusti R, Aielli F, et al. Management of cancer pain in adult patients: ESMO Clinical Practice Guidelines. Annals of Oncology 2018; 29: iv166–iv191.
4. Deandrea S, Corli O, Consonni D, et al. Prevalence of breakthrough cancer pain: A systematic review and a pooled analysis of published literature. Journal of Pain and Symptom Management 2014; 47: 57–76.
5. Løhre ET, Klepstad P, Bennett MI, et al. From 'breakthrough' to 'episodic' Cancer Pain? A European Association for Palliative Care Research Network Expert Delphi Survey Toward a Common Terminology and Classification of Transient Cancer Pain Exacerbations. J Pain Symptom Manage 2016; 51: 1013–19.
6. Bennett MI, Eisenberg E, Ahmedzai SH, et al. Standards for the management of cancer-related pain across Europe—A position paper from the EFIC Task Force on Cancer Pain. European Journal of Pain (United Kingdom) 2019; 23: 660–68.

7. Canal-Sotelo J, Trujillano-Cabello J, Larkin P, et al. Prevalence and characteristics of breakthrough cancer pain in an outpatient clinic in a Catalan teaching hospital: incorporation of the Edmonton Classification System for Cancer pain into the diagnostic algorithm. BMC Palliat Care. 2018 May 28;17(1):81.
8. Campagna S, Sperlinga R, Milo A, et al. The Circadian Rhythm of Breakthrough Pain Episodes in Terminally-ill Cancer Patients. Cancers (Basel). 2018 Dec 24;11(1):18.
9. Friedrichsdorf SJ, Finney D, Bergin M, et al. Breakthrough Pain in Children with Cancer. J Pain Symptom Manage 2007; 34: 209–16.
10. Mercadante S, Portenoy RK. Breakthrough cancer pain: Twenty-five years of study. Pain 2016; 157: 2657–63.
11. Mercadante S, Marchetti P, Cuomo A, et al. IOPS-MS Study Group. Factors Influencing the Clinical Presentation of Breakthrough Pain in Cancer Patients. Cancers (Basel). 2018 Jun 1;10(6):175.
12. Hagen NA, Stiles C, Nekolaichuk C, et al. The Alberta Breakthrough Pain Assessment Tool for Cancer Patients: A Validation Study Using a Delphi Process and Patient Think-Aloud Interviews. J Pain Symptom Manage 2008; 35: 136–52.
13. Webber K, Davies AN, Zeppetella G, et al. Development and validation of the breakthrough pain assessment tool (BAT) in cancer patients. J Pain Symptom Manage 2014; 48: 619–31.
14. Hansen RB, Frost CØ, Sonne NM, et al. Exploring the Patients' Perception of Background and Breakthrough Pain: A McGill Pain Questionnaire Inquiry in Patients with Bone Cancer Pain. J Palliat Med 2019; 22: 881–83.
15. Gonella S, Sperlinga R, Sciannameo V, et al. Characteristics of Breakthrough Pain and Its Impact on Quality of Life in Terminally Ill Cancer Patients. Integr Cancer Ther. 2019 Jan-Dec; 18:1534735419859095.
16. George B, Minello C, Allano G, et al. Opioids in cancer-related pain: current situation and outlook. Supportive Care in Cancer 2019; 27: 3105–18.
17. Løhre ET, Thronæs M, Klepstad P. Breakthrough cancer pain in 2020. Current Opinion in Supportive and Palliative Care 2020; 14: 94–9.
18. World Health Organization. WHO guidelines for the pharmacological and radiotherapeutic management of cancer pain in adults and adolescents. Geneva 2018.
19. Singh V, Gillespie TW, Lane O, et al. A dose-escalation clinical trial of intranasal ketamine for uncontrolled cancer-related pain. Pharmacotherapy 2022; 42: 298–310.

Chapter 10

# Role of Radiotherapy in Oncology

• Anil Tibdewal • Amiya Agrawal

Radiotherapy plays a crucial role in the management of cancer, either as a standalone mode of treatment or in combination with other treatment modalities such as surgery and chemotherapy. Its primary objective is to target and destroy cancer cells while preserving the surrounding healthy tissues.

In recent years, advancements in radiation therapy techniques and technology have further enhanced its effectiveness and reduced potential side effects. These developments have expanded the scope of radiotherapy, making it an increasingly integral component of multidisciplinary cancer care.

As our comprehension of the complex processes involved in cancer progresses, the significance of radiotherapy in the field of oncology also keep advancing. With ongoing research and innovation, the future holds great promise for further maximizing the therapeutic benefits of radiotherapy while minimizing its limitations.

Radiotherapy is often utilized as a curative treatment for localized cancers, where the main goal is to eradicate the cancer cells and achieve long-term remission. It can be used as the primary treatment modality, particularly when surgery is not a viable option or when the tumor is located in a critical or hard-to-access area. In cases where surgical resection is incomplete or there is a high-risk of recurrence, radiotherapy serves as an essential adjuvant strategy to target any remaining cancerous cells and reduce the likelihood of relapse.

Furthermore, radiotherapy is frequently employed in concurrence with other treatment modalities like chemotherapy, to enhance the overall therapeutic effect. This multidisciplinary approach aims to maximize the chances of eradicating the cancer and preventing recurrence, underscoring the pivotal role of radiotherapy in achieving curative outcomes for cancer patients.

Given its ability to target cancerous cells with utmost precision and conformity, radiotherapy continues to be a cornerstone in the curative management of various malignancies, contributing significantly to improving the survival and quality of life (QoL) of patients.

The importance of radiotherapy also extends its role in palliative care. Radiation therapy administered to enhance the QoL for patients, rather than aim for a cure, is known as palliative radiation therapy.[1] It constitutes a significant portion of the treatment provided by radiation oncologists. About 40 to 50% of the treatments given in radiation oncology facilities are intended for palliation. For patients with advanced cancer, radiotherapy helps to alleviate symptoms commonly pain, bleeding, and pressure, improving their quality of life (Table 10.1).

**Table 10.1: Site-wise indications of palliative radiotherapy**

| Site | Symptoms | Probable causes |
|---|---|---|
| Brain | Headache, vomiting, blurring of vision, seizures, neurological deficits | Brain metastases, recurrent inoperable gliomas, brainstem tumors |
| Head and neck | Pain, bleeding, nerve compression, fungation | Large nodal mass, carotid invasion, inoperable recurrent disease |
| Esophagus | Chest pain, grade 3 or more dysphagia, obstruction | Locally advanced/progressive disease, post stenting dysphagia |
| Lung | Shortness of breath, hemoptysis, chest pain, lung collapse, neuropathic chest wall pain | Superior vena caval obstruction, large nodal mediastinal mass, endobronchial mass, chest wall mass |
| Abdomen | Abdominal and back pain, hematemesis, biliary obstruction, gastric outlet obstruction | Coeliac plexus invasion, inoperable pancreatic/gastric mass, large liver mass |
| Genitourinary | Hematuria, obstructive, hydroureteronephrosis, urinary outlet obstruction, pelvic pain | Recurrent/inoperable bladder or urethra tumors with/without involvement of VUJ |
| Gynecological | Pelvic pain, limb edema, uncontrolled bleeding PV | Frozen pelvis due to advanced cervical disease, involvement of pelvic walls |
| Rectum/Anus | Bleeding requiring transfusions, obstruction, pelvic pain | Highly vascular or large rectal/anal mass not amenable for definitive therapy |
| Bone and spine | Pain with or without neuropathy, risk of pathological fracture, neurological deficits, diminished mobility, spinal instability | Lytic bone metastases with or without soft tissue component, compression of the spinal cord and other skeletal related events (SREs) |

## MECHANISM OF ACTION

Likely, the primary ways that radiotherapy functions are through the reduction of tumor size and the suppression of pain-related chemical mediator release. This leads to pain relief and gives a durable response, especially in responsive tumors like carcinoma of breast and prostate.[2] Radiotherapy has different biological actions at different doses. Conventional and hypo-fractionated regimens of radiotherapy have an anti-proliferative effect that causes tumor shrinkage keeping in mind the 5 Rs of radiobiology.

The 5Rs of basic radiobiology in radiotherapy are **R**epair, **R**eassortment, **R**epopulation, **R**eoxygenation and **R**adiosensitivity. The ability of cells to recover from DNA damage caused by radiation is referred to as repair. The biological effects of dose rate and fractionation depends on the ability of cells to repair themselves . Reassortment involves variations in the cell cycle phases affecting their susceptibility to radiation. Repopulation is the re-proliferation of surviving tumor cells during and after each fraction of radiotherapy. Reoxygenation is the process whereby cells in a tumor that are hypoxic after a dose of radiation become oxygenated again as the tumor shrinks. Finally, radiosensitivity determines the intrinsic response of cells to radiation.[3]

Ablative doses of radiation (>10 Gy) causes endothelial cell death and activates the ceramide and acid sphingomyelinase pathway **(Fig. 10.1)**. Combination of these results

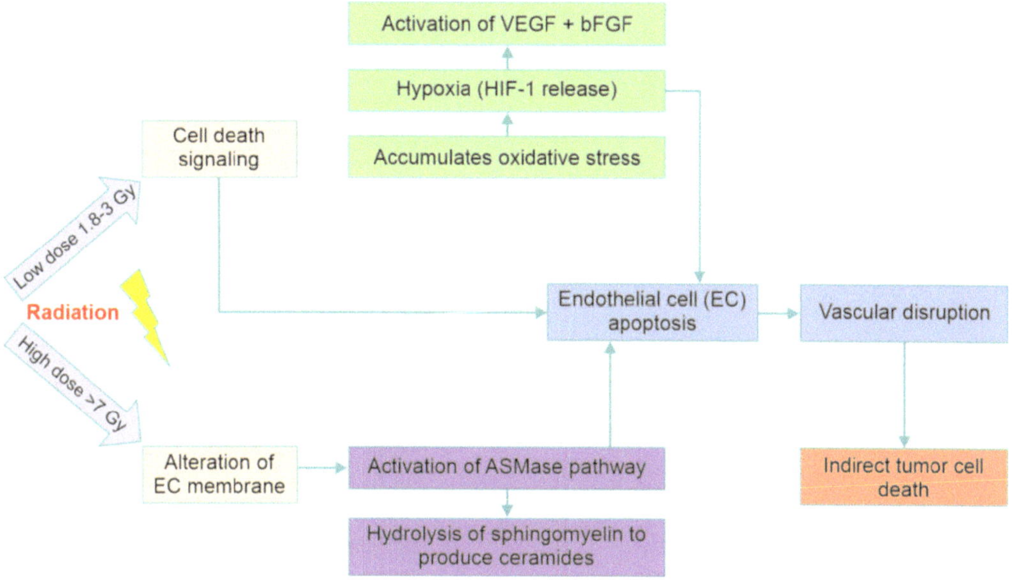


**Fig. 10.1:** Mechanism of cell death with radiation

in DNA damage and death of cancer cells.[4] However, the exact mechanism of action is not known with certainty.

The swift onset of pain relief frequently experienced within 24 hours following single-fraction local or hemi-body irradiation, along side the occasionally observed lack of direct correlation between initial pain reduction and tumor shrinkage, hints at the influence on inflammatory chemical mediators. For bone metastases, it has been suggested that radiotherapy may affect the host cells that generate substances causing pain or bone destruction, directly impacting the activity of bone-resorbing cells like osteoclasts, or alter the neural pathways that transmit pain signals.[5]

Contrary to high dose RT, the anti-inflammatory properties shown by low dose RT (LDRT) has been shown to provide relief in benign inflammatory disorders like osteoarthritis.[6] Low-dose radiation therapy markedly influences macrophages by suppressing the pathway that produces nitric oxide, specifically by suppressing the enzyme responsible for its synthesis. Additionally, it lowers the release of pro-inflammatory signaling molecules from white blood cells exposed to radiation and enhances the programmed cell death (apoptosis) of cancer cells.[7]

## TECHNIQUES AND DOSE-FRACTIONATION

Different techniques of external beam radiation therapy are utilized for treatment ranging from non-conformal to highly precise volumetric radiotherapy with image guidance. Two-dimensional and three-dimensional conformal radiation therapy (2D-RT and 3D-CRT) are frequently chosen for patients who are expected to have a limited life. More advanced modes of treatment delivery include intensity-modulated radiation therapy (IMRT), volumetric modulated arc therapy (VMAT), and tomotherapy. These improve the accuracy of tumor targeting while reducing damage to surrounding healthy tissue, thus drastically minimizing the potential side effects of the therapy. Additionally,

**Table 10.2: Factors determining radiotherapy technique and dose schedule**

| Tumor related | Patient related | Logistics related |
|---|---|---|
| 1. Aggressiveness of tumor histology<br>2. Synchronicity of development of metastases<br>3. Oligometastatic vs polymetastatic status<br>4. Time to development of neurological deficits | 1. Age<br>2. Karnofsky performance status (KPS)<br>3. Clinical circumstances such as pain intensity, risk of fractures, cord compression, uncontrolled bleed<br>4. Life expectancy<br>5. Compliance and willingness for daily treatment | 1. Duration of treatment<br>2. Family support and socio-economic status<br>3. Time taken to commute to hospital<br>4. Cost of treatment<br>5. Reimbursement issues |

sophisticated approaches like stereotactic body radiation therapy (SBRT) and stereotactic radiosurgery (SRS) are becoming more prevalent, particularly for delivering very high radiation doses with precision to well-defined tumor sites in certain patient populations. The selection of a specific radiation technique and treatment schedule for an individual patient is determined by a range of factors (Table 10.2).[8]

Multiple randomized controlled trials assessing single fraction versus multiple fractions of radiation therapy for palliation face many challenges with broad applicability. In randomized and non-randomized studies, there was no meaningful or significant variation in the overall response rate (ORR )and complete response rates (CRR) when comparing single fraction (SFRT) to multiple fraction (MFRT) radiotherapy. The impressive efficacy of SFRT treatments has been demonstrated in many non-randomized trials, which are more indicative of routine clinical practice than randomized trials.[9]

## BONE METASTASES

Approximately half of all individuals diagnosed with cancer will experience metastasis to the bones. The likelihood of developing bone metastasis in breast, prostate, and lung cancers is around 85%. Bone pain can arise from the growth of a tumor into nearby tissue, causing changes in the bone's microenvironment (altering the balance between osteoblasts and osteoclasts activity and leading to bone structure breakdown), invasion into nerve roots, or from an augmented production of inflammatory substances that activate nerve fibers. Radiotherapy is the most effective approach for treating bone metastasis.[10,11]

Many RCTs and observational trials have focused on finding the optimal choice of the dose-fractionation regimen for pain relief. They demonstrated equivalent pain relief and durability of a single fraction of 8 Gray (Gy) with multiple fractionation schedules, which included 30 Gy/10 fractions, 24 Gy/6 fractions, or 20 Gy/5 fractions.[9,12] Single fraction RT is associated with a higher rates of re-treatment to the same painful treated site as compared to protracted treatment. But single fraction may be more convenient and sensible for patients, especially with a limited life expectancy.

To evaluate the pain response, the international bone metastases consensus response criteria (IBMCC) using Numeric Pain Rating Scale (NPRS) and oral morphine equivalent dose (OMED) is used in combination.[13] The ORR with radiotherapy is between 50% and 80% with complete response of approximately 30%.[14] When comparing conventional

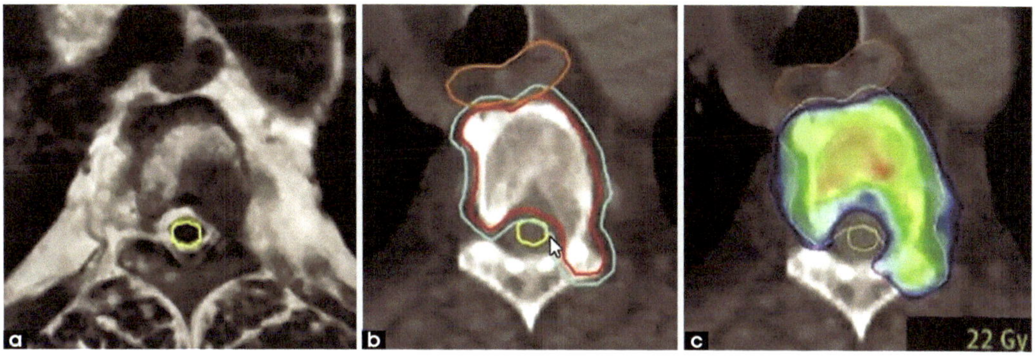


Figs 10.2a to c: Radiotherapy for vertebral metastases. (a) Lytic lesion in thoracic vertebral body on MRI spine, (b) Clinical target volume (CTV) for radiotherapy planning, (c) Isodose coverage of 22 Gy with VMAT planning technique

radiotherapy of 20 Gy in 5 fractions with SBRT (stereotactic body radiotherapy) using 24 Gy in 2 fractions, SBRT is found to be superior in improving CRR in terms of pain.[15] A prospective observational study from TMH, Mumbai, that studied the "long-term outcomes of conventional palliative radiotherapy in bone metastases of lung cancer" highlighted that 8 Gy single fraction confers an excellent overall response rate of 80% even after 6 months of radiotherapy.[16]

For complicated bone metastases like epidural spinal cord compression (Figs 10.2a to c), impending fracture of weight-bearing bones, the first step is to consider need for an immediate surgical decompression along with administration of high dose dexamethasone (10–16 mg/day). An urgent referral for palliative RT is strongly advised.[17] Protracted course of RT is usually preferred but 8 Gy in single fraction can also be administered in patients whose PS is poor.[18] The rades prognostic score may serve as a predictor for the restoration of walking ability following radiotherapy treatment.[19]

## BRAIN METASTASES

Patients experiencing symptoms from brain metastases, should undergo local treatment, irrespective of the systemic therapy being administered. The survival estimates have been studied in different histologies and compiled in a diagnosis-specific graded prognostic assessment (ds-GPA). This helps in choosing the ideal radiotherapy treatment schedule for the patient.[20]

For those with brain metastases without symptoms (asymptomatic), local therapy should not be postponed unless otherwise indicated. The choice to delay local therapy ought to be made based on a collaborative assessment by a multi-disciplinary team, weighing the potential advantages and risks for the patient.

Current recommendations for management of brain metastases in patients with non-small-cell lung cancer (NSCLC), breast cancer, and melanoma, etc. include a variety of treatment plans. For patients who have one to four brain metastases that have not been surgically removed and do not have small-cell lung carcinoma, and who lack options for systemic therapy if they are asymptomatic, stereotactic radiosurgery alone (18 Gy in single fraction to 30 Gy in 5 fractions) is the suggested treatment (Fig. 10.3). For

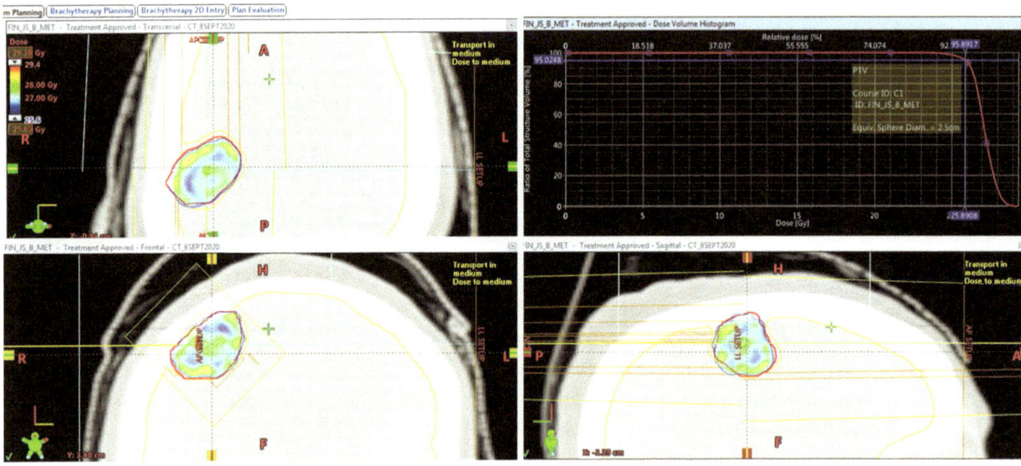


Fig. 10.3: "Stereotactic radiosurgery plan" for solitary brain metastases

those with one to two brain metastases that have been surgically removed, SRS to the post-surgical cavity alone is recommended. A combination of SRS, whole brain radiation therapy (WBRT), or both, is considered a reasonable approach for other cases.

Patients undergoing WBRT who donot have lesions in the hippocampal region and an expected survival of four months or more should also be considered for memory-sparing techniques like use of memantine and avoidance of the hippocampus.[21] The dose of WBRT can range from 20 Gy/5 fractions to 40 Gy/15 fractions with or without a simultaneous integrated boost to brain lesions. However, patients who have been incidentally diagnosed with asymptomatic brain metastases, who either have a KPS of 50 or lower, or KPS under 70 without any systemic therapy options available, are not likely to benefit from radiotherapy.

Most patients with brain metastases from NSCLC histology do not experience significant advantages from WBRT in terms of extended survival, enhanced quality of life, or decreased reliance on steroids. QUARTZ study suggests that providing the best supportive care alone with dexamethasone is not inferior to combining it with WBRT for clinical treatment.[22]

## BLEEDING

Hypofractionated palliative radiotherapy aimed at controlling bleeding is highly potent and should be a part of personalized care for cancer management.[23] Hemostatic radiotherapy is commonly applied to a range of cancers such as those in the head and neck, particularly cancers of base of the tongue, as well as in cases of fungating and hemorrhagic neck nodes, and lung or bronchial tumors causing hemoptysis. It is also used in pelvic tumors like cervical cancer causing heavy vaginal bleeding. Radiotherapy doses like 40 Gy/15 fractions, 30 Gy/10 fractions, 20 Gy/5 sessions, and a single dose of 4 to 8 Gy have all been found to be comparably successful in achieving hemostasis. However, longer treatment periods are discouraged to minimize the risk of patients discontinuing treatment and improving compliance.[24]

## OLIGOMETASTATIC DISEASE

The landscape of treatment for metastatic cancer has transformed significantly, due to the advent of new therapeutic approaches and technological innovations. There is now a diverse array of treatment possibilities, which has altered the prognosis of metastatic disease from being an immediate fatality to one with potential for extended life expectancy. With in-depth genetic profiling, biomarker harvesting, and the administration of specialized systemic treatments, the primary aim is to prolong the patient's survival.[25]

About 30 years ago, Hellman and Weichselbaum introduced the concept of the oligometastatic state, suggesting a phase of limited metastatic spread that sits somewhere between confined disease and extensive tumor distribution (polymetastases).[26]

In individuals with less than or equal to 5 metastatic sites, in at least 3 organs, a robust performance status, and a 6 month life expectancy or longer, the SABR-COMET trial showed a significant lasting improvement in survival when all known disease areas were treated.[27]

Stereotactic ablative body radiotherapy (SABR) is a highly conformal type of external beam radiotherapy which non-invasively delivers very high dose to the metastatic site. There is a strong radiobiological basis for its effectiveness. High dose radiotherapy (>7 Gy per fraction) causes substantial destruction of tumor cells caused by its direct impact on the cells' DNA, as well as its indirect effect on the blood vessels, which results in a release of tumor-related antigens and numerous pro-inflammatory cytokines. This activates an immune response against the tumor and causes cell death.[28]

SABR successfully addresses the problem of natural radio-resistance encountered in certain tumor types. Metastases from traditionally radioresistant cancers like colorectal, renal cell carcinoma, sarcoma and melanoma exhibit comparable rates of local control to those seen in patients with cancers typically more sensitive to radiation, such as breast, lung, liver and prostate cancers.[29] Dose escalation to safe yet ablative levels has been achieved in most organ sites with the use of SBRT.[30]

### Advantages and Disadvantages

The benefits of using radiotherapy for pain management in palliative care are diverse and far-reaching. They are as follows:

1. *Rapid pain relief:* Radiotherapy can provide rapid pain relief, often within a few days of treatment initiation. This quick onset of action can drastically improve the patient's comfort and provide quality of life.
2. *Non-invasive approach:* Unlike some surgical interventions, radiotherapy is non-invasive, making it a favorable option for those who are not suitable for surgery due to their overall health status or other medical considerations.
3. *Symptom control:* Radiotherapy can effectively alleviate symptoms such as bleeding, obstruction, and neurological deficits, thereby addressing a range of distressing manifestations associated with advanced cancer.
4. *Precision in targeting tumors:* With advanced techniques such as IMRT and image-guided radiation therapy (IGRT), radiotherapy can accurately target tumors and at the same time avoids radiation exposure to surrounding healthy tissues, and thus the risk of adverse effects.

5. *Enhanced quality of life:* By amelioriating pain and associated symptoms, radiotherapy contributes to an enhanced overall QoL for patients undergoing palliative care, addressing not only physical discomfort but also emotional and psychological well-being.

While radiotherapy offers significant benefits in palliative pain management, it is essential to acknowledge and understand the potential drawbacks associated with radiotherapy. These include:

1. *Acute side effects:* Radiotherapy can lead to acute side effects such as fatigue, skin reactions, pain flare at the treatment site. Although these effects are usually temporary and manageable, they can cause additional discomfort for patients already dealing with the burden of their illness.
2. *Increase hospital visits:* For patients with terminal stage cancer who may already be undergoing other treatments or experiencing fatigue and reduced mobility, the need to attend multiple radiotherapy sessions can be burdensome and may impact their overall well-being.
3. *Delayed onset of action:* While radiotherapy gives rapid relief from pain for majority patients but some may experience a delayed onset of action, requiring patience and understanding during the initial phase of treatment.
4. *Long-term side effects:* In very few cases, radiotherapy can cause lasting side effects, including damage to body tissues, which may affect a patient's life quality over time.

It is essential for healthcare providers to weigh the potential drawbacks of radiotherapy against its benefits and consider them keeping in mind each patient's individual circumstances and goals of treatment. The decision to incorporate radiotherapy into a palliative care plan should involve discussions with the patient and their caregivers with empathy and compassion to ensure that their concerns and preferences are addressed, making sure that the potential impact on their QoL is carefully considered.

## RADIOISOTOPES

To treat metastatic bone pain, there are radioisotopes that specifically target the bone lesions such as phosphorus-32 (P-32) and strontium-89 (Sr-89) can be injected to systemically deliver radiation inside the body. They are integrated into tumor cells, where DNA damage caused by the deposition of radioactive molecules kills the cells, ultimately reducing the tumor.

Radionuclide therapy can be administered on its own or alongside chemotherapy or radiotherapy to improve pain management and delay the emergence of new pain. The ideal candidates for treatment aimed at alleviating pain from bone lesions are individuals with multiple sites involvement which demand escalating dosages of analgesics or are resistant to pain medication.

223Ra is a type of radionuclide that emits alpha particles and accumulates in bone because it mimics calcium. The alpha radiation from high linear energy transfer (LET) from causes breaks in the double-stranded cellular DNA. Presently, its use is limited to patients who suffer from symptomatic bone-metastases particularly in castration-resistant prostate cancer (CRPC).

However, it is less exact in delivering particular amounts of radiation than external beam radiotherapy because the dosage is administered at a low dose rate over a long span of time. Its therapeutic application is limited due to hematological toxicity caused by bone marrow destruction.[31]

## Conclusion

As a vital component of multidimensional palliative care, the integration of radiotherapy in pain management provides patients with advanced cancer the opportunity to receive comprehensive and tailored support to enhance their comfort, function, and dignity during the course of their illness. With ongoing advancements in technology and research, the future of radiotherapy in oncology holds promise for further enhancing its efficacy and reducing its side effects. Radiotherapy will continue to solidify its place as an indispensable component of comprehensive cancer care.

## References

1. Indications, barriers and paths to advancement in palliative radiation oncology | Applied Radiation Oncology [Internet]. [cited 2024 Feb 26]. Available from: https://www.appliedradiationoncology.com/articles/indications-barriers-and-paths-to-advancement-in-palliative-radiation-oncology
2. Arcangeli G, Giovinazzo G, Saracino B, D'Angelo L, Giannarelli D, Arcangeli G, et al. Radiation therapy in the management of symptomatic bone metastases: the effect of total dose and histology on pain relief and response duration. Int J of Radia Onco Biol Phys. 1998 Dec;42(5):1119–26.
3. Herskind C, Ma L, Liu Q, Zhang B, Schneider F, Veldwijk MR, et al. Biology of high single doses of IORT: RBE, 5 Rs, and other biological aspects. Radiation Oncology. 2017 Jan 19;12(1):24.
4. Brown JM, Carlson DJ, Brenner DJ. The Tumor Radiobiology of SRS and SBRT: Are More Than the 5 Rs Involved? Int J of Radi Onco Biol Phys. 2014 Feb;88(2):254–62.
5. Price P, Hoskin PJ, Easton D, Austin D, Palmer SG, Yarnold JR. Prospective randomised trial of single and multifraction radiotherapy schedules in the treatment of painful bony metastases. Radiotherapy and Oncology. 1986 Jan;6(4):247–55.
6. Trott KR, Kamprad F. Radiobiological mechanisms of anti-inflammatory radiotherapy. Radiotherapy and Oncology. 1999 Jun 1;51(3):197–203.
7. Dove APH, Cmelak A, Darrow K, McComas KN, Chowdhary M, Beckta J, et al. The Use of Low-Dose Radiation Therapy in Osteoarthritis: A Review. Int J of Radia Onco Biol Phys. 2022 Oct;114(2):203–20.
8. Sierko E, Hempel D, Zuzda K, Wojtukiewicz M. Personalized Radiation Therapy in Cancer Pain Management. Cancers. 2019 Mar 19;11(3):390.
9. Chow R, Hoskin P, Schild SE, Raman S, Im J, Zhang D, et al. Single vs multiple fraction palliative radiation therapy for bone metastases: Cumulative meta-analysis. Radiotherapy and Oncology. 2019 Dec;141:56–61.
10. Lutz S, Balboni T, Jones J, Lo S, Petit J, Rich SE, et al. Palliative radiation therapy for bone metastases: Update of an ASTRO Evidence-Based Guideline. Practical Radiation Oncology. 2017 Jan;7(1):4–12.
11. Cheon PM, Wong E, Thavarajah N, Dennis K, Lutz S, Zeng L, et al. A definition of "uncomplicated bone metastases" based on previous bone metastases radiation trials comparing single-fraction and multi-fraction radiation therapy. Journal of Bone Oncology. 2015 Mar;4(1):13–7.
12. Behroozian T, Navarro I, Hoskin P, Johnstone C, Recht A, Menten J, et al. Update on the systematic review/meta-analysis of uncomplicated bone metastases treated with external beam radiation. Radiotherapy and Oncology. 2022 Sep;174:109–10.
13. Chow E, Hoskin P, Mitera G, Zeng L, Lutz S, Roos D, et al. Update of the International Consensus on Palliative Radiotherapy Endpoints for Future Clinical Trials in Bone Metastases. Inter Jour of Radi Onco Biol Phys. 2012 Apr;82(5):1730–7.
14. Saito T, Yamaguchi K, Toya R, Oya N. Single-Versus Multiple-Fraction Radiation Therapy for Painful Bone Metastases: A Systematic Review and Meta-analysis of Nonrandomized Studies. Advances in Radiation Oncology. 2019 Oct;4(4):706–15.
15. Sahgal A, Myrehaug SD, Siva S, Masucci GL, Maralani PJ, Brundage M, et al. Stereotactic body radiotherapy versus conventional external beam radiotherapy in patients with painful spinal

metastases: an open-label, multicentre, randomised, controlled, phase 2/3 trial. The Lancet Oncology. 2021 Jul;22(7):1023–33.

16. Long Term Outcomes of Conventional Palliative Radiotherapy in Bone Metastases of Lung Cancer: A Prospective Study - International Journal of Radiation Oncology, Biology, Physics [Internet]. [cited 2024 Feb 28]. Available from: https://www.redjournal.org/article/S0360-3016(23)05227-6/fulltext
17. Oldenburger E, Brown S, Willmann J, van der Velden JM, Spałek M, van der Linden YM, et al. ESTRO ACROP guidelines for external beam radiotherapy of patients with complicated bone metastases. Radiotherapy and Oncology. 2022 Aug;173:240–53.
18. Effect of Single-Fraction vs Multifraction Radiotherapy on Ambulatory Status Among Patients With Spinal Canal Compression From Metastatic Cancer: The SCORAD Randomized Clinical Trial | Neurology | JAMA | JAMA Network [Internet]. [cited 2024 Feb 28]. Available from: https://jamanetwork.com/journals/jama/fullarticle/2756290
19. Rades D, Fehlauer F, Schulte R, Veninga T, Stalpers LJA, Basic H, et al. Prognostic Factors for Local Control and Survival After Radiotherapy of Metastatic Spinal Cord Compression. JCO. 2006 Jul 20;24(21):3388–93.
20. Survival in Patients With Brain Metastases: Summary Report on the Updated Diagnosis-Specific Graded Prognostic Assessment and Definition of the Eligibility Quotient - PubMed [Internet]. [cited 2024 Feb 28]. Available from: https://pubmed.ncbi.nlm.nih.gov/32931399/
21. Vogelbaum MA, Brown PD, Messersmith H, Brastianos PK, Burri S, Cahill D, et al. Treatment for Brain Metastases: ASCO-SNO-ASTRO Guideline. J Clin Oncol. 2022 Feb 10;40(5):492–516.
22. Mulvenna P, Nankivell M, Barton R, Faivre-Finn C, Wilson P, McColl E, et al. Dexamethasone and supportive care with or without whole brain radiotherapy in treating patients with non-small cell lung cancer with brain metastases unsuitable for resection or stereotactic radiotherapy (QUARTZ): results from a phase 3, non-inferiority, randomised trial. The Lancet. 2016 Oct 22;388(10055):2004–14.
23. Song J, Brown C, Dennis K, Gaudet M, Haddad A. Palliative Radiotherapy for Haemostasis in Malignancy: a Systematic Review. Clinical Oncology. 2023 Sep 1;35(9):e478–88.
24. Hemostatic Radiotherapy: Journal of Radiation and Cancer Research [Internet]. [cited 2024 Feb 29]. Available from: https://journals.lww.com/jrcr/fulltext/2021/12030/hemostatic_radiotherapy.4.aspx
25. Tsai CJ, Gomez DR, Yang TJ. Metastatic Disease as a Distinct Discipline in Radiation Oncology. JAMA Oncology. 2021 Jan 1;7(1):21–2.
26. Foster CC, Pitroda SP, Weichselbaum RR. Definition, Biology, and History of Oligometastatic and Oligoprogressive Disease: The Cancer Journal. 2020;26(2):96–9.
27. Stereotactic ablative radiotherapy versus standard of care palliative treatment in patients with oligometastatic cancers (SABR-COMET): a randomised, phase 2, open-label trial - PubMed [Internet]. [cited 2024 Feb 27]. Available from: https://pubmed.ncbi.nlm.nih.gov/30982687/
28. Song CW, Glatstein E, Marks LB, Emami B, Grimm J, Sperduto PW, et al. Biological Principles of Stereotactic Body Radiation Therapy (SBRT) and Stereotactic Radiation Surgery (SRS): Indirect Cell Death. International Journal of Radiation Oncology × Biology × Physics. 2019 Mar; S0360301619302913.
29. Tree AC, Khoo VS, Eeles RA, Ahmed M, Dearnaley DP, Hawkins MA, et al. Stereotactic body radiotherapy for oligometastases. Lancet Oncol. 2013 Jan;14(1):e28-37.
30. Solberg TD, Fraass A, Potters L. Quality and Safety Considerations in Stereotactic Radiosurgery and Stereotactic Body Radiation Therapy. Practical Radiation Oncology. 2011;49.
31. Pandit-Taskar N, Mahajan S. Targeted Radionuclide Therapy for Bone Metastasis. In: Volterrani D, Erba PA, Strauss HW, Mariani G, Larson SM, editors. Nuclear Oncology: From Pathophysiology to Clinical Applications [Internet]. Cham: Springer International Publishing; 2020 [cited 2024 Feb 27]. p. 1–33. Available from: https://doi.org/10.1007/978-3-319-26067-9_27-2.

Chapter 11

# Neurolysis in Cancer Pain Management

• Aparna Chatterjee • M Naga Sailaja

Pain is a symptom that is highly prevalent in cancer and feared by all who suffer from this illness. The WHO ladder was framed in 1986 with the aim to administer analgesics to the patients based on pain intensity (discussed in detail in Chapter 7). The ladder has stood the test of time and till date is used widely. When analgesia is administered as per the ladder, approx 85–90% patients receive acceptable pain relief. The remaining 10–15% who may have poorly controlled pain or unacceptable side effects may require interventional procedures to control pain.[1] Interventional procedures have now been proposed as the 4th step of the ladder.[2] Procedures namely, peripheral nerve and plexus blocks, central neuraxial blocks, sympathetic and neurolytic blocks, intrathecal drug delivery systems, neuromodulation and ablative neurosurgical procedures are performed to provide pain relief. These procedures help interrupt the transmission of pain along pathways either temporarily or permanently. Neurolysis is one such interventional procedure which aims to deliberately injure or disrupt the nerve by either physical or chemical means to bring about degenerative changes in the nerve and interrupt transmission of pain impulses.[3]

## HISTORY

Neurolysis has been described and practiced for over a century. Chemical neurolysis was first demonstrated by Luton in 1863, wherein he injected irritant chemicals subcutaneously in patients suffering from sciatic neuralgia.[4] He used silver nitrate and saline solutions with varying success. The irritant would be injected between the trochanter and ischium. He also described the injection of sodium chloride over the anterior portion of maxilla for infraorbital neuralgia. Subsequently, in 1874, Bartholow demonstrated the use of subcutaneous injections of chloroform in patients with trigeminal neuralgia and Baccelli in 1888, advocated subcutaneous injections of phenol for neuralgias. Alcohol neurolysis for trigeminal neuralgia was performed and reported for the first time by Schlosser in 1904. This method gained in popularity and was widely practiced. The coeliac plexus block was first described by Kappis in 1919 while, Boas in 1978 explained the distinction between retrocrural and transcrural needle placement blocking the splanchnic and the celiac plexus nerve fibers, respectively.[5]

Radiofrequency ablation ( RFA) was described in early 20th century. It was first used for chronic pain conditions by Rosomoff and Mullan who introduced the percutaneous cervical cordotomy in 1965. RFA lesioning was thereafter attempted in cases of unilateral cervical cancer pain, post herpetic neuralgia and phantom limb pain.[6]

Over time, with better understanding of pathophysiology, refinement of techniques and especially with the advances in the field of imaging in recent times has greatly improved the precision with which neurolysis can be performed, with better efficacy and safety profile.

## PATHOPHYSIOLOGY OF NEUROLYSIS

Neurolysis results in Wallerian degeneration which is a form of nerve injury wherein the destructive lesion leads to degeneration of the axon distal to it.

The afferent neuronal pathways or corresponding sympathetic ganglia are destroyed interrupting pain pathways and transmission of impulses thereby providing targeted pain relief to the patient.

However, as long as the axolemma is intact, nerve regeneration can occur in 3–6 months. The effects therefore last for around the same time period.[7]

Neurolysis was especially thought to be useful when disease has progressed to a point where the pain was intractable and other pain management options were not effective.[6] This misunderstanding that interventions were an option once other options were exhausted has led to late referals for neurolysis. In the current scenario, with greater safety and efficacy, interventions earlier in the course of the disease can provide effective pain relief in cases with intractable pain.[8] This was demonstrated by Akhan, et al in the case of a neurolytic celiac plexus block where >50% invasion of the fat planes by the tumor, correlated with little pain relief.[9]

### Advantages

Neuroablative procedures help minimise or reduce pain intensity thereby:

- Improve the overall quality of life
- Reduce analgesic doses and possible side effects especially of opioids
- Improve day to day functioning of the patient and reduce total hospital visits.

Neurolysis can be performed at any level of the pain pathway. This begins at the peripheral nerve carrying pain impulses and ends in the central nervous system. The nerves that can be targeted with neurolysis include:

*Peripheral nerves:* Peripheral nerves are mixed nerves and run the risk of motor weakness, hence neurolysis of peripheral nerves is rarely done. Neurolysis of peripheral nerves on the trunk such as intercostal nerves is performed, since less likely to cause any weakness of extremities.

*Sympathetic ganglia:* The paired sympathetic chains extend from the base of the skull to the coccyx , placed on either side just lateral to the vertebral column. The sympathetic chain makes up the thoracolumbar outflow of the Autonomic nervous system. The visceral sensory afferents are mixed with autonomic efferent fibers in the thoracic, abdominal, and pelvic cavities and these are the ganglia that are blocked in cancer pain management.[10]

### Contraindications[3]

- Patient refusal
- *Infection:* Both local or systemic
- Deranged coagulation

- Drug allergy
- Uncertain diagnosis
- Uncooperative patient
- Lack of expertise
- Neutropenia (relative)
- Neurological deficits (relative)

## Techniques of Neurolysis

Neurolysis is performed by placing a needle in close proximity to the nerve to be damaged either by injecting a chemical substance or applying heat or cold to the nerve as mentioned below.

### *1. Physical Methods*

*Radiofrequency ablation (RFA):* Radiofrequency ablation involves application of high frequency alternating current (50–500 kHz) through the uninsulated tip of the RF probe into the tissues due to which ionic agitation and resistive heating of the tissues occurs.[11] The RFA system creates a closed-loop circuit consisting of an electrical generator, a needle electrode, a patient (a resistor), and large dispersive electrodes (or "grounding pads") which helps generate and maintain the current.

RFA is used to ablate specific nerves or pain pathways in the trigeminal ganglion, dorsal root entry zone, dorsal root ganglion, sympathetic chain, facet joints, and peripheral nerves. The advantage that RFA offers is that it is more precise, reproducible and effective to a greater extent.

RFA is performed by inserting a specialized needle through the skin, under fluoroscopy, ultrasound or computerized tomography (CT) guidance to position the tip with precision close to the target nerve, after which the lesion is created. The tip of the needle is uninsulated and the current delivered is concentrated here resulting in localized heating of an area of up to 5 mm around the distal 5–10 mm of the needle. In conventional RFA, the needle tip is heated to 80–90°C for 60–90 sec, whereas in pulsed RFA, the temperature is maintained below 43°C by the use of 2Hz, 20 ms pulses of alternating current for 3–5 min. The temperature above which the human protein starts to denature and tissue damage occurs is 43°C. Pulsed RFA is known to result in less tissue damage, dysaesthesia, motor block and deafferentation pain. Another form of RFA is the cooled RFA, wherein a continuous flow of water helps to actively cool the tip and prevent the current from reaching high temperatures; this allows more spherical and larger lesioning.

In cancer pain, RFA can be used to ablate medial branch nerve, Gasserian ganglion as well as for percutaneous cordotomy, rhizotomy and sympathectomy. Ablation of pain pathways can result in pain relief which lasts for 3–12 months until the axonal regeneration occurs.

Studies comparing chemical neurolysis with RFA, found RFA to act faster, provide much longer duration of analgesia and more effective in a higher proportion of patients with a better safety profile.[12,13]

RF procedures are also associated with complications depending on the site ablated, such as; post-lesioning neuritis/neuralgia, numbness, motor paralysis, pneumothorax, Horner's syndrome and incomplete pain relief.[14]

*Cryoablation:* Specialized cryoprobes produce rapid tissue cooling, reaching –20 to 25°C within a few seconds by the rapid expansion of argon under pressure. It is then thawed by introducing helium gas into the cryoprobes. The lesion size can be monitored in real time. Cryoablation disrupts the vasa nervorum leading to axonal destruction by producing endoneural edema.

The probe and the entire system is a closed one, such that the gas used for the procedure does not escape into the patient's tissues. The size of the ice ball also depends on the probe, a 2.0 mm probe forms a 5.5 mm ice ball while the 1.4 mm probe forms a 3.5 mm ice ball. Precise gas flows are necessary for safe and effective cryoablation; inadequate gas flows will not produce an ice ball while excessive flows can cause freezing proximally up the probe which may increase the risk of skin burns.[15]

The application of cold to tissues creates a conduction block, similar to that of local anesthetics. At 10°C, the larger myelinated fibers stop conducting, whereas all nerve fibers stop conducting impulses at –20°C. The extent and duration of the effect is therefore a function of the degree of cold produced.

The extent of the freezing depends on the following factors:

1. How close the probe is to the nerve.
2. The size of the probe
3. The size of the ice ball formed
4. The rate of freezing and its duration.
5. The temperature of the tissues around the probe which is affected by local heat from the blood vessels, etc.

Cryotherapy is contraindicated when the lesion is located within a centimetre delicate structures such as the spinal cord, a major motor nerve, the artery of Adamkiewicz, as wellas the bowel and bladder.

Complications such as accidental spinal cord injury, neuritis, vessel injuries, impaired motor or sensory function, fistulas, hematoma, infection and rarely bone fractures when large areas are treated are possible with cryotherapy.

### *2. Chemical Neurolysis*[16,17]

Chemical neurolysis can be performed with a variety of agents such as alcohol, phenol, glycerol, ammonium salts as well as hypertonic saline. Alcohol and phenol are the most commonly used.

*Alcohol:* It is used in concentration of 50–100%. Causes intense pain on injection and hence preferable to inject local anesthetic prior to neurolysis with alcohol. Alcohol destroys the nerve tissue by precipitation of cell membrane proteins, extraction of lipid compound and demyelination. Injection of alcohol in close proximity to a nerve is associated with severe burning pain almost immediately along the nerve's distribution, and followed thereafter by a warm, numb sensation. Denervation is usually complete after 1 week. Alcohol spreads rapidly from the injection site, and is completely oxidised by the liver. Cardiac arrhythmias, hypotension, non-target tissue necrosis could occur.

*Alcoholic neuropathy:* When mixed nerves are targeted, presents with hypoaesthesia, neuritis, deafferentation pain and motor deficits can occur. Alcohol is also used for intrathecal neurolysis in advanced cancers with refractory pain, and is hypobaric in comparison with the cerebrospinal fluid (CSF).

- *Phenol:* Phenol is available as a 3–12% solution. Phenol is more viscous, and does not diffuse freely into the tissues on injection as compared to alcohol. Phenol has local anesthetic action and, therefore, does not cause any pain on injection but has a warmth sensation followed by numbness. It is known to have a greater affinity for vascular tissues. Phenol is also hyperbaric in comparison with CSF when prepared in an oil base.
- Ammonium salts cause nonspecific axonopathy but are used rarely, while glycerol has been used for neurolysis and demyelination of the gasserian ganglion.[18]

## NEUROLYTIC PROCEDURES IN VARIOUS CANCER PAIN SYNDROMES

### 1. Head and Neck Cancers

Pain is one of the most distressing of symptoms in patients with head and neck cancers and is usually present even at diagnosis.[19] This pain is difficult and challenging to treat since it is usually dynamic and worsens with mastication and deglutition. When the pain is not relieved adequately with analgesics, the option of neuroablation such as of the trigeminal, glossopharyngeal, occipital, sphenopalatine ganglia and the cervical plexus offers hope and can be performed where necessary.

Occipital nerve blocks can help reduce pain and headaches due to skull base invasion by malignancies.[20] RFA of the pain in the distribution of the trigeminal nerve and its branches, glossopharyngeal nerve and the sphenopalatine ganglion is also amenable to RFA.

#### *Trigeminal Nerve RFA*

***Anatomy:*** Trigeminal nerve is the fifth (V) cranial nerve and the largest of the twelve cranial nerves in the body. It is a mixed nerve, that is it has both sensory and motor fibers and has a wide area of distribution. It originates in the brainstem (pons) and innervates various structures of the head and face. It is a paired nerve, and each nerve innervates ipsilateral half of the head and face. Each trigeminal nerve has three main branches; the ophthalmic (V1), maxillary (V2) and mandibular (V3) and hence the name trigeminal (from Latin word "trigeminus" which means three twins).

Depending on the distribution of pain in the trigeminal area, RFA can either target the gasserian ganglion of the trigeminal nerve or any of its branches. The most common method is the intracranial approach to the gasserian ganglion. Extracranial approach for targeting specific branches has also been described.[21]

The procedure is performed under fluoroscopy guidance with the patient in the supine position and head extended. An oblique submental view to visualize the foramen ovale is obtained by tilting and moving the C-arm. The entry point of the probe is ~2–3 cm lateral to the angle of the mouth on the side which is affected. The trajectory of the needle follows the line directed towards the pupil when observed from the front and passes 3 cm anterior to the external auditory meatus when observed from the side **(Fig. 11.1)**.

A 22-gauge, 10 cm RFA cannula with a 5 mm tip is often used for this procedure. Local anesthesia is administered after which the cannula is advanced in towards the foramen ovale in the same axis as the X-ray beam. A finger is be placed in the oral cavity to ensure that the buccal mucosa has not been penetrated. When the cannula enters the

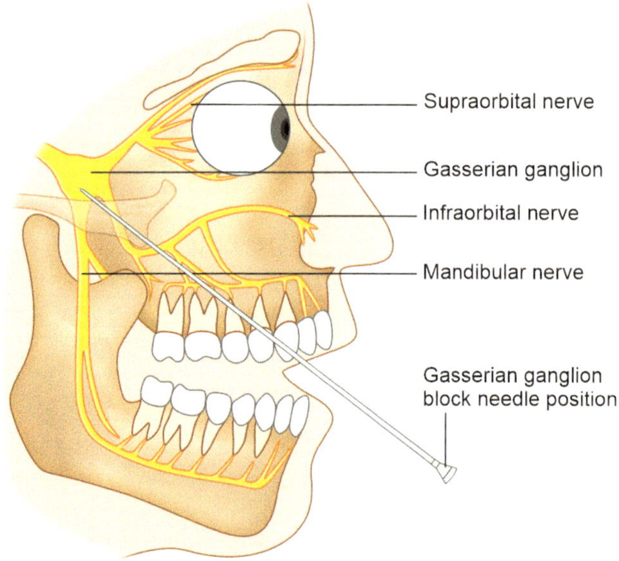


**Fig. 11.1:** Trigeminal nerve block/ RFA, needle direction and positioning

foramen ovale, the depth of the cannula inside the Meckel's cavity is deciphered on a lateral fluoroscopic view.

The electrode is then advanced approximately 2–4 mm further through the canal of the foramen ovale such that the tip of the electrode reaches the junction of the petrous ridge of the temporal bone and the clivus. The stylet is then removed, and the cannula is aspirated to ensure that there is no CSF or blood following which 0.5 ml of contrast is injected to confirm that the needle has not penetrated the dura.[21,22] A test stimulation is mandatory before any RFA lesioning.

The mandibular nerve lies in the lateral portion of the foramen ovale. If the nerve is stimulated at 2 Hz or between 0.1 and 1.5 Hz, lower jaw muscle contraction may be observed which confirms that the needle has passed through the foramen ovale and the tip is on the roots of the trigeminal nerve.

After confirming the needle position as mentioned, 0.5 ml of 0.25% bupivacaine with 40 mg of triamcinolone is injected. Around 30 sec later, RFA lesioning at 60°C is carried out for 60 sec. The needle can be repositioned to repeat the lesioning if more than one branch of the trigeminal nerve is to be ablated. Both, targeted approach and gasserian ganglia approach have been found to be equally effective in pain relief.[22]

Complications such as diminished corneal reflex, masseter weakness and paralysis, dysesthesia, anesthesia dolorosa, keratitis, and transient paralysis of cranial nerves III and VI have been reported.

#### *Glossopharyngeal Neuroablation*

In the past, neuroablation of the glossopharyngeal nerve was performed either surgically or with alcohol. It is indicated for pain in the base of tongue, pharynx, and tonsils. As this nerve is a mixed nerve, in recent times, pulsed RFA is recommended and preferred. There are two approaches to the glossopharyngeal nerve, the extraoral

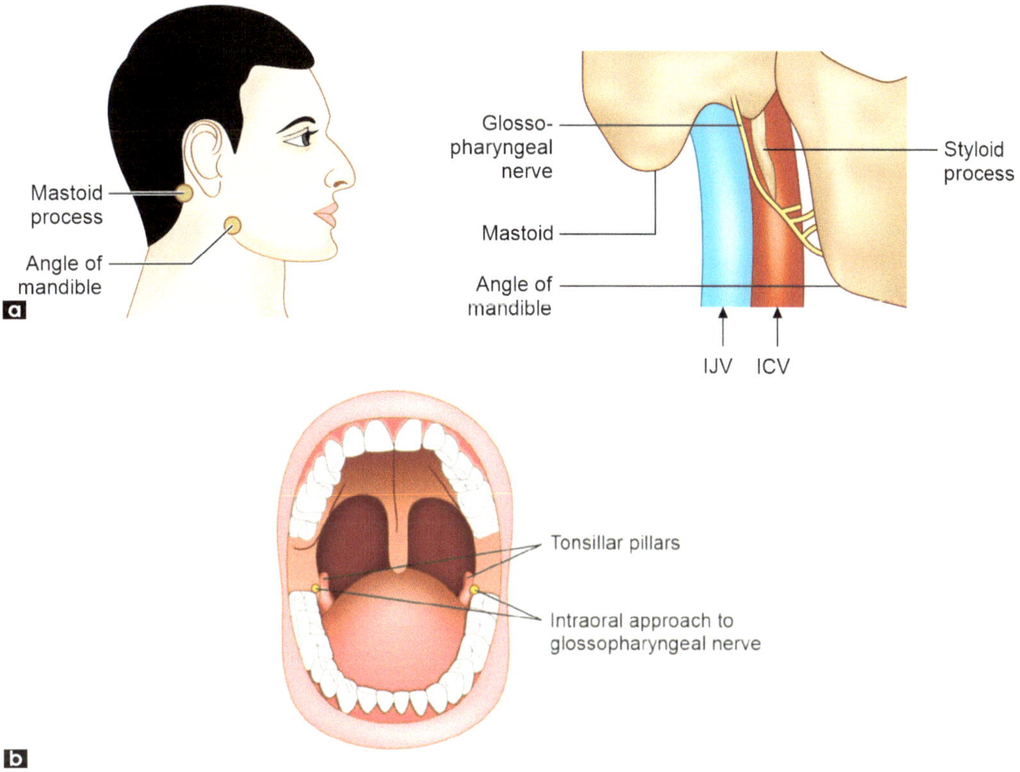


**Figs 11.2a and b:** Approaches to the glossopharyngeal nerve block

and the intraoral approach. The extraoral procedure is performed under fluoroscopy guidance with the RFA needle placed at the midpoint of the line joining the angle of the mandible and the mastoid process **(Fig. 11.2a)** till it contacts the styloid process at a depth of approximately 3 cm.

a. Extraoral approach
b. Intraoral approach

After ruling out the presence of blood or cerebrospinal fluid (CSF) by negative aspiration, a current of 50Hz at 0.5 V is delivered to produce the pain as a method of diagnosing the source of pain and confirming it. Stimulation is done with 2Hz at 0.5–2V which should not result in contraction of the stylopharyngeus. Lesioning done at 42°C for 3 cycles of 120 seconds each.

An alternative is the transoral approach, which is relatively easy. The operator's left hand should be placed over the line joining the mastoid process to the mangle of mandible and the styloid process is to be palpated. The tongue is retracted medially and away from the ipsilateral tonsillar pillar. A 7–8 cm needle with the end bent at 45° is attached to a syringe with local anesthetic. The needle is held with a pen grasp and inserted gently into the area between the base of the ipsilateral anterior and posterior tonsillar pillars **(Fig. 11.2b)**. At a depth of not more than 0.5 cm, after negative aspiration for blood, 1–2 ml of the local anesthetic can be injected for providing pain relief.

## 2. Chest Wall Tumors

Chest wall tumors can result in intractable pain. In these patients the disease is incurable and pain relief is one of the palliation options available. The condition can be dealt with intercostal blocks (ICB) either neurolytic or pulsed RFA or an implantable intrathecal pump.

Neurolytic ICB is performed under radiologic guidance. The needle is inserted proximal to the angle of the rib at its lower border and advanced a few millimetres after encountering bone. A water soluble contrast 0.5 ml is injected at the point to confirm placement in the intercostal groove. Blocks with local anesthetic are performed similarly at three levels to identify the nerve involved in the generation of the pain. This acts as a diagnostic block prior to neurolysis. Once confirmed, neurolysis is performed at the same points with 6–10% phenol as motor block is not of concern. Pain relief is usually immediate. Some patients however, do present with neuritis or deafferentation pain, but this incidence is low.[23] Pneumothorax is a very rare complication.

## 3. Abdominal Cancer Pain

Pancreatic cancer most often gets diagnosed in an advanced stage, the disease is such that there is a high incidence of neural invasion. The patients usually suffer excruciating pain in the upper abdomen with at times the upper back. Diffuse, crampy, poorly localized, deep seated pain which worsens on lying down and relieved with bending forward is commonly reported. The pain is amenable to opioids though associated with adverse events such as nausea, vomiting, constipation, drowsiness and dry mouth. The pain aggravates with disease progression and is transmitted via the splanchnic nerves and the celiac plexus. Neurolysis of these structures plays a very important role and is effective in reducing the need for opioids and to improve pain relief.

*Anatomy:* The splanchnic nerves are preganglionic sympathetic fibers which lie retrocrural at the level of T12 vertebra. They consist of the greater (T5–T10), lesser (T10–T11) and the least (T12) splanchnic nerves. They pass through the crura of the diaphragm and synapse into the celiac plexus which lies anterior to the aorta near the origin of the celiac trunk.

The celiac plexus itself is a group of 1–5 ganglia located anterocrurally anywhere between T12 and L2 vertebral bodies **(Fig. 11.3)**.[24] It consists of the pregangionic, post-ganglionic, parasympathetic and visceral afferent sensory fibers. The celiac plexus innervates the upper abdominal organs such as the pancreas, liver, spleen, biliary tract, gallbladder, adrenals, kidneys, mesentery, stomach, and bowel to the level of the proximal transverse colon, as well as the blood vessels of the abdomen.

A neurolytic celiac plexus block (NCPB) is indicated for cancer pain arising from abdominal organs such as the pancreas, stomach, gallbladder, liver, small intestine, large intestine up to the transverse colon, spleen, kidneys and the proximal ureters. Chronic pancreatitis is the only non-malignant condition wherein a celiac plexus block is performed, usually with steroids and rarely a with a neurolytic agent.

The block is highly effective with a 80% success rate especially if performed earlier in the course of treatment as the celiac axis is free.[3] Several RCTs have demonstrated the success of a NCPB.[25] Once >50% of the fat planes are invaded by the disease, success rate is poor.[26] Contraindications include, refusal by patient, deranged coagulation, local or systemic sepsis.

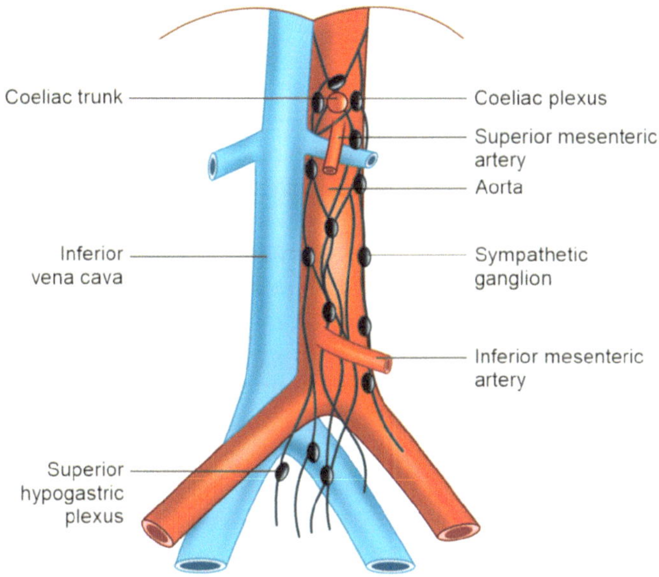


**Fig. 11.3:** Sympathetic nerves and the plexus

The traditional or classic posterolateral approach was the original technique described by Kappis. Here the patient is placed in a prone position with a pillow placed at the midsection of the abdomen to reduce the lumbar lordosis and improve patient comfort. In case patient is unable to provide this position due to pain, then intravenous analgeiscs may have to be administered to help assist the patient. The patient's arms are kept underneath his/her head or allowed to hang off the table. An intravenous line should be secured and a suitable intravenous fluid should be on flow. Routine monitors such as NIBP, $SpO_2$ and ECG monitors must be attached. The classic technique involves use of 2 needles or a 2 needle technique. The procedure can be performed under fluoroscopy

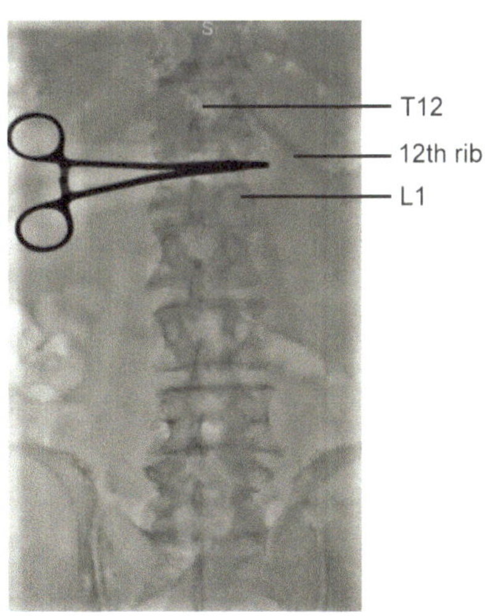


**Fig. 11.4:** Locate L1 vertebra and identify the structures

or CT guidance. The landmarks include the 12th ribs, T12, 12th thoracic) and L1 (1st lumbar) vertebral body (Fig. 11.4).

Under strict aseptic precautions, the L1 vertebral body is identified. Skin wheals with local anesthetic are raised at a distance of 6–8 cm from the midline at the level of L1 vertebrae. Ususally corresponds to the junction of the paraspinal muscles with the 12th rib. Two 15 cm, 22 G spinal needles/biopsy needles can be used and inserted at the site of the wheals directed 45 degrees to the coronal plane and 15 degrees cephalad to contact the body of L1 vertebrae. The needle is then slightly withdrawn and redirected an additional 10 degrees till it finally walks off the vertebral body. The final position should be 1–1.5 cm anterior to the vertebral body. The needle on the left pulsates indicating its proximity to the aorta. 2–3 ml of water soluble contrast is administered through each needle after confirming negative aspiration for blood. It will help confirm if the needle is placed retrocrural (1–1.5 cm ahead of the L1 vertebral body), transcrural or anterocrural. In case of a transcrural or anterocrural approach, the final needle position will be an additional 1–2 cm ahead of the retrocrural position (Fig. 11.5).

If the contrast hugs the L1 body, likely to be retrocrural. Anteroposterior (Fig. 11.6) and lateral fluoroscopic views (Fig. 11.5) help confirm position of the needles. The contrast gets washed away if in a vessel, if muscle striations are seen, it indicates that the needle is in the diaphragm and needles should be advanced a cm and contrast injection repeated.

Once the final position of the needles is confirmed, 4–5 ml of local anesthetic (0.25% Bupivacaine or 1% lignocaine) is administered through each needle. This works as a diagnostic block and confirms the correct positioning further with a reduction in pain intensity prior to injecting the neurolytic agent as well as provides analgesia prior to injection of the neurolytic (alcohol) which otherwise is painful. This is followed by injection of 15–20 ml of 50% alcohol through each needle along with repeated aspiration to rule out any blood. In case the procedure is performed under CT guidance much less volume of the neurolytic agent can be used (8–10 ml) as the needles are placed with greater precision. Alcohol is the preferred neurolytic agent here since it does not have a greater affinity for vascular tissue like phenol. While withdrawing the needles, inject

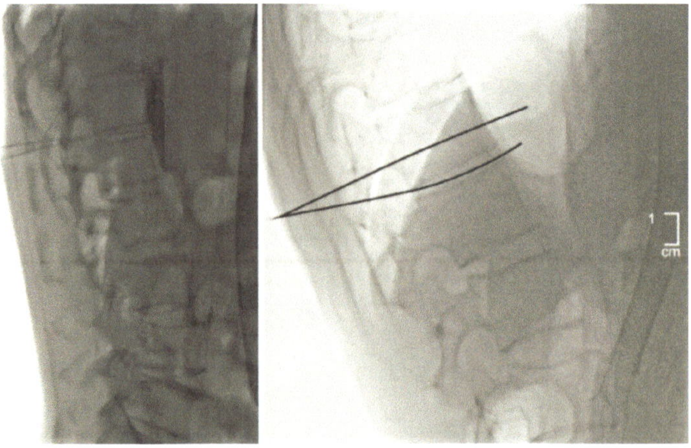


Fig. 11.5: Spread of the contrast hugging the L1 body (retrocrural) {L} and needles placed anterocrural {R}

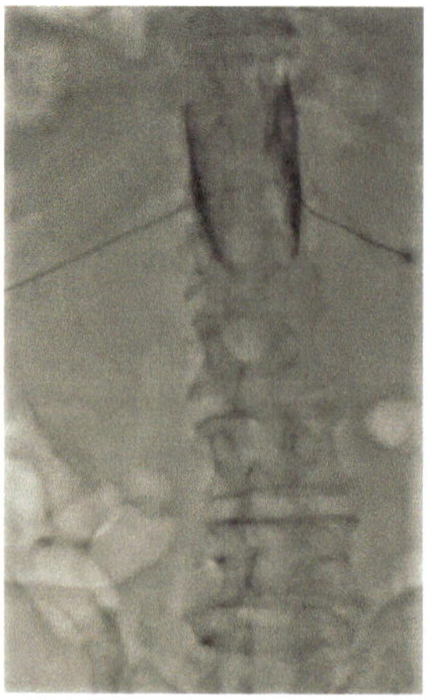

Fig. 11.6: Spread of contrast in AP view

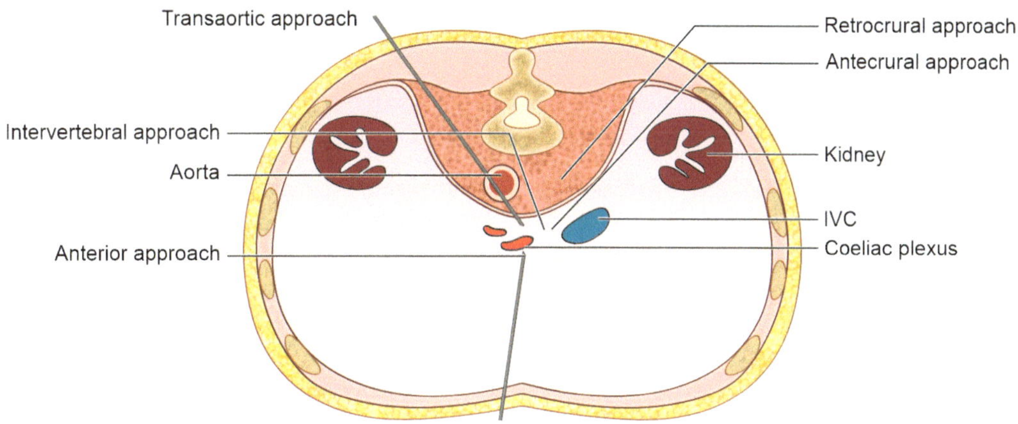


Fig. 11.7: Approaches to the celiac plexus

local anesthetic or saline through them so as to not allow the neurolytic agent to remain in the tract which can cause skin necrosis.

There are several other approaches for the NCPB such as the anterocrural, retrocrural, transaortic, transdiscal, anterior and endoscopic. Needle positions and advantages of each are mentioned below (Fig. 11.7).

- *Transaortic posterolateral approach:*[27] The patient in prone position and a single needle on the left side is used for the technique. The needle is placed just ahead of the anterior wall of the aorta. Hence, the position of the needle is as close to the ganglia as is possible. The neurolyic agent covers the aorta and encircles it. In advanced disease, the tumour is known to invade through all tissues including nerves and the celiac ganglia may be engulfed in tumor mass and thus not reachable. This approach may possibly overcome this problem
- *Transdiscal:*[28] Approach is posterolateral and patient in prone position. The needle is passed through the T12–L1 disc. Was developed to minimise the risk of organ perforation in case of organomegaly. The risk of pneumothorax was lower, and the target was the splanchnic nerves primarily. Not commonly used technique. The risks involve discitis, disc degeneration, etc.
- *Anterior approach*: With patient in supine position. A single needle is introduced through the epigastrium till it touches L1 body and then withdrawn by 1–2 cm. Can be performed under ultrasound guidance as well as fluoroscopic or CT guidance. Patient comfort is a distinct advantage. Especially useful if patient cannot lie prone. Also only a single needle is used.[26]
- *Endoscopic approach:*[29] The patient in left lateral position in the endoscopy suite. The needle is placed anterior to the lateral aspect of the aorta at the level of the celiac trunk . Precision is much improved with Doppler guidance of the interposed vessels. It is an easy technique.

The main adverse events are transient hypotension due to splanchnic vasodilation, diarrhea due to unopposed parasympathetic tone and needle site pain. Other complications include; paresthesia, paresis, pneumothorax, hematuria, shoulder pain, hemorrhagic gastritis, duodenitis, and rarely death.

The procedure must be performed under imaging either under ultrasound (anterior approach)/fluoroscopy/CT guidance for precision and safety. CPB is relatively safe and effective and has the best quality of evidence among neurolytic blocks with a reduction in opioid use and better patient satisfaction.[30]

*4. Pelvic Cancer Pain*

***Superior hypogastric block:***[31,32] Pelvic cancers can result in lower abdominal pain, which when unrelenting can be managed with superior hypogastric plexus (SHP). The nerves innervating the pelvic viscera such as the bladder, uterus, vagina, prostate, testes, urethra, descending colon and the rectum, relay in the superior hypogastric plexus. The SHP lie bilaterally in front of the L3 to S1 intervertebral discs in the retroperitoneum between the origins of the common iliac arteries and just inferior to the origins of the internal iliac arteries from the aorta. A neurolytic SHP block is indicated in pelvic visceral pain, pelvic cancer pain, endometriosis (a non-cancer indication) and refractory penile pain.

Classic approach for the block is a posterior approach under fluoroscopy guidance to locate L4–L5 interspace **(Fig. 11.8)**. Under strict aseptic technique and local analgesic wheal raised at a distance of 5–7 cm from the midline, two needles (15 cm, 22 G) are inserted bilaterally. The needles are directed 30 degree caudad towards the anterolateral aspect of L5 vertebral body. Obstacles in placement of the needle include the large iliac crest, the L5 tranverse process and the L5 vertebral body. Once the L5 vertebral body is contacted, the needles are walked off the body. The aim is to advance the needles to approximately 1 cm ahead of the vertebral body, where one may notice a 'pop' as the needle traverses the anterior fascia of the psoas muscle. This occurs at a depth of approximately 8–12 cm. The needle tip positioning is confirmed after injection of 3–5 ml of a water soluble contrast medium. The dye should be seen spreading smoothly in front of the L5 vertebral body and the sacral promontory. This is followed by an injection of 8–10 ml of 0.25% bupivacaine or 1% lignocaine for confirming the pain relief. Once confirmed, 15 ml of 50% alcohol can be injected in aliquots through each needle after confirming negative aspiration.

Several variations to the original technique have been developed such as the transdiscal approach where the needle is passed through the L5–S1 disc or the transarterial approach, where the needle is passed through the Iliac artery till blood is no longer aspirated. This suggests that the needle lies just anterior to the artery which is retroperitoneal and in the same plane as the SHP. Most of the variations were carried out to overcome the procedural difficulty.

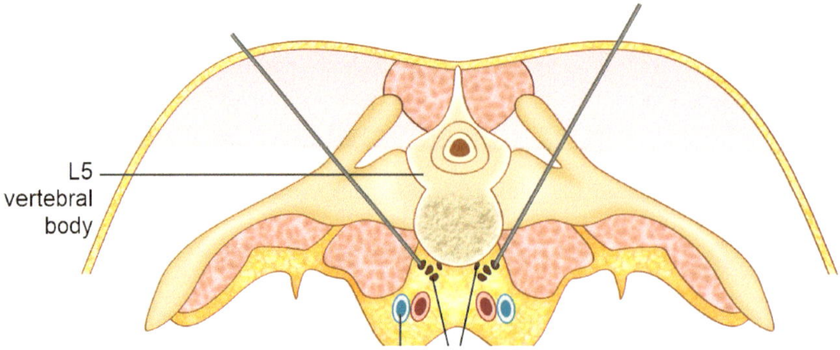


**Fig. 11.8:** Superior hypogastric plexus approach

Common complications which can occur during this block include, injury to the common iliac vessels, pelvic viscera, L5 nerve root and discitis in the transdiscal approach.

*Ganglion impar block*[33,34]

The ganglion impar is a solitary ganglion formed at the termination of the bilateral paravertebral sympathetic chains which fuse in the midline at this point. It is retroperitoneal and located behind the rectum, in the midline or just to the side of the sacrococcygeal joint (SCJ) or coccyx. The ganglion relays innervation to the perineum, coccyx, anus, distal rectum, vulva/scrotum, urethra and vagina. Patients in whom this block would benefit usually present with complaints of perineal and perianal burning sensation, urinary or rectal urgency, tenesmus. Other indications include radiation proctitis, coccydynia which is the only non-malignant indication for the block. The block is performed under fluoroscopy guidance.

The original technique described by Plancarte[35] was the anococcygeal approach, with patient in lateral position where a bent needle was passed through the anococcygeal membrane with a finger placed in the rectum to guide the needle and prevent any rectal injury. Other approaches such as the Trans-sacrococcygeal and the transdiscal approaches have since been described.

The trans-sacrococcygeal approach is performed with the patient in the prone position, with a pillow under the lower abdomen.

A 25-G spinal needle is inserted under fluoroscopic guidance through the sacrococcygeal disc. The needle is placed just anterior to the sacrococcygeal junction in the precoccygeal space (Fig. 11.9). The position is confirmed by injection of 1–2 ml of water soluble contrast. The ideal spread is in the form of a "comma". Local anesthetic, either lignocaine or bupivacaine 1–2 ml can be injected as a diagnostic block followed by the neurolytic agent usually phenol 6% (2–8 ml).

The block is relatively safe, however there is risk of rectal injury and neuritis. RF ablation of the ganglion has also been described.[36]

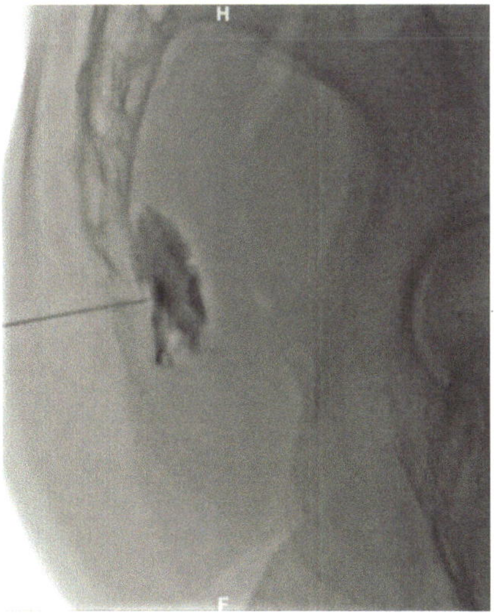


**Fig. 11.9:** Ganglion impar contrast spread ( trans-sacrococcygeal approach)

*Intrathecal neurolysis:*[18] May be used to provide pain relief in malignant pelvic or perineal pain syndromes as well as in chest wall or abdominal wall disease when the pain is refractory. Such neurolysis should always be preceded by a diagnostic block with a local anesthetic. Neurolytic agents used for such a procedure are either phenol or alcohol. Phenol is hyperbaric and thus settles down in the CSF, thus is useful in perineal or pelvic pain. Alcohol is hypobaric and thus rises in the CSF and is beneficial for pain at the thoracic level. Thus positioning a patient appropriately is extremely crucial in this setting.

In case of perineal/pelvic pain. Phenol is used, patient is kept in sitting position with a posterior tilt of 45°. The dura is punctured in the midline at L5/S1 level, and 0.1–0.3 ml increments of phenol are injected to a maximum of 3 ml.

The position prevents spread of the drug anteriorly and reduces the risk of motor block and limit sensory loss in areas unaffected by pain. It is preferred that the patient stays in this position for approximately 6 hours. Loss of bladder, bowel function and lower limb weakness are a risk, and hence the procedure is usually offered only to those who are already incontinent, wheelchair-bound, or both.

In those situations where the procedure is performed for chest wall or abdominal disease, the patient position is equally important. Mainly to prevent spillage of the alcohol or phenol to ventral nerve roots **(Fig. 11.10)**.

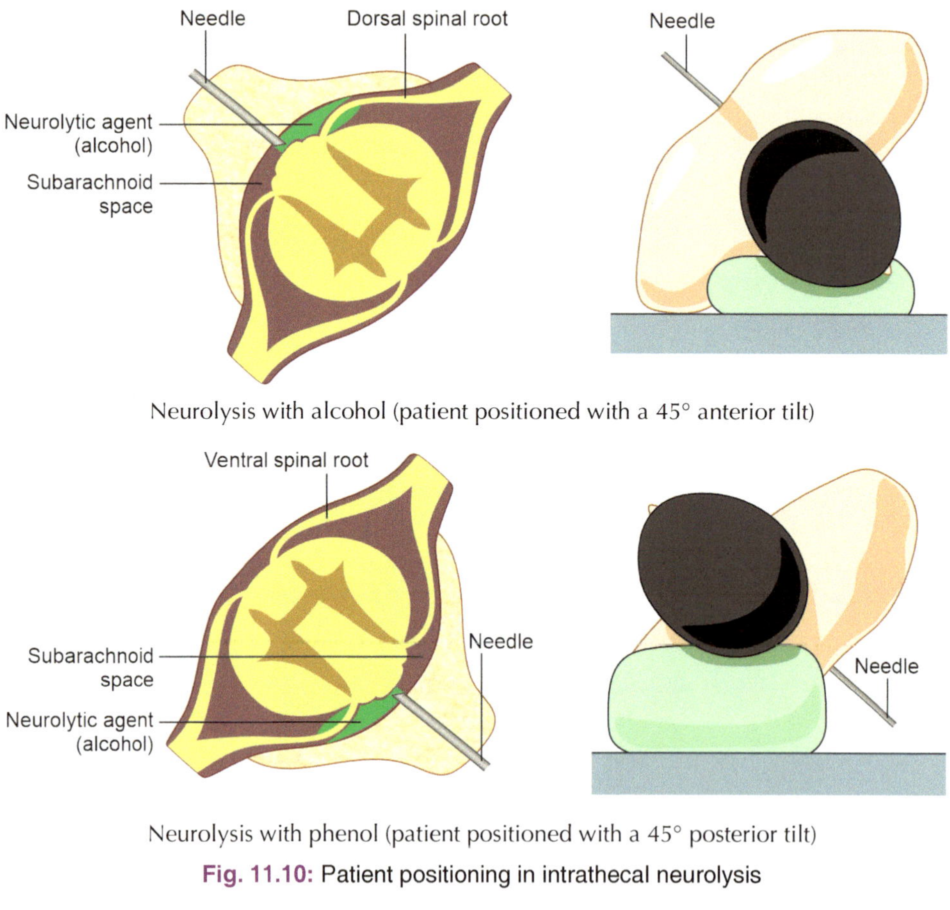


**Fig. 11.10:** Patient positioning in intrathecal neurolysis

Here, neurolysis of the dorsal root is performed where it exits the spinal cord. The needle tip placed at vertebral level where the dorsal root which is to be targeted, leaves the spinal cord and not where it passes through the intervertebral foramen.

*Epidural neurolysis:* A less often performed procedure for neuraxial neurolysis. Can be considered in cases where pain is limited to a few dermatomes in the thorax or abdominal wall. Especially if patient cannot be optimally positioned for intrathecal neurolysis.

The epidural catheter is placed close to the vertebral level corresponding to the dermatomal distribution of pain. The epidural catheter is left in place and repeat slow injections of 1–2 ml of 50% alcohol are performed over a few days. There is a risk of weakness of extremities or bowel/bladder paresis. Rarely performed nowadays.

*Cordotomy:* Prior to the WHO ladder, most patients with cancer pain underwent surgical neuroablation. These procedures were meant to disrupt neural pathways in the brain and spinal cord especially in patients with terminal cancer to provide relief from intractable pain. Most of these procedures have since been discontinued due to poor evidence or lack of it.

Midline myelotomy is used in rare cases of intractable visceral pain. Median tractotomy and thalamotomy too are very seldom carried out. Dorsal root entry zone (DREZ) lesions are currently still performed occasionally in few centers for pain which occurs due to traumatic brachial plexus avulsion rather than for cancer pain.[37]

Cordotomy first described in 1889, involves lesioning of the lateral spinothalamic tract on the contralateral side and is usually performed for patients with intractable cancer pain. It is an irreversible and invasive procedure. Can be performed percutaneously, open, endoscopic or via transdiscal approaches. Percutaneous cordotomy in those days was the most commonly performed procedure and is till date practised in very few centers.[38]

The lateral spinothalamic tract is disrupted by a radiofrequency lesion at C1–2 level for managing unilateral pain below C4.

Common indications are intractable pain from brachial plexus or chest wall invasion, malignant pleural mesothelioma and tumor infiltration of ilium or the lumbosacral plexus.

When effective, it provides good analgesia and about 30% of patients may come off their opioid doses. Previously performed under fluoroscopy guidance but nowadays is performed under CT guidance.

The endoscopic-guided technique where the lesioning is performed under direct vision has apparently a better safety profile.[39]

Complications include cord edema with ipsilateral motor weakness, pain on the side of cordotomy and failure of the procedure. Lesioning of the spinocerebellar/corticospinal tract can lead to ataxia and paresis, of the reticulospinal tract can result in respiratory failure, in addition there is risk of sympathetic dysfunction, bladder dysfunction or Horner's syndrome due to unintentional lesions.

In the current era, with advances in oncological treatment, over 50% of cancer patients survive beyond ten years. Role of neuroablative procedures in such a scenario would be limited and possibly could be replaced by implantable neuromodulation systems such as for spinal cord stimulation, DRG stimulation, and peripheral nerve stimulation, etc. for managing intractable pain.[40] The compatibility with investigations such as a MRI which is routinely necessary for monitoring progress in cancer patients had in the past limited the use of such devices in cancer patients.[41]

## Neuromodulation

It is the process which involves the inhibition, stimulation, modification, regulation or therapeutic alteration of activity, electrically or chemically. The use of neuromodulation is associated with (1) a reduction in opioid and adjunct medication consumption and (2) a reduction in pain severity and pain interference scores.[42]

The techniques may be invasive or non-invasive. They can alter neural activity by electrical, magnetic, optical or acoustic stimuli. When used as a treatment, neuromodulation offers higher specificity than medication, and noninvasive neuromodulation further provides more reversibility than surgical alternatives. Neuromodulation techniques such as spinal cord stimulation (SCS) and dorsal root ganglion stimulation (DRGS) are interventional procedures used frequently in chronic pain conditions such as post-laminectomy syndrome, complex regional pain syndrome, and peripheral neuropathy. These techniques are slowly being adopted for the treatment of various cancer-related pain.[42]

*Spinal cord stimulators (SCS):* Have been established for treating persistent pain such as in complex regional pain syndromes and refractory spinal pain. Involves stimulation of the dorsal columns of the spinal cord by means of electrodes which are placed in the epidural space. Thought to modulate neuronal function and reverse maladaptive changes which occur as a result of persistent pain. Conventional SCS use 60–200 Hz frequency whereas the more recent high frequency SCS use 10,000Hz frequency. Mechanism postulated for pain relief include a decrease in central sensitization and hyperpolarization of the dorsal horn neurons.

Spinal cord stimulators have been successfully used in treatment of chemotherapy induced neuropathic pain and also for localized cancer pain.[43]

*Peripheral nerve stimulation (PNS):* Indicated where SCS is contraindicated or the area is more amenable to PNS. A small lead electrode is inserted subcutaneously close to the peripheral nerve and connected to an implantable pulse generator. Works similar to acupuncture and transcutaneous electrical nerve stimulation (TENS) thus modulating the neuronal activity. Application to cancer pain has not as yet been proven and the evidence is poor. One series which reports positive outcomes in 7 out of 12 cancer patients in whom the pain not adequately managed with other options.[44]

*Acupuncture:* Acupuncture though considered a "complementary therapy" should be considered a form of neuromodulation. It predates the use of electrical stimulation. There is currently some evidence for use of acupuncture in cancer pain. A RCT, trialing electroacupuncture using thoracic paravertebral needles in 60 patients with pancreatic cancer has reported a significant reduction in pain scores in the acupuncture group.[45]

## Conclusion

Intractable cancer pain unrelieved by the administration of analgesics as per the WHO ladder or those who suffer excessive side effects of the analgesics could benefit from Neurolysis, which is documented to relieve pain and improve quality of life of such patients. With advances in imaging, these procedures can be performed precisely and have become much more safer than in the past. This, as well as the fact that these procedures fail when fat planes are invaded significantly by the tumor, encourages the use of neurolysis at much earlier stages of the disease. However, for improving the safety profile, proper patient selection, trained professionals and proper infrastructure are of utmost importance.

## References


1. Wiffen PJ, Wee B, Derry S, Bell RF, Moore RA. Opioids for cancer pain—an overview of Cochrane reviews. Cochrane Database of Systematic Reviews 2017, Issue 7. Art. No.: CD012592. DOI: 10.1002/14651858.CD012592.pub2.
2. World Health Organization. WHO's pain relief ladder. Available from: http://www.who.int/cancer/palliative/painladder/en/.
3. Bhatnagar S, Gupta M. Evidence-based clinical practice guidelines for interventional pain management in cancer pain. Indian journal of palliative care. 2015 May;21(2):137
4. Swerdlow M. The history of neurolytic block. In Techniques of neurolysis 1989 (pp. 1–11). Boston, MA: Springer US.
5. Vig S, Bhan S, Bhatnagar S. Celiac plexus block–an old technique with new developments. Pain Physician. 2021;24(5):379.
6. Koyyalagunta D, Burton AW. The role of chemical neurolysis in cancer pain. Current pain and headache reports. 2010 Aug;14:261–7.
7. Gordon T. Peripheral Nerve Regeneration and Muscle Reinnervation. Int J Mol Sci. 2020 Nov 17;21(22):8652. doi: 10.3390/ijms21228652. PMID: 33212795; PMCID: PMC7697710.
8. Bhaskar A. Interventional pain management in patients with cancer-related pain. Postgrad Med. 2020 Nov;132(sup3):13–16. doi: 10.1080/00325481.2020.1807796. Epub 2020 Oct 22. PMID: 32799614
9. Akhan O, Ozmen MN, Basgun N, Akinci D, Oguz O, Koroglu M, Karcaaltincaba M. Long-term results of celiac Ganglia block: correlation of grade of tumoral invasion and pain relief. AJR Am J Roentgenol. 2004 Apr;182(4):891–6. doi: 10.2214/ajr.182.4.1820891. PMID: 15039160
10. Wehrwein EA, Orer HS, Barman SM. Overview of the Anatomy, Physiology, and Pharmacology of the Autonomic Nervous System. Compr Physiol. 2016 Jun 13;6(3):1239–78. doi: 10.1002/cphy.c150037. PMID: 27347892.
11. Tatli S, Tapan Ü, Morrison PR, Silverman SG. Radiofrequency ablation: technique and clinical applications. Diagnostic and Interventional Radiology. 2012 Sep 1;18(5):508.
12. Amr SA, Reyad RM, Othman AH, Mohamad MF, Mostafa MM, Alieldin NH, Hamed FA. Comparison between radiofrequency ablation and chemical neurolysis of thoracic splanchnic nerves for the management of abdominal cancer pain, randomized trial. European Journal of Pain. 2018 Nov;22(10):1782–90.
13. Elkomos PM, Zakhary LE, Daniel SH. Comparative study between knee genicular nerve ablation by thermal radiofrequency vs thermal radiofrequency plus alcohol neurolysis for treatment of symptomatic knee osteoarthritis. Ain Shams Medical Journal. 2023 Dec 1;74(4):979–85.
14. Rowe DS. Neurolytic techniques for pain management. Pain Clin. 1995;8:107–5.
15. Trescot AM. Cryoanalgesia in interventional pain management. Pain physician. 2003;6(3):345.
16. Viswanathan A, Sharma M. Cervical cordotomy. Practical Management of Complex Cancer Pain. 2022 Feb 3:197.
17. Collantes Celador, Enrique, Jan Rudiger, and Alifia Tameem (eds). Essential Notes in Pain Medicine (Oxford, 2022; online edn, Oxford Academic, 1 June 2022), https://doi.org/10.1093/med/9780198799443.001.0001, accessed 24 Mar. 2024.
18. J Scott-Warren, Arun Bhaskar, Cancer pain management: Part II: Interventional techniques, Continuing Education in Anaesthesia Critical Care & Pain, Volume 15, Issue 2, April 2015, Pages 68–72.
19. Ing JW. Head and neck cancer pain. Otolaryngol Clin N Am. 2017;50(4):793–806.

20. Ghei A, Khot S. Pain management in patients with head and neck carcinoma. Otorhinolaryngol Clin. 2010;2:69–75. doi: 10.5005/jp-journals-10003-1019.
21. Lin H, Cao G, Jin G, Yang Z, Huang C, Shao J, Yao M, Huang B. Extracranial non-gasserian ganglion application of radiofrequency thermocoagulation on the mandibular branch of the trigeminal through the foramen ovale for trigeminal neuralgia. Pain Physician. 2021;24(4):E425.
22. Bharti N, Sujith J, Singla N, Panda NB, Bala I. Radiofrequency thermoablation of the Gasserian ganglion versus the peripheral branches of the trigeminal nerve for treatment of trigeminal neuralgia: a randomized, control trial. Pain Physician. 2019;22(2):147.
23. Aggarwal A, Suresh V, Gupta B, Sonthalia S. Post-herpetic Neuralgia: A Systematic Review of Current Interventional Pain Management Strategies. J Cutan Aesthet Surg. 2020 Oct-Dec;13(4):265–274. doi: 10.4103/JCAS.JCAS_45_20. PMID: 33911406; PMCID: PMC8061658
24. Araújo Santana JG, Nogueira Aquino Á, Lins Serafim J, Pereira de Oliveira AD, di Cássia de Oliveira Angelo R. Morphological Variations of the Celiac Plexus and its Clinical Implications: a literature Review. Journal of Morphological Sciences. 2021 Jan 1;38.
25. Zhong W, Yu Z, Zeng JX, Lin Y, Yu T, Min XH, et al. Celiac plexus block for treatment of pain associated with pancreatic cancer: A meta-analysis. Pain Pract. 2014;14:43–51
26. Principles and Practice of Pain Medicine, 2nd Edition. By Carol A. Warfield and Zahid H. Bajwa. New York, NY, McGraw-Hill, 2004. ISBN: 0-07-144349-5.
27. Lieberman RP, Waldman SD. Celiac plexus neurolysis with the modified transaortic approach. Radiology. 1990 Apr;175(1):274–6. doi: 10.1148/radiology.175.1.2315494. PMID: 2315494
28. Ina H, Kitoh T, Kobayashi M, Imai S, Ofusa Y, Goto H. New technique for the neurolytic celiac plexus block: the transintervertebral disc approach. Anesthesiology. 1996 Jul;85(1):212–7. doi: 10.1097/00000542-199607000-00028. PMID: 8694369
29. Seicean A. Celiac plexus neurolysis in pancreatic cancer: the endoscopic ultrasound approach. World J Gastroenterol. 2014 Jan 7;20(1):110–7. doi: 10.3748/wjg.v20.i1.110. PMID: 24415863; PMCID: PMC3885999
30. Hochberg U, Ingelmo P, Solé E, Miró J, Rivera G, Perez J. Early Interventional Treatments for Patients with Cancer Pain: A Narrative Review. J Pain Res. 2023;16:1663–71.
31. Urits I, Schwartz R, Bangalore Siddaiah H, Kikkeri S, Chernobylsky D, Charipova K, Jung JW, Imani F, Khorramian M, Varrassi G, Cornett EM, Kaye AD, Viswanath O. Inferior Hypogastric Block for the Treatment of Chronic Pelvic Pain. Anesth Pain Med. 2021 Feb 16;11(1):e112225. doi: 10.5812/aapm.112225. PMID: 34221944; PMCID: PMC8241820
32. Yoham AL, Bordoni B. Anatomy, Abdomen and Pelvis: Inferior Hypogastric Plexus. In: StatPearls. StatPearls Publishing, Treasure Island (FL); 2023. PMID: 33620788.
33. Sharma, Gaurav; Mahalle, Apurv1; Banode, Pankaj2; Chandak, Aruna3. Ganglion Impar Neurolysis in Chronic Perineal Pain. Journal of Datta Meghe Institute of Medical Sciences University 15(4):p 578–581, Oct–Dec 2020. | DOI: 10.4103/jdmimsu.jdmimsu_301_20
34. Malhotra N, Goyal S, Kumar A, Kanika, Singla V, Kundu ZS. Comparative evaluation of transsacrococcygeal and transcoccygeal approach of ganglion impar block for management of coccygodynia. J Anaesthesiol Clin Pharmacol. 2021 Jan-Mar;37(1):90–96. doi: 10.4103/joacp.JOACP_588_20. Epub 2021 Apr 10. PMID: 34103830; PMCID: PMC8174441
35. Plancarte R, Amescua C, Patt RB, Allende S. Presacral blockade of the ganglion of walther (ganglion impar). Anesthesiology 1990; 73:A751.doi: 10.1097/00000542-199009001-00749
36. Usmani H, Dureja G, Andleeb R, Tauheed N, Asif N. Conventional radiofrequency thermocoagulation vs pulsed radiofrequency neuromodulation of ganglion impar in chronic perineal pain of nononcological origin. Pain Med 2018; 19:2348–2356. doi: 10.1093/pm/pnx244
37. Bhaskar A. Interventional pain management in patients with cancer-related pain. Postgrad Med. 2020 Nov;132(sup3):13–16. doi: 10.1080/00325481.2020.1807796. Epub 2020 Oct 22. PMID: 32799614
38. Ischia, Stefano1; Luzzani, Aldo; Ischia, Alberto; Faggion, Sergio. A new approach to the neurolytic block of the coeliac plexus: The transaortic technique. Pain 16(4):p 333–341, August 1983. | DOI: 10.1016/0304-3959(83)90148-3

39. Jain P, Dutta A, Sood J. Coeliac plexus blockade and neurolysis: an overview. Indian journal of anaesthesia. 2006 May 1;50(3):169–77.
40. Yasuda I and Wang HP, Endoscopic ultrasound-guided celiac plexus block and neurolysis. Digestive Endoscopy, 2017;29:455–462. https://doi.org/10.1111/den.12824
41. Candido KD, Kusper TM, Knezevic NN. New Cancer Pain Treatment Options. Curr Pain Headache Rep. 2017 Feb;21(2):12. doi: 10.1007/s11916-017-0613-0. PMID: 28265859
42. Yu K, Niu X, He B. Neuromodulation management of chronic neuropathic pain in the central nervous system. Advanced Functional Materials. 2020 Sep;30(37):1908999.
43. Cruccu G, Garcia-Larrea L, Hansson P, Keindl M, Lefaucheur JP, Paulus W, Taylor R, Tronnier V, Truini A, Attal N. EAN guidelines on central neurostimulation therapy in chronic pain conditions. Eur J Neurol. 2016 Oct;23(10):1489–99. doi: 10.1111/ene.13103. Epub 2016 Aug 11. PMID: 27511815
44. Mainkar O, Sollo CA, Chen G, et al. Pilot study in temporary peripheral nerve stimulation in oncologic pain. Neuromodulation 2020;23:819–26.
45. Chen H, Liu TY, Kuai L, et al. Electroacupuncture treatment for pancreatic cancer pain: A randomized controlled trail. Pancreatology 2013; 13:594–97.

Chapter 12

# Interventional Radiology in Cancer Pain

• Nitin S Shetty • Suyash Kulkarni
• Kunal Gala • Monish GK

Scan this QR code to gain free online access to the photographic illustration of this chapter in high resolution.

## INTRODUCTION

Interventional radiology (IR) is a diagnostic and therapeutic subspecialty in medicine that comprises a large variety of minimally invasive therapeutic procedures, with the key differentiator being the performance of each relying on image guidance.[1] Armed with this unique skillset, the interventional radiologist can access pain generators throughout the body and target them to provide long-lasting and effective pain relief. This role is critical as it has been shown that integrated supportive care, which includes pain management, significantly reduces in-patient stays and thus reduces overall costs with better patient experience, particularly in patients with cancer.[2] The pain associated with oncologic diseases has now been included in the International Classification of Diseases (ICD-11) due to increasing opioid dependence in the Western world. It has now spurred interest in non-pharmacological treatments, including those offered by interventional radiologists.[3]

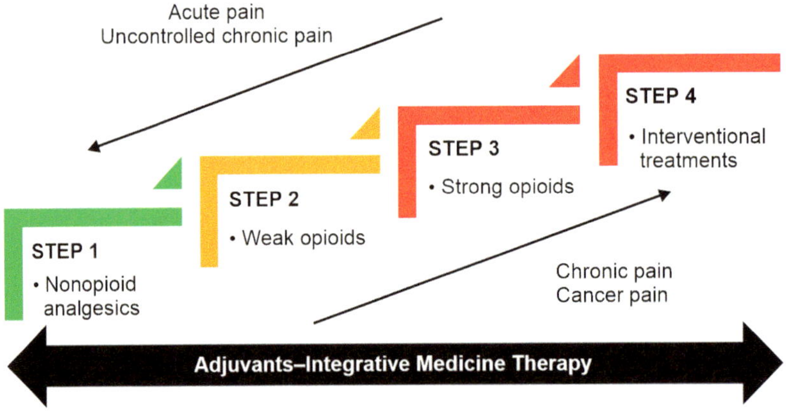


**Fig. 12.1:** Analgesic ladder (*Adapted from* Francois, et al)

According to the analgesic ladder **(Fig. 12.1)**, when opioid analgesics fail to control the pain adequately, or if the pain is localisable and amenable to local therapies, then intervention should be offered. A multidisciplinary team decision has also been shown to be better for optimally managing refractory pain.[4] It is suggested that the third step of the pain ladder be skipped, given the rising opioid abuse crisis now plaguing the Western hemisphere, and to intervene earlier.[5]

Table 12.1: Interventional pain palliation procedures based on pain origin (IR: Interventional radiology)

| Cause of pain | IR procedures |
|---|---|
| Spinal | Vertebral augmentation (cementing)<br>Radiofrequency ablation<br>Cryoablation |
| Non-spinal | *Musculoskeletal related:*<br>Tumor embolization<br>Ablation<br>Peripheral nerve blocks and chemical ablation |
| | *Visceral related:*<br>Celiac plexus block<br>Catheter directed therapy |

The approach to the patient with cancer-related pain can be broadly divided into spinal and non-spinal related causes. The major interventions that can be offered depend on the cause, feasibility, safety and anatomical factors (Table 12.1).

The most common interventions performed for pain palliation include vertebral augmentation, ablation, and angioembolisation, described in the subsequent paragraphs.

## Vertebral Augmentation (VA)

Radiation is one of the most common modality used to treat painful bone metastases. External beam radiotherapy (EBRT) is commonly used, but maximum pain relief is manifested only after about 4 weeks after treatment. Even suggestive of, only 50% of patients have pain relief at two weeks, and not all tumors are radiosensitive6. Vertebral augmentation is used in patients who have painful spinal fractures and provides quicker and more sustained pain relief—neoplastic or otherwise and involves the injection of PMMA—polymethyl methacrylate-bone cement into the fractured vertebral body (vertebroplasty) or inflation of balloons within them to increase the height and reduce the compressive deformity followed by PMMA injection (kyphoplasty).[7] Pain relief after cementoplasty in the treatment of metastatic bone tumors occurs both from the stabilisation of microfractures and via the toxic effect that the exothermic reaction of polymethylmethacrylate has on nociceptors.[8]

Conventionally, the treatment for neoplastic vertebral fractures has been with analgesics and supportive care. Radiotherapy, along with SBRT (stereotactic body radiation therapy), has now been used to provide pain relief to these patients with good results. The main disadvantage of radiotherapy is the slower onset of pain relief—this can be of particular importance in patients who have severe refractory pain related to the cancer and require early relief. There have been numerous contradictory studies about which modality performs better, but older studies have been primarily limited due to patient selection bias and issues with randomisation.[9–11] The evidence favours vertebral augmentation for quicker and more sustained pain relief from vertebral compression fractures. Surgery is the standard of care for pathological vertebral compression fractures complicated by spinal instability.[12] The spinal instability neoplastic score (SINS) is a prognostic tool for decision-making regarding spinal stability.

*Selection criteria:* Painful vertebral compression fracture, relatively stable spine (as SINS score). Patients are selected for vertebroplasty based on pain score with/without analgesics and, depending on the SINS score, calculated on pre-procedure planning contrast-enhanced MRI (CE-MRI) of the whole spine (Fig. 12.2). Cases with significant intradural extension and posterior cortical wall breach are considered relative contraindications to vertebral augmentation due to the risk of damage to the underlying spinal structures. Grossly unstable spinal fractures with SINS >9, with cord compression symptoms or rapidly progressing neurological deficits, are better treated by emergent open surgical fixation.[13,14]

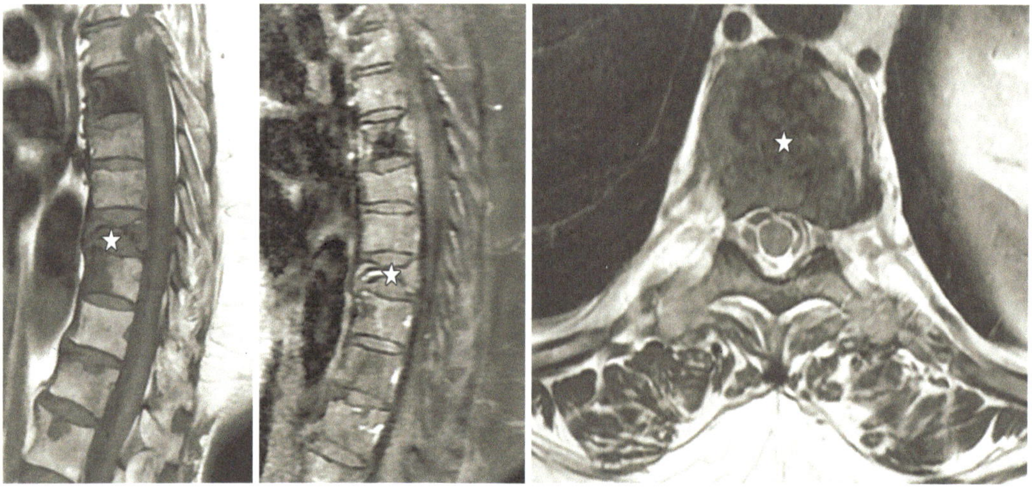

Fig. 12.2: Sagittal T1, sagittal post-contrast T1 and axial T2 images at the D9 level of the spine (from left to right) show multiple metastatic spinal lesions in a patient with metastatic breast carcinoma with >50% collapse of the vertebral body at T9 level (star). The prevertebroplasty pain score was 7/10, and the spinal tenderness was maximum at the T9 level

*Exclusion criteria:* The only absolute contraindications are coagulopathy which is uncorrectable and active infection/sepsis.

*Procedure:* Cementoplasty is done under fluoroscopic guidance in the IR suite with the patient in the prone position. Typically, the site of most localized spinal tenderness is targeted for optimum outcomes. A transpedicular approach is used and two bone biopsy needles are placed with the tip at the junction of the posterior one-third and anterior two-thirds of the body (Fig. 12.3). PMMA cement is then prepared and injected under controlled fluoroscopic guidance to make sure the cement does not spillover into the posterior spinal canal. Small amounts of cement extravasation into the disc space or canal are usually inconsequential but can cause neurological deficits such as paraparesis, and due diligence must be exercised. A rare complication that can happen is pulmonary cement embolism the mechanism is postulated to be due to the intravasation of cement through the vertebral epidural plexus into the pulmonary system.[15]

In cases with a significant soft tissue component along with the fracture, as in metastatic lesions, the underlying soft tissue is ablated first to create a cavity, followed by cementoplasty. Combined ablation and cementoplasty are done for lesions primarily in load-bearing bones (such as the spine, hip, and knee, Fig. 12.5). Pain relief is also better

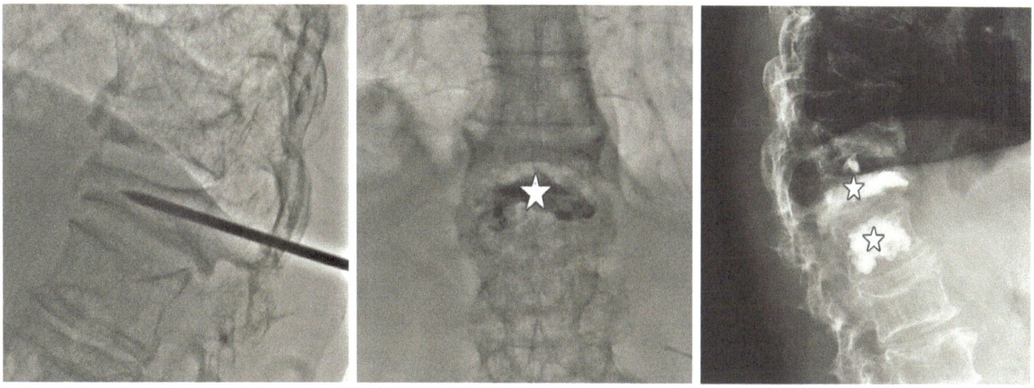

Figs 12.3: Left fluoroscopic spot image showing the positioning of needles (arrow) with middle and right radiographs showing good cement deposition(star) in the involved D12 and D11 vertebra (star). Post vertebroplasty pain score was down to 3/10 from 7/10 with no neurological deficit

when ablation is combined with vertebroplasty rather than with vertebroplasty alone.[16] Ablation methods are usually heat-based for cancer-related pain, as in radiofrequency ablation (RFA), but cryoablation can also be used as it is generally less painful.[17]

### Sacroplasty

Sacral insufficiency fractures are associated with severe and debilitating pain–these can be due to a variety of causes, including but not limited to osteoporosis, steroid therapy, radiation therapy to the pelvis and rheumatoid arthritis.[18] Sacral metastases are another cause of significant morbidity to the patient, resulting in considerable movement restriction in day-to-day activities.

Essentially, cementoplasty of the sacrum, sacroplasty can be performed with a short-axis or long-axis approach (Fig. 12.4). Regardless of approach, the procedure provides significant pain relief with a quick onset duration.[19–22] More importantly, studies have found that sacroplasty offers better pain relief than conservative management or surgical fixation, especially in the acute period. Hospital stays are also lower in sacroplasty viz-a-viz surgical fixation.[23] Kyung-Chul, et al. (2018) also found that patients could do more activities of daily living (ADL) post-procedure than before.[24]

The efficacy of percutaneous vertebroplasty has been debated since its conception, with multiple conflicting results.[25,26] A recent meta-analysis involving 1351 patients in 2018 showed a 2.83-fold decrease in pain among the case-control studies and a significant reduction in pain in single-arm studies.[27] The 2022 update of the ACR (Americal College of Radiology) appropriateness criteria suggests vertebroplasty and balloon kyphoplasty are equally effective in pain palliation, while ablation is typically for treating painful spinal metastases.[28] A multi-society position statement concluded that the vertebral augmentation of vertebral compression fractures was beneficial in providing short term pain relief and likely to sustain the same long-term.[29] Given the evidence that it is more effective than prolonged medical treatment in achieving analgesia, improving function in patients with painful fractures and avoiding the complications of narcotic use, the threshold for performing vertebral augmentation has declined.[30]

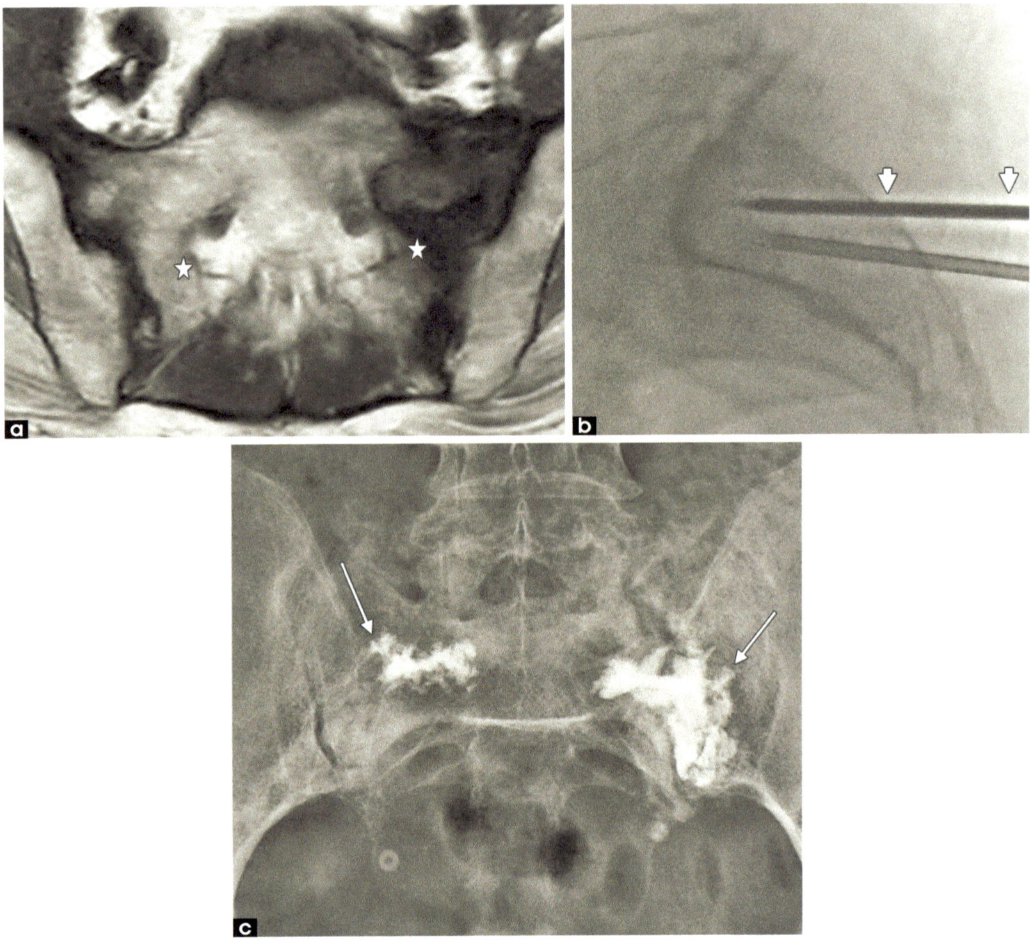

Figs 12.4a to c: Axial T1 image (a) showing bilateral sacral insufficiency fractures in a case of metastatic CA cervix post-radiation therapy. Spot radiographic image (b) showing needle placement with long axis approach—(arrowheads), with post-procedure radiograph (c) showing good cement deposition

## Ablation

Pain is the most common presentation of patients with skeletal metastases. Furthermore, these patients are usually undertreated with analgesics before starting anti-neoplastic therapy.[31] Given the relatively slow pain relief in radiotherapy, ablation has emerged as a minimally invasive modality that provides excellent pain relief, which is quicker and provides sustained relief, particularly when combined with cementoplasty.[32]

Ablation refers to tissue destruction caused by heat or any chemical substance. Ablation is typically used in the palliative setting to debulk large tumors and decrease pain. Still, ablation can be curative for smaller lesions (such as osteoid osteoma), provided a good zone is achieved. Temperature >60°C is maintained in thermal ablation until the tumor cells are killed. This can be achieved by the use of radiofrequency waves, microwaves or high-frequency ultrasound–labelled radiofrequency ablation (RFA), microwave ablation (MWA) and high-intensity focused ultrasound (HIFU),

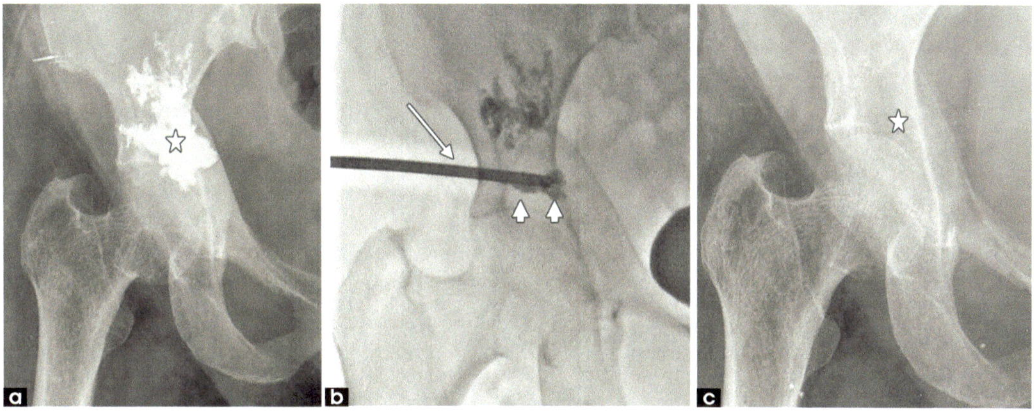

**Figs 12.5a to c:** Patient with lung carcinoma metastasis to the right acetabulum. (a: hip radiograph) Lytic metastatic lesion involving the left ilium and acetabulum (star); (b: fluoroscopic spot image) showing needle inserted into the acetabular roof (arrow) with the injection of cement (arrowheads); (c: post-procedure follow-up radiograph) Pelvic radiograph showing good cement deposition (star) in the right acetabular roof post acetabuloplasty. The patient had good palliation of pain—pain score decreased from 9/10 to 4/10 post-procedure

respectively.[33] Thermal ablation also includes cryoablation, in which tumor necrosis is achieved by freezing the tumor cells to <20°C.[34] Appropriate patient selection is critical to achieving good outcomes with ablation. The various technical differences between the ablation modalities are illustrated in Table 12.2. In the IR suite, ablation is performed with imaging guidance–usually, CT is the workhorse because of the multiplanar imaging,

**Table 12.2: Table comparing the technical principles of the various available ablation modalities**

| Parameter | RFA | MWA | IRE | Cryo-ablation |
|---|---|---|---|---|
| Principle | Hyperthermia | Hyperthermia | Non-thermal-Membrane poration | Hypothermia |
| Applicator | Unipolar electrode (RITA) | Bipolar electrode (Covidien) | Unipolar electrodes (Nanoknife) | Cryo probe (IceCure) |
| Disadvantages | Heat sink effect | Requires cooling | High precision needed<br>Small area | Long ablation time<br>Cryo-shock (rare)– systemic inflammatory response due to cytokine storm |
| Abscopal effect | Yes | No | +/– | Yes |
| Advantages | Simpler, probe variety | Effective near vessels | Less susceptible to produce vascular and bowmage | Relatively painless |

but ultrasound and even fluoroscopy can be used. Care must be taken to target the lesion correctly and adjust the machine parameters based on the required zone of ablation, typically per the manufacturer's recommendations. The abscopal effect is spontaneous distant tumor regression induced by releasing various immunomodulating factors. Ablation has been shown to produce a therapeutically effective antitumor response when combined with appropriate immunomodulators, which is of particular interest in the setting of metastatic disease.[35]

*Inclusion criteria for ablation for patients with skeletal metastases include:* A pain score nadir more than 4/10 per day using the brief pain inventory-short form typically filled in the 24 hours before treatment,[36] not more than two sites of painful skeletal metastases with pain (i.e. oligometastatic disease), life expectancy of at least or more than 2 months, platelet counts more than 75,000/microliter and international normalised ratio less than 1.5.

*Exclusion criteria:* Distant and multiple painful metastases and whenever there is impending fracture of the targeted bone (surgery may be preferred).

With the addition of ablation to vertebroplasty, radiological local tumor response rates of up to 70% have been described one year after treatment.[37] This sustained and early pain relief makes combination therapies enticing as pain palliative procedures.[38,39]

Given the significant benefit and minimal invasiveness, the indications for ablation have expanded to include not only metastatic lesions but also small primary tumors. Primary malignant bone tumors <3 cm can be treated in patients who refuse surgery/ in whom surgery would be quite morbid **(Figs 12.6 and 12.7)**. Multiple benign tumors such as osteoid osteoma, osteoblastoma, chondroblastoma **(Fig. 12.8)** and eosinophilic granuloma have also been treated with ablation with curative intent.[5,40–42] Cryoablation is preferred for the ablation of painful primary bone lesions since the zone of ablation—the 'iceball'–can be directly visualised as it forms under CT or USG guidance **(Fig. 12.9)**. This dynamic process helps assess the required ablation zone correctly and limits damage to nearby structures. The other main advantage is that it has better intrinsic analgesic properties than thermoablation and can preserve a tissue's collagenous structure, which results in less peri-ablational inflammation.[43,44]

Ablation can also be used to debulk large lesions, which can aid in pain palliation. This applies to both benign and malignant lesions. Fibromatosis is a benign disease which follows a highly variable course. While the primary treatment is to 'wait and watch', ablation has earned credit in treating cases with new-onset pain or progressing size, causing patient discomfort in those situations wherein the disease does not respond to systemic therapy as a form of local control.[45]

## Angioembolisation

Angioembolisation refers to purposeful blockage of the vessels with embolic agents–embolic agents currently include gel foam, polyvinyl alcohol particles and stainless steel coils.[46] Angioembolisation for pain palliation of metastatic disease was described back in 1979 by Chuang, et al. wherein they did angioembolisation for painful bony metastases from renal cell carcinoma.[47] Angioembolisation for painful lesions is typically done in a palliative setting for those with intractable pain, or it can be done as a primary treatment/combined with immunotherapy for slow-growing lesions which are not amenable to surgical management.

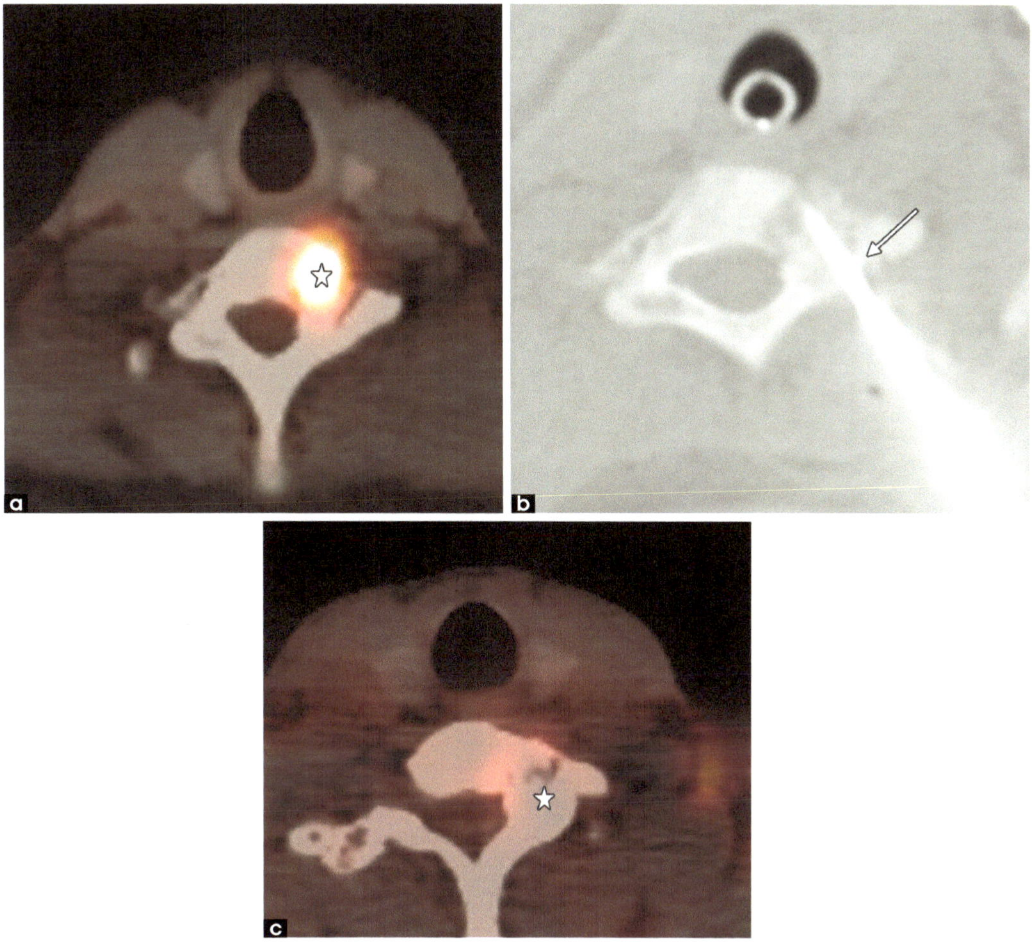

Figs 12.6a to c: (a) Axial PET-CT image showing FDG avid C7 osteoblastoma (star); (b) showing placement of RFA electrode within the lesion (arrow); (c) post-procedure PET image showing post-ablation PET scan with no significant FDG uptake within the lesion. The pre-procedure pain score was 7/10. The pain score decreased to 2/10 within 48 hours after ablation.

The axial location of any giant cell tumor (GCT) of bone makes surgical resection all but impossible due to proximity to vital structures and possible nerve injury, which could result in bladder or bowel dysfunction. Many cases also invade the spinal canal, preventing en bloc resection.[46] These patients also have significant pain due to the location of the tumor and, in some cases, due to neural involvement.[48] Due to this reason, immunotherapy with Denosumab and selective arterial embolisation has emerged as conservative options promising disease control and pain relief. Angioembolisation of GCT and sacral metastases effectively treats pain associated with unresectable lesions and produces good local response rates as well (Fig. 12.10).[49,50] Embolization, while associated with a durable and reliable response, usually has to be repeated if and when the disease recurs or is associated with new-onset pain.[51,52]

Embolization of hypervascular bone metastases—such as those from renal or thyroid primaries—has also been performed with a palliative intent to relieve pain (Fig. 12.11).

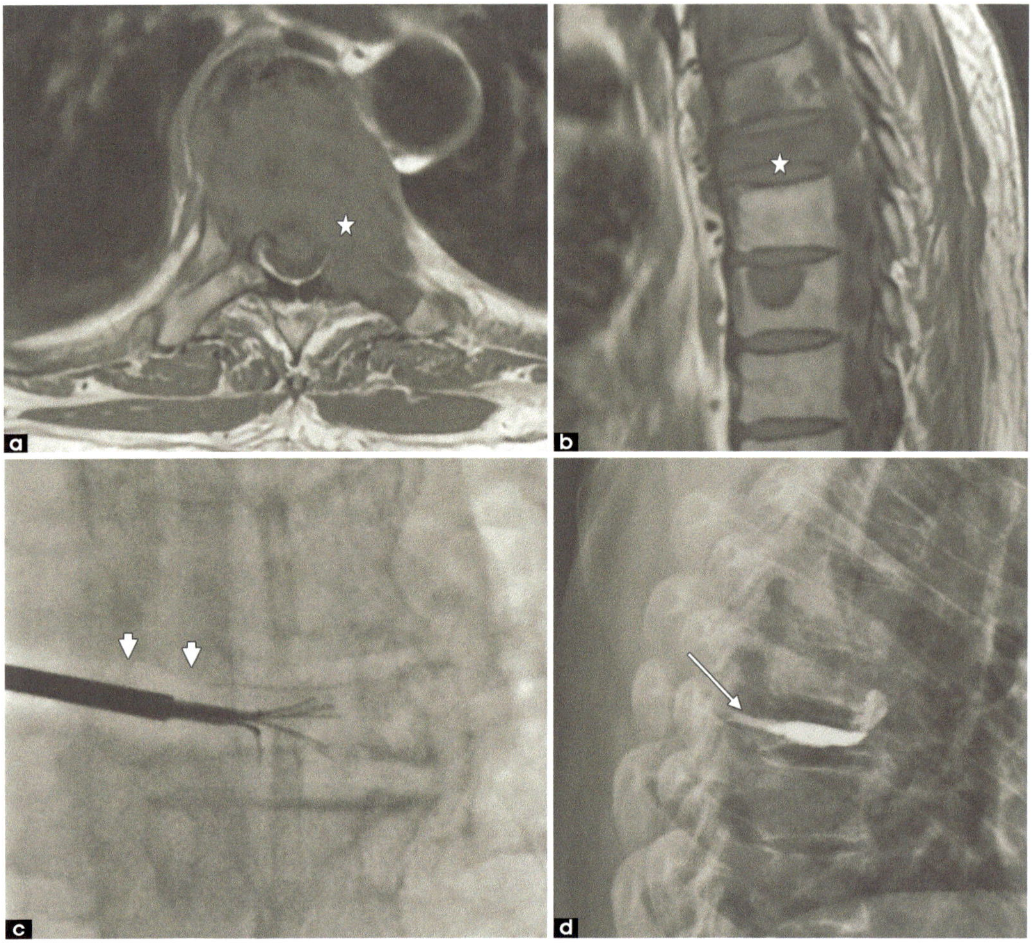

Figs 12.7a to d: (a) Axial T1 MRI at D7 level; (b) Sagittal T1 mid spine showing metastatic soft tissue at D7 with vertebral collapse (star); (c) A fluoroscopic spot image of RFA was done with a RITA Starburst 15 cm needle (arrowheads), followed by cementoplasty; (d) Post-procedure spine radiograph showing good cement deposition in the collapsed vertebra (arrow) The pre-procedure pain score was 7/10, which improved to 3/10 on post-procedure follow-up

Preoperative embolization of these vascular metastases when they occur in the spine and present with cord symptoms is essential to reduce surgical blood loss.[52] Given the much lesser incidence of complications with the advent of newer, smaller microcatheters and selective embolization, it certainly seems this modality will be a part of pain palliation in metastatic disease.

## Conclusion

Interventional radiology has grown manifold in the last decade by introducing new hardware and techniques. The application of the broad spectrum of IR techniques to pain palliation has resulted in a paradigm shift away from opioid abuse for analgesia.[7] The combination of a pain physician and an interventional radiologist should be considered essential in any patient presenting with intractable pain, given the variety of pain sites the interventionalist can target, whether percutaneously or endovascularly. It stands

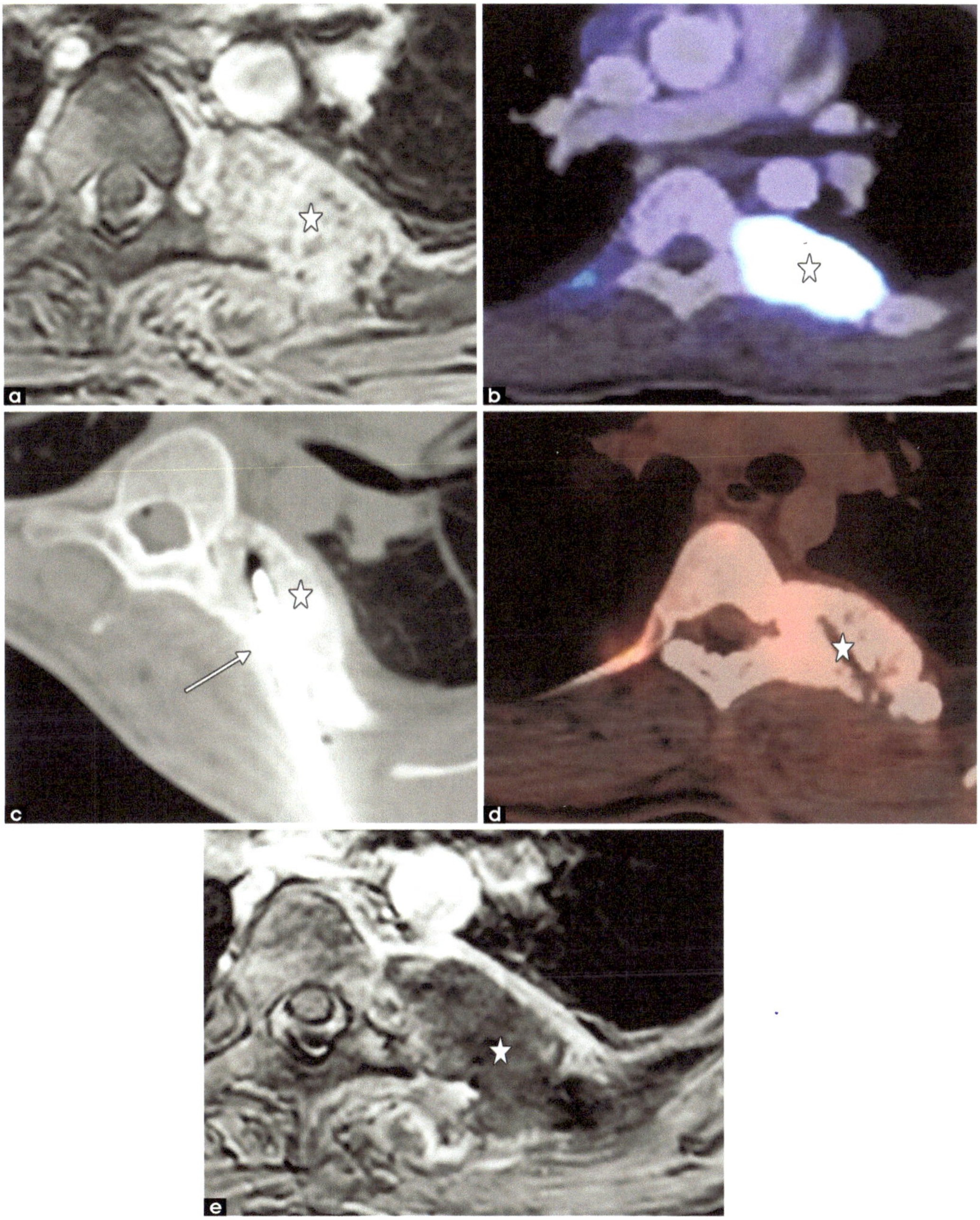


**Figs 12.8a to e:** (a) Axial post-contrast MRI showing enhancing osteoblastoma involving the left 5th rib (star); (b) Axial PET-CT showing tumoral FDG avidity; (c) Axial CT obtained during ablation shows the cryoprobe (arrow) placed within the lesion. Overlapping ablations were done to ensure complete coverage of margins; (d) Post-procedure PET-CT showing no residual FDG avidity; (e) Follow-up contrast MRI after 3 months shows no enhancing component within the lesion

to reason that IR will continue to play an even more significant role in the future of cancer pain management.

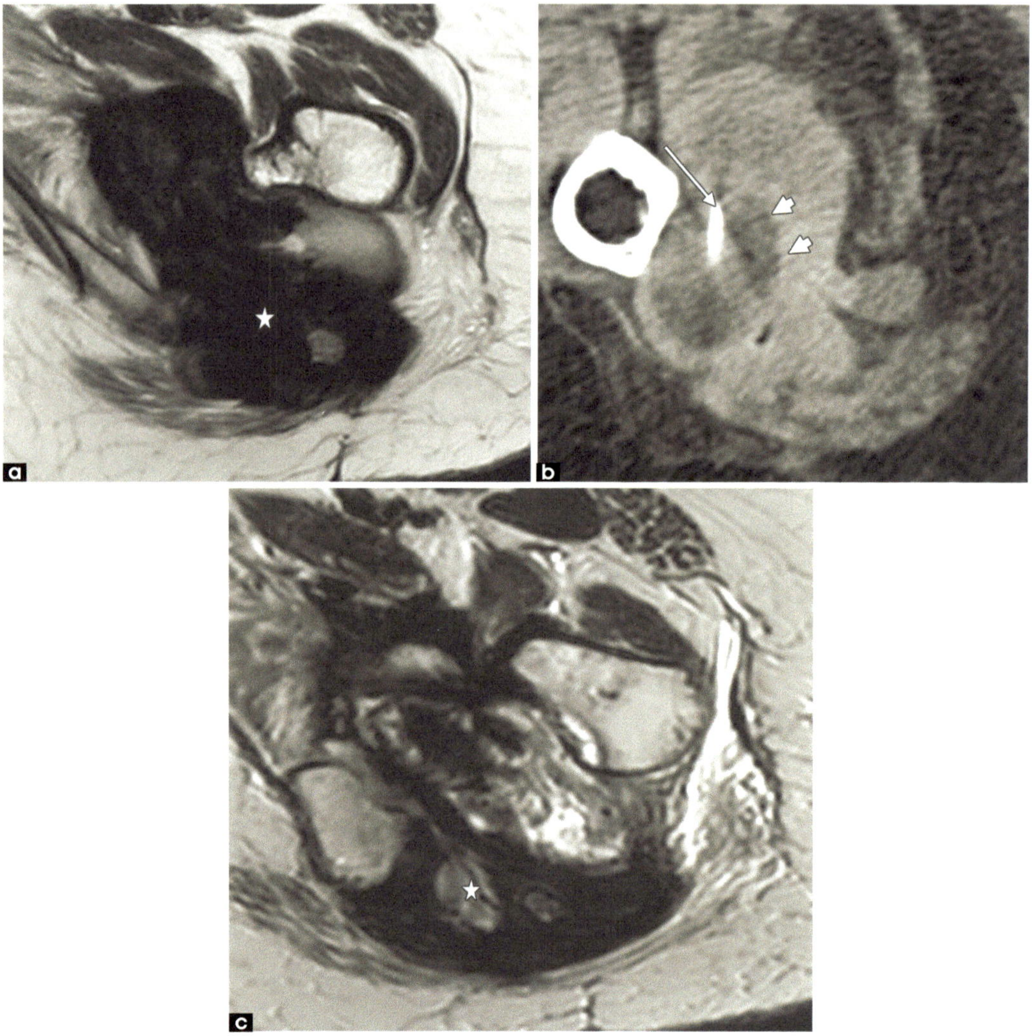


Figs 12.9a to c: (a) T2 weighted axial MRI image showing hypointense fibromatosis (star) in the right upper thigh; (b) CT image during cryoablation shows the cryoprobe within the lesion (arrow) and surrounding hypodense ice-ball (arrowheads); (c) Post-procedure follow-up T2 weighted MRI image shows cystic changes within the lesion indicating good response. Patient had significant improvement of pain post- procedure with decrease in pain score from 7/10 to 1/10

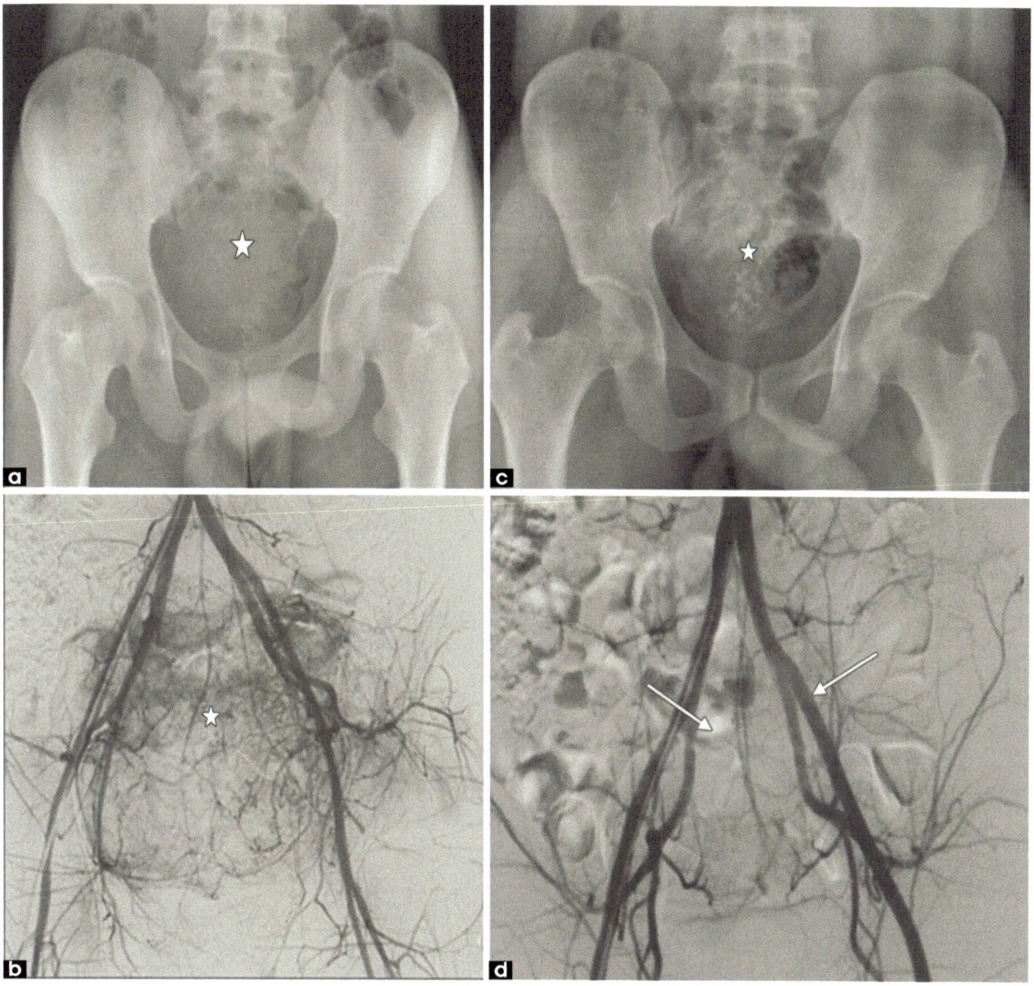


**Figs 12.10a to d:** (a and b) Pre-embolisation plain pelvic radiograph and angiographic run showing lytic lesion in the sacrum (in a known case of sacral GCT ) with significant vascularity; (c and d) Response pelvic radiograph and angiographic image showing significant radiological response as sclerosis and significantly decreased residual tumor blush (arrows) respectively

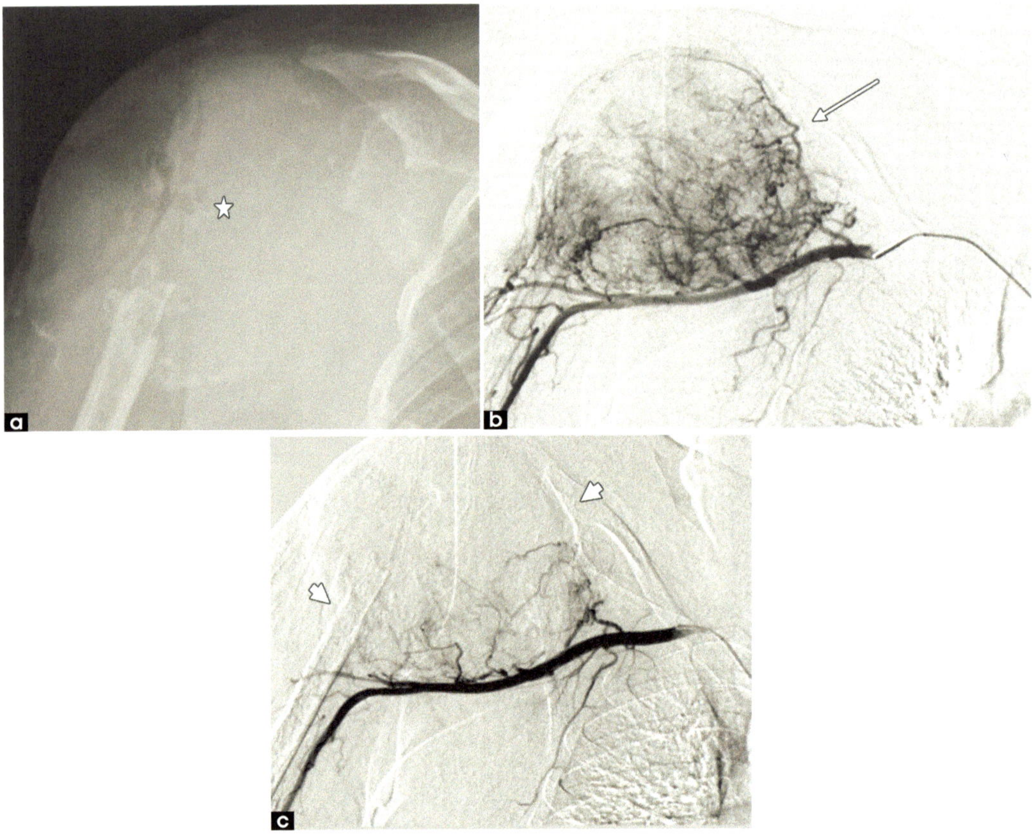


Figs 12.11a to c: (a) Right upper arm radiograph showing a large lytic metastasis from renal cell carcinoma (star). Pre-embolization (b) and post-embolization (c) angiograms of hypervascular (arrow) right humeral metastases from renal cell carcinoma demonstrating a significant reduction in tumor blush post-angioembolization (arrowheads). On six weeks follow-up, the patient had sustained a decrease in pain score from 8/10 to 4/10

## References

1. Bluemke DA, Liu S. Chapter 41 - Imaging in Clinical Trials. In: Gallin JI, Ognibene FP, editors. Principles and Practice of Clinical Research (Third Edition) [Internet]. Boston: Academic Press; 2012. p. 597–617. Available from: https://www.sciencedirect.com/science/article/pii/B9780123821676000412
2. Kaltman J, Sun CL, Loscalzo MJ, Kronstadt E, Goodspeed E, Qamar S, et al. The impact of early integrated supportive care on length of stay at an NCI-designated cancer center. J Clin Oncol. 2020 May 20;38(15_suppl):2024–2024.
3. Mestdagh F, Steyaert A, Lavand'homme P. Cancer Pain Management: A Narrative Review of Current Concepts, Strategies, and Techniques. Curr Oncol. 2023 Jul 18;30(7):6838–58.
4. Allano G, George B, Minello C, Burnod A, Maindet C, Lemaire A. Strategies for interventional therapies in cancer-related pain-a crossroad in cancer pain management. Support Care Cancer Off J Multinatl Assoc Support Care Cancer. 2019 Aug;27(8):3133–45.
5. Ryan A, Byrne C, Pusceddu C, Buy X, Tsoumakidou G, Filippiadis D. CIRSE Standards of Practice on Thermal Ablation of Bone Tumours. Cardiovasc Intervent Radiol. 2022 May 1;45(5):591–605.

6. Janjan N, Lutz ST, Bedwinek JM, Hartsell WF, Ng A, Pieters RS, et al. Therapeutic guidelines for the treatment of bone metastasis: a report from the American College of Radiology Appropriateness Criteria Expert Panel on Radiation Oncology. J Palliat Med. 2009 May;12(5):417–26.
7. Fletcher A, Moore KJ, Stensby JD, Hulbert A, Saemi AM, Davis RM, et al. The Pain Crisis: Interventional Radiology's Role in Pain Management. Am J Roentgenol. 2021 Sep;217(3):676–90.
8. Sabharwal T, Katsanos K, Buy X, Gangi A. Image-guided ablation therapy of bone tumors. Semin Ultrasound CT MR. 2009 Apr;30(2):78–90.
9. Calmels V, Vallée JN, Rose M, Chiras J. Osteoblastic and mixed spinal metastases: evaluation of the analgesic efficacy of percutaneous vertebroplasty. AJNR Am J Neuroradiol. 2007 Mar;28(3):570–4.
10. Chew C, Craig L, Edwards R, Moss J, O'Dwyer PJ. Safety and efficacy of percutaneous vertebroplasty in malignancy: a systematic review. Clin Radiol. 2011 Jan;66(1):63–72.
11. Dalbayrak S, Onen MR, Yilmaz M, Naderi S. Clinical and radiographic results of balloon kyphoplasty for treatment of vertebral body metastases and multiple myelomas. J Clin Neurosci Off J Neurosurg Soc Australas. 2010 Feb;17(2):219–24.
12. Fisher CG, DiPaola CP, Ryken TC, Bilsky MH, Shaffrey CI, Berven SH, et al. A Novel Classification System for Spinal Instability in Neoplastic Disease: An Evidence-Based Approach and Expert Consensus From the Spine Oncology Study Group. Spine. 2010 Oct 15;35(22):E1221.
13. Chen Y, He Y, Zhao C, Li X, Zhou C, Hirsch FR. Treatment of spine metastases in cancer: a review. J Int Med Res. 2019 Dec 26;48(4):0300060519888107.
14. Evidence reviews for invasive interventions: Spinal metastases and metastatic spinal cord compression: Evidence review. 2023 [cited 2024 Feb 11]; Available from: https://www.ncbi.nlm.nih.gov/books/NBK595813
15. Nairn RJ, Binkhamis S, Sheikh A. Current Perspectives on Percutaneous Vertebroplasty: Current Evidence/Controversies, Patient Selection and Assessment, and Technique and Complications. Radiol Res Pract. 2011 May 21;2011:e175079.
16. SY, Mg B, UR, AA, IC. Role of radiofrequency ablation and cement injection for pain control in patients with spinal metastasis. BMC Musculoskelet Disord [Internet]. 2021 Oct 29 [cited 2024 Feb 25];22(1). Available from: https://pubmed.ncbi.nlm.nih.gov/34715849/
17. The condition, current treatments and procedure | Radiofrequency ablation as an adjunct to balloon kyphoplasty or percutaneous vertebroplasty for palliation of painful spinal metastases | Guidance | NICE [Internet]. NICE; 2023 [cited 2024 Feb 11]. Available from: https://www.nice.org.uk/guidance/ipg759/chapter/2-The-condition-current-treatments-and-procedure
18. De Smet AA, Neff JR. Pubic and sacral insufficiency fractures: clinical course and radiologic findings. AJR Am J Roentgenol. 1985 Sep;145(3):601–6.
19. Tian QH, Liu HF, Wang T, Cheng YS, Wu CG. Percutaneous Sacroplasty for Painful Sacral Metastases Involving Multiple Sacral Vertebral Bodies: Initial Experience with an Interpedicular Approach. Korean J Radiol. 2019 Jun;20(6):939–46.
20. Kortman K, Ortiz O, Miller T, Brook A, Tutton S, Mathis J, et al. Multicenter study to assess the efficacy and safety of sacroplasty in patients with osteoporotic sacral insufficiency fractures or pathologic sacral lesions. J Neurointerventional Surg. 2013 Sep 1;5(5):461–6.
21. Mahmood B, Pasternack J, Razi A, Saleh A. Safety and efficacy of percutaneous sacroplasty for treatment of sacral insufficiency fractures: a systematic review. J Spine Surg. 2019 Sep;5(3):365–71.
22. Butler CL, Given CA, Michel SJ, Tibbs PA. Percutaneous Sacroplasty for the Treatment of Sacral Insufficiency Fractures. Am J Roentgenol. 2005 Jun;184(6):1956–9.
23. Briggs P, King SW, Staniland T, Gopal S, Shah R, Chimutengwende-Gordon M, et al. A Systematic Review of Sacral Insufficiency Fractures: Treatment Modalities and Outcomes. Cureus [Internet]. 2023 Jul 11 [cited 2024 Feb 28];15(7). Available from: https://www.cureus.com/articles/166430-a-systematic-review-of-sacral-insufficiency-fractures-treatment-modalities-and-outcomes
24. Choi KC, Shin SH, Lee DC, Shim HK, Park CK. Effects of Percutaneous Sacroplasty on Pain and Mobility in Sacral Insufficiency Fracture. J Korean Neurosurg Soc. 2017 Jan 1;60(1):60–6.

25. Aebi M. Vertebroplasty: about sense and nonsense of uncontrolled "controlled randomized prospective trials." Eur Spine J Off Publ Eur Spine Soc Eur Spinal Deform Soc Eur Sect Cerv Spine Res Soc. 2009 Sep;18(9):1247–8.
26. Wali AR, Martin JR, Rennert R, Resnick DK, Taylor W, Warnke P, et al. Vertebroplasty for vertebral compression fractures: Placebo or effective? Surg Neurol Int. 2017;8:81.
27. Qi L, Li C, Wang N, Lian H, Lian M, He B, et al. Efficacy of percutaneous vertebroplasty treatment of spinal tumors: A meta-analysis. Medicine (Baltimore). 2018 Jan;97(3):e9575.
28. Khan MA, Jennings JW, Baker JC, Smolock AR, Shah LM, Pinchot JW, et al. ACR Appropriateness Criteria® Management of Vertebral Compression Fractures: 2022 Update. J Am Coll Radiol. 2023 May 1;20(5, Supplement):S102–24.
29. Jensen ME, McGraw JK, Cardella JF, Hirsch JA. Position statement on percutaneous vertebral augmentation: a consensus statement developed by the American Society of Interventional and Therapeutic Neuroradiology, Society of Interventional Radiology, American Association of Neurological Surgeons/Congress of Neurological Surgeons, and American Society of Spine Radiology. J Vasc Interv Radiol JVIR. 2007 Mar;18(3):325–30.
30. Van Meirhaeghe J, Bastian L, Boonen S, Ranstam J, Tillman JB, Wardlaw D, et al. A randomized trial of balloon kyphoplasty and nonsurgical management for treating acute vertebral compression fractures: vertebral body kyphosis correction and surgical parameters. Spine. 2013 May 20;38(12):971–83.
31. Janjan NA, Payne R, Gillis T, Podoloff D, Libshitz HI, Lenzi R, et al. Presenting symptoms in patients referred to a multidisciplinary clinic for bone metastases. J Pain Symptom Manage. 1998 Sep;16(3):171–8.
32. Grönemeyer DHW, Schirp S, Gevargez A. Image-guided radiofrequency ablation of spinal tumors: preliminary experience with an expandable array electrode. Cancer J Sudbury Mass. 2002;8(1):33–9.
33. Santiago FR, del Mar Castellano García M, Montes JLM, García MR, Fernández JMT. Treatment of bone tumours by radiofrequency thermal ablation. Curr Rev Musculoskelet Med. 2009 Jan 7;2(1):43–50.
34. Silverman SG, Tuncali K, Adams DF, vanSonnenberg E, Zou KH, Kacher DF, et al. MR imaging-guided percutaneous cryotherapy of liver tumors: initial experience. Radiology. 2000 Dec;217(3):657–64.
35. Takaki H, Cornelis F, Kako Y, Kobayashi K, Kamikonya N, Yamakado K. Thermal ablation and immunomodulation: From preclinical experiments to clinical trials. Diagn Interv Imaging. 2017 Sep;98(9):651–9.
36. Daut RL, Cleeland CS, Flanery RC. Development of the Wisconsin Brief Pain Questionnaire to assess pain in cancer and other diseases. Pain. 1983 Oct;17(2):197–210.
37. Wallace AN, Tomasian A, Vaswani D, Vyhmeister R, Chang RO, Jennings JW. Radiographic Local Control of Spinal Metastases with Percutaneous Radiofrequency Ablation and Vertebral Augmentation. Am J Neuroradiol. 2016 Apr 1;37(4):759–65.
38. Bagla S, Sayed D, Smirniotopoulos J, Brower J, Neal Rutledge J, Dick B, et al. Multicenter Prospective Clinical Series Evaluating Radiofrequency Ablation in the Treatment of Painful Spine Metastases. Cardiovasc Intervent Radiol. 2016 Sep;39(9):1289–97.
39. Levy J, Hopkins T, Morris J, Tran N, David E, Massari F, et al. Radiofrequency Ablation for the Palliative Treatment of Bone Metastases: Outcomes from the Multicenter OsteoCool Tumor Ablation Post-Market Study (OPuS One Study) in 100 Patients. 2020 Nov 1;
40. Tordjman M, Perronne L, Madelin G, Mali RD, Burke C. CT-guided radiofrequency ablation for osteoid osteomas: a systematic review. Eur Radiol. 2020 Nov;30(11):5952–63.
41. Becce F, Theumann N, Rochette A, Larousserie F, Campagna R, Cherix S, et al. Osteoid osteoma and osteoid osteoma-mimicking lesions: biopsy findings, distinctive MDCT features and treatment by radiofrequency ablation. Eur Radiol. 2010 Oct;20(10):2439–46.
42. Beyer T, van Rijswijk CSP, Villagrán JM, Rehnitz C, Muto M, von Falck C, et al. European multicentre study on technical success and long-term clinical outcome of radiofrequency

ablation for the treatment of spinal osteoid osteomas and osteoblastomas. Neuroradiology. 2019 Aug;61(8):935–42.

43. Image-guided ablation of painful metastatic bone tumors: a new and effective approach to a difficult problem | Skeletal Radiology [Internet]. Available from: https://link.springer.com/article/10.1007/s00256-005-0003-2
44. Cazzato RL, Garnon J, Ramamurthy N, Koch G, Tsoumakidou G, Caudrelier J, et al. Percutaneous image-guided cryoablation: current applications and results in the oncologic field. Med Oncol. 2016 Nov 11;33(12):140.
45. Yan YY, Walsh JP, Munk PL, Mallinson PI, Simmons C, Clarkson PW, et al. A Single-Center 10-Year Retrospective Analysis of Cryoablation for the Management of Desmoid Tumors. J Vasc Interv Radiol. 2021 Sep 1;32(9):1277–87.
46. Kamath N, Agarwal J, Gulia A. Axial giant cell tumor—current standard of practice. J Clin Orthop Trauma. 2019;10(6):1027–32.
47. Chuang VP, Wallace S, Swanson D, Zornoza J, Handel SF, Schwarten DA, et al. Arterial occlusion in the management of pain from metastatic renal carcinoma. Radiology. 1979 Dec;133(3 Pt 1):611–4.
48. Patel S, Chiu RG, Rosinski CL, Ansari D, Chaker AN, Nunna RS, et al. Incidence, Management, and Outcomes of Spinal Giant Cell Tumor of Bone in Adult Patients: A National Cancer Database Analysis. World Neurosurg. 2020 Dec 1;144:e296–305.
49. Lin PP, Guzel VB, Moura MF, Wallace S, Benjamin RS, Weber KL, et al. Long-term follow-up of patients with giant cell tumor of the sacrum treated with selective arterial embolization. Cancer. 2002;95(6):1317–25.
50. Puri A, Gupta SM, Gulia A, Shetty N, Laskar S. Giant cell tumors of the sacrum: is non-operative treatment effective? Eur Spine J. 2021 Oct 1;30(10):2881–6.
51. Giant cell tumor of the spine - PubMed [Internet]. Available from: https://pubmed.ncbi.nlm.nih.gov/18156047/
52. Owen RJT. Embolization of Musculoskeletal Bone Tumors. Semin Interv Radiol. 2010 Jun;27(2):111–23.

Chapter 13

# Sleep and Cancer Pain

• Aparna Chatterjee • Nitin Satish

## DEFINITION OF SLEEP AND PAIN, SLEEP DISTURBANCES, INSOMNIA

Sleep is a complex, recurring, reversible neuro-behavioral state of relative perceptual disengagement from and unresponsiveness to the environment, characterized by closed eyes, behavioral quiescence, and perceptual disengagement from surroundings.[1,2]

Sleep is fundamental for the health and well-being of a person. It is necessary for their cognitive, emotional, mental, and physical well-being, as well as their metabolic, cardiovascular, and cerebrovascular health. It helps partially isolate a person from their external environment and allows repair. Long-term sleep restriction, short-term sleep deprivation, circadian misalignment, and untreated sleep disorders can all have a significant and negative effect on mood, mental health, and physical health.[3] Recent research has strengthened known and suspected links between insufficient sleep and a variety of disorders, including hypertension, obesity, diabetes, impaired immune function, cardiovascular disease and arrhythmias, mood disorders, neurodegeneration, and dementia.[4] Since sleep is necessary for immune system function, any disruption or limitation in sleep can cause a delay in healing following cancer surgery. Patients with poor sleep quality on the first postoperative night were found to have longer hospital stays, an increased risk of nosocomial infections, and postoperative delirium.[5]

The American Academy of Sleep Medicine (AASM) terminology uses the terms N for NREM sleep stages, N1 and N2 instead of stage 1 and stage 2, N3 to indicate the sum of stage 3 and stage 4 (often referred to as slow-wave sleep in human literature), and R to refer to REM sleep.

A nightly pattern of sleep in mature humans sleeping on a regular schedule includes several consistent characteristics: Sleep starts in NREM and advances through deeper non-rapid eye movement (NREM) stages (stages 2, 3, and 4 in the classic definitions, or stages N2 and N3 in the updated definitions) before the first episode of REM sleep roughly 80 to 100 minutes later. After that, NREM and REM sleep cycles repeat several times, each lasting about 90 minutes. NREM stages 3 and 4 (also known as stage N3) concentrate in the early NREM cycles, and REM sleep episodes lengthen throughout the night.[2]

NREM sleep can be roughly defined as a relatively inactive but actively regulating brain in a moving body. It is usually linked to minimal or fragmentary mental activity. NREM (pronounced "non-REM") sleep is conventionally subdivided into four stages. The EEG patterns during NREM sleep are typically described as synchronous, with predictable waveforms such as sleep spindles, K-complexes, and high-voltage slow waves. Arousal thresholds are normally lowest in stage 1 and highest in stage 4 sleep. In contrast, REM sleep is distinguished by EEG activation, muscle atonia, and episodic bursts of rapid eye movements accompanied by muscle twitches and cardiorespiratory irregularities. Human REM sleep is associated with dreaming, with vivid dream recall reported in approximately 80% of arousals during this stage. REM sleep can thus be considered an activated brain in a paralysed body.[2]

While individual sleep requirements vary, the American Academy of Sleep Medicine (AASM) and the Sleep Research Society (SRS) recommend that the average adult sleep 7 or more hours per night on a regular basis for ideal health.[6]

The master clock, located in the hypothalamus's suprachiasmatic nuclei, regulates the circadian rhythm of sleep and wakefulness. The neuroanatomical substrates of NREM sleep are primarily seen in the ventrolateral preoptic nucleus of the hypothalamus, whereas those of REM sleep are discovered in the pons.[7]

Excessive daytime somnolence (EDS), insomnia, irregular movements or behaviors during sleep, and inability to sleep at the desired time are the four most common sleep-related complaints reported by patients.[7]

Insomnia is a common problem characterized by difficulty initiating, maintaining, or obtaining high-quality sleep. The *Diagnostic and Statistical Manual of Mental Disorders* (DSM) defines insomnia as dissatisfaction with sleep quantity or quality, along with difficulty initiating, maintaining, or early awakening from sleep with a duration of symptoms occurring at least three days a week for at least three months, and there must be daytime impairment to meet diagnostic criteria.[8] The reported prevalence in the general population ranges from 2 to 48% due to differences in methodologies for defining and assessing insomnia in study populations. Cancer-related insomnia is almost three times more common than in the general population. According to various studies, 30–50% (up to 95%) of cancer patients experience severe sleep problems, such as insomnia symptoms or insomnia syndromes.[9] Even after adjusting for potential confounding factors such as depression and anxiety, chronic insomnia patients report frequent chronic health conditions such as hypertension, heart disease, chronic pain, cancer, and diabetes.[10] Sleep disorders in cancer patients can occur at the initial stage of diagnosis, in the postoperative period, during chemotherapy and/or radiotherapy and immunotherapy, or in the advanced stages of the cancer.[11]

The international classification of sleep disorders, second edition (ICSD) diagnostic criteria for primary insomnia require:

i. A predominant complaint of difficulty initiating or maintaining sleep, or non-restorative sleep, for at least one month.

ii. Sleep disturbance (or associated daytime fatigue) causes clinically significant distress or impairment in social, occupational, or other important areas of functioning,

iii. Sleep disturbance does not occur exclusively during the course of another sleep disorder (e.g. narcolepsy, breathing-related sleep disorder, etc.).

iv. Disturbance is not due to the direct physiological effects of a substance (e.g. a drug of abuse or medication) or another psychiatric or general medical condition.[12]

The duration criteria for chronic insomnia disorder was revised by the ICSD-3 to three months, and a frequency criterion (at least three times per week) was added.[13] Short-term insomnia (ICSD-3) or episodic insomnia (DSM-5) follows the same criteria as chronic insomnia but lasts less than three months.[14]

However, there is no established criterion for determining the amount of wakefulness or the amount of sleep that is abnormal and/or indicative of insomnia.

However, most clinicians and researchers regard ≥30 minutes to fall asleep and/or ≥30 minutes of wakefulness after sleep onset and a total sleep time of ≤6.5 hours per night as the threshold between normal and abnormal sleep.[12]

Unlike people who do not have cancer, cancer patients usually experience pain from one or more sources, such as cancer-related pain, treatment-related pain (e.g. chemotherapy, radiotherapy), and/or pain unrelated to the tumor or treatment interventions.[13] Chronic pain has a prevalence of 10 to 40%, which is similar to the prevalence of sleep disorders (10–36%).[15] Thus, both chronic pain and sleep deprivation are common problems in the general population. Sleep disturbances are twice as common in recently diagnosed or treated cancer patients, with reported prevalence rates ranging from 30 to 75% compared to the general population. Insomnia symptoms in cancer vary between studies, with rates ranging from 30 to 50%. Patients with lung cancer had the highest or second-highest overall prevalence of sleep problems, whereas breast cancer patients had a high prevalence of insomnia and fatigue.[16] According to Gallaway, et al.'s analysis of data from a telephonic survey of 12,019 cancer survivors in the United States, approximately 10% of cancer survivors reported pain that persisted for years after initial diagnosis and were more likely to report a lack of sleep. Furthermore, cancer survivors who reported sleeping less than 7 hours per night (15.0%) experienced more physical pain than those who slept 7 hours or more per night (9.1%).[17] Sleep disturbances have been reported to be very common in patients with advanced cancer, despite having received much less attention.[16] According to Fortner, et al.'s study, 61% of breast cancer patients had significant sleep deficits, as measured by the Pittsburgh sleep quality index. The sleep of breast cancer patients in this study showed a marked reduction in total sleep time. They also showed that insufficiencies in pain-related quality of life were linked with poor sleep. In other words, breast cancer patients who reported a lower pain-related quality of life were more likely to have difficulty sleeping.[18]

## Subjective and Objective Methods to Evaluate Sleep Quality

### *Objective*

- *Polysomnography (PSG):* Gold standard; inconvenient, elaborate system of electronic sensors and needs to be completed in a laboratory.
- *Actigraphy:* Fairly inexpensive and non-invasive setup for estimating sleep-wake rhythms over extended periods (days to months); limited precision in distinguishing wakefulness during sleep episodes; and fails to provide data on sleep architecture.

*Subjective methods:* Self-reported questionnaires such as:

- Pittsburgh Sleep Quality Index (PSQI): Most frequently used, recognized as a reference or gold standard for self-perceived sleep quality
- Sleep Severity Index (ISI)
- Sleep Severity Scale (AIS)
- Mini Sleep Questionnaire (MSQ)
- Leeds Sleep Assessment Questionnaire (LSEQ)
- Epworth Sleep Scale (ESS)
- Jenkins Sleep Scale (JSS)[19]

## ASSOCIATION BETWEEN SLEEP AND PAIN

Numerous studies have shown a relationship between sleep and pain.[20–23] Chronic pain patients have been seen to have a reduction in total sleep time (TST) and sleep efficiency (SE), as well as an increase in sleep onset latency (SOL) and wakefulness after sleep onset (WASO), suggesting that they sleep less, take a longer time to fall asleep, and spend more time awake.[24] Sleep efficiency (SE) is the ratio of total sleep time to total time in bed. It has been observed that people who suffer from chronic pain often have difficulty sleeping, and those who do not get enough sleep may experience more pain. Pain has been recognized as one of the most important contributors to sleep difficulties in cancer patients, with 45% associating much of their sleep problems with pain. Pain can affect both overall sleep quality and specific sleep parameters, like sleep onset latency. Prolonged sleep latency, difficulty falling asleep, and feeling tired (i.e. daytime sleepiness) have all been linked to cancer-related pain. A recent study discovered that prolonged sleep onset latency, described as the inability to fall asleep within 30 minutes, is a common clinical affliction among cancer patients (approximately 40%).[13] Disturbed sleep contributes to overall patient disability and distress in multiple forms.

Sleep physiology disruptions have been linked to musculoskeletal pain, fatigue, mood swings, decreased mental alertness, and depressive symptoms.[20]

In a study conducted by McCracken, et al. 88.9% of chronic pain patients documented at least one complaint related to a disrupted sleep and wake cycle. The study also found that an unsettled sleep and rest pattern was linked to augmented pain, depression, physical and psychosocial disability, and less daily active time. They established the frequently observed clinical finding that sleep and rest are commonly disrupted in chronic pain patients. Likewise, other studies have discovered that chronic pain causes emotional despair that interferes with sleep. As a result, sleep, emotional distress, pain perception, and daily activity appear to form a feedback loop, with each contributing to the other.[20]

The literature on the relationship between pain and sleep problems reveals a bidirectional relationship between the two (Fig. 13.1), with evidence indicating that pain predicts sleep disturbance and, conversely, poor sleep quality exacerbates pain, particularly among those with chronic pain.[25,26] This can lead to a vicious cycle in which pain worsens due to a lack of sleep, and the lack of sleep exacerbates the pain.

Epidemiological, pharmaceutical, clinical, and experimental studies have all demonstrated a reciprocal relationship between sleep and pain. For example, 50–88% of patients with chronic pain also have sleep problems. Alternatively, over 40% of insomnia patients experience chronic pain.[15]

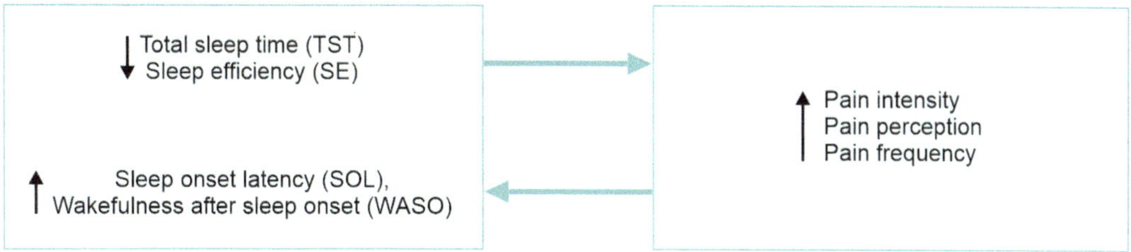


Fig. 13.1: The bidirectional association between sleep and pain

Yet, only a few studies investigate this specific outcome in the context of some of the most common sleep disturbances.

Schrimpf, et al. confirmed the effect of sleep deprivation on pain perception in a meta-analysis. The between-group analysis showed a medium effect (SMD = 0.62), while the within-group analysis had a large effect (SMD = 1.49). Sleep deprivation has been linked to increased self-reported pain and altered evoked pain responses, as measured by somatosensory testing protocols (e.g. heat pain thresholds, pressure pain thresholds, or laser-evoked pain).[15]

A study conducted on 139 adolescents suffering from cancer pain evaluated the pain, sleep quality, and fatigue symptoms. They discovered a moderate to high negative correlation between the pain characteristics of the adolescents involved in the study and their fatigue levels, as well as a moderate to high positive correlation between the pain characteristics and sleep quality.[27]

It is thus, equally essential to address both sleep and pain issues simultaneously, as improving one can positively impact the other.

Sleep disorders, according to the prospective studies reviewed, increase the possibility of new-onset chronic pain in pain-free individuals, worsen the long-term prognosis of existing chronic pain, and influence daily variation in clinical pain. Moreover, good sleep appears to improve the long-term prognosis of people suffering from tension headaches, migraines, and chronic musculoskeletal pain. According to research into bidirectional relationships, sleep disturbances may predict pain to a greater extent than pain can predict sleep disorders. The significance of the effect was stronger for the sleep pain direction than for the opposite direction, especially in cancer patients.[28]

## Mechanism

There is currently a lack of understanding of the mechanisms underlying the relationship between pain and sleep. Suggested theories include the influence of neurotransmitters such as dopamine, serotonin, or endogenous opioids in mediation. Other hypotheses include the proximity of pain, sleep, and negative affect neural pathways.

Sleep disturbances are thought to impair repair processes, contributing to the development of chronic pain, which could be linked to dopamine, endogenous opioid signaling pathways, and negative affect.[28] Possible theories include:

### *1. Dopaminergic Signaling*

Dopamine (DA) is the primary neurotransmitter in the forebrain reward system, which is a complex network of mesolimbic and nigrostriatal circuitry that underpins the human behavioral drive to seek pleasure. DA plays an important role in the promotion and maintenance of arousal states and is, therefore, closely related to sleep-wake regulation. Foo and Mason[29] proposed that serotonergic raphe cells that signal alertness may become dysregulated during chronic pain, promoting more extended periods of sleep deprivation and greater disarrangement of sleep continuity. Given the plenitude of DA receptors in that region of the brainstem and the well-known interaction of serotonergic and dopaminergic neurotransmission, pain-induced DA signaling changes may influence the raphe nuclei's modulation of sleep and wake. Additional research is needed to determine how sleep deprivation alters DA and whether these changes are associated with concurrent changes in pain sensitivity. Also, more clinical studies are required to demonstrate the behavioral consequences of sleep disturbance on reward processing and how these changes affect coping with chronic pain.[28]

### 2. Opioidergic Signaling

An abundance of cross-disciplinary research indicates that opioid peptides play an important role in descending pain modulatory systems. Sleep deprivation has been shown in preclinical studies to disrupt endogenous opioid systems and diminish the effectiveness of μ-opioid receptor agonists for analgesia. Opioid receptors are located in a variety of nuclei that actively regulate sleep and pain, including the preoptic suprachiasmatic nuclei, which control sleep-wake cycles, and the periaqueductal gray, which is paramount for descending pain inhibition. Sleep deprivation has been shown in animal studies to affect μ- and δ-opioid receptor function in mesolimbic circuits, lowering basal endogenous opioid levels and downregulating central opioid receptors.[28]

### 3. Negative and Positive Affect

Mediation analyses have revealed that increases in negative affect (e.g. moods or emotions) may account for a significant portion of the variance in the directional relationships between sleep disturbance and pain in non-clinically depressed samples. Several studies have found links between sleep, pain, and negative mood, but little is known about the temporal dynamics of these associations. Affect may be considered as a term that comprises both moods, which are longer-duration, lower-intensity affective states, as well as emotions, which are shorter-duration, higher-intensity affective states.[28] Among cancer patients, the experience of chronic stress, negative emotions, and pain may have important health-related implications. Chronic, long-term negative emotional states and pain may lead to hypothalamic pituitary adrenal (HPA) axis dysregulation and downstream glucocorticoid and cytokine dysregulation, which facilitates tumorigenesis.[13]

### 4. Relationship with Inflammatory and Immune Biomarkers (Table 13.1)

*Natural killer cell activity (NKCA):* Shakhar, et al. and Irish, et al. investigated the relationship between sleep quantity changes and natural killer cell activity (NKCA). Low levels have been linked to certain pain conditions, such as fibromyalgia, and may contribute to an exaggerated pain response in some people with chronic pain.[30]

*Cortisol levels:* Chronic pain has been linked to a sustained stress response and, as a result, raised cortisol levels. Rueggeberg, et al. discovered that a reduction in sleep quantity (by one standard deviation) during the first two years of their study was associated with an increase in diurnal cortisol secretion over the four-year follow-up period. However, increased sleep quantity had no significant effect on cortisol levels.[30]

*Interleukin-6 (IL-6) and C-reactive protein (CRP) levels:* Systemic inflammation markers are activated in response to infections. They also have a pain-facilitating effect, which can affect pain modulation and processing. Persistently elevated levels of these markers have been observed in several chronic illnesses, and they have been linked to the development, maintenance, and severity of chronic pain. An elevation of IL-6 in post-surgical cancer patients with sleep disturbances has been proposed as a mechanism for patients with poorer preoperative sleep having higher postoperative pain scores than those who reported good sleep. Ferrie, et al. analysed data from the UK Whitehall study

**Table 13.1: The impact of sleep deprivation on neurobiological mediators: Sleep deficiency's effect on systems/mediators is represented by up- and down-arrows, with up-arrows representing an activating influence and down-arrows representing a deactivating influence**

| Mediator | Effect of sleep deficiency | Activating/deactivating |
|---|---|---|
| Opioid | Reduced responsivity | ↓ |
| Monoaminergic-dopamine | D2 receptor activating | ↓ |
| Monoaminergic norepinephrine | NE transported mRNA in LC and NE levels in blood | ↑ |
| Orexin signaling | In hypothalamus, plasma, bone marrow<br>In hypothalamus, LC, cortex, CSF | ↓<br>↑ |
| Melatonin | In blood | ↓ |
| Endocannabinoids | In blood | ↑ |
| Monoaminergic-serotonin | Serotonin 1A receptor sensitivity<br>Extracellular in basal fore brain | ↓<br>↑ |
| HPA axis | Cortisol | ↑ |
| Adenosine signaling | Adenosine (A2A receptor mediated) | ↑ |
| Nitric oxide signaling | NO in basal forebrain, PAG, cortex | ↑ |
| Immune system | Prostaglandins (PGE2)<br>Cytokine (IL-1, IL-6, TNF) | ↑<br>↑ |

NE: Norepinephrine; LC: Locus coeruleus; CSF: Cerebrospinal fluid; HPA: Hypothalamus-pituitary adrenal; NO: Nitric oxide, PAG: Periaqueductal gray; IL: Interleukin; TNF: Tumor necrosis factor

and found no link between increased sleep quantity and changes in IL-6 and CRP levels. However, they discovered that a five-year decrease in sleep quantity was associated with increased levels of inflammatory markers. In a fully adjusted analysis that controlled for age, gender, occupation, blood pressure, BMI, cholesterol level, and diabetes status, each 1-hour decrease in sleep quantity was associated with a 2.7% increase in IL-6.[30]

The association between pain and sleep implies that, while treating chronic pain, sleep should possibly be simultaneously targeted for a better benefit. This was suggested by Vitiello, et al. in a study of patients with osteoarthritis and insomnia, which found that short-term (2 months) improvement in sleep predicted long-term (9 and 18 months) improvement across multiple measures of sleep factors, chronic pain, and fatigue episodes.[31]

## Management

### *Non-pharmacological Approaches*

***Cognitive-behavioral therapy (CBT):*** CBT is recommended as a non-pharmacological multimodal combination of therapy for the management of sleep problems, as well. as a first-line treatment for insomnia. Cognitive behavioral therapy (CBT) is also the most commonly used psychological approach to treat chronic pain (CP).[24] To improve sleep, the National Cancer Institute (NCI) recommends cognitive behavioral therapy for insomnia (CBT-I) in conjunction with a regular sleep schedule, relaxing before bedtime, and limiting caffeine consumption.[5]

A randomized controlled trial (RCT) showed that CBT for insomnia (CBT-1) was more efficacious than CBT for pain (CBT-P). Although neither treatment enhanced pain or mood in the RCT, they resulted in clinically meaningful, immediate pain reductions in one-third of patients. Improvements in CBT-I lasted, indicating that it may deliver better long-term pain alleviation than CBT-P.[32] A systematic review and network meta-analysis also established that CBT-I may be the most useful treatment choice for people suffering from comorbid insomnia and chronic pain.[33] CBT-I was significantly more effective than the control and CBT-P in terms of post-treatment pain, disability, and depression, as well as sleep at follow-up. CBT-P and the control demonstrated no significant differences in effectiveness for any of the outcomes. Nonetheless, given the small sample size and the high-risk of bias in the studies included in the meta-analysis, the findings should be interpreted with caution.[33] There is also evidence that CBT, specifically CBT-1, can improve sleep efficiency, total wake time, and time to sleep onset in patients who have undergone breast or gynecologic cancer surgery.[5]

*Alternative and complementary approaches:* Although not yet recommended by current guidelines, many complementary and alternative therapies are popular. These include aromatherapy, music therapy, acupuncture massage, etc.

### Pharmacological Approaches

#### *1. Targeting Sleep*

*Benzodiazepine receptor agonists (BzRAs):* The most well-known and commonly. prescribed medication for treating sleep disorders, as well as adjuvant therapy for pain relief. However, special care should be taken when prescribing BzRAs alongside opioids for CP and insomnia, which is common in clinical practice. For example, BzRAs combined with buprenorphine can cause severe respiratory depression.[24] They are indicated for short-term insomnia symptoms (i.e. not more than three weeks), as long-term therapies are less effective (most likely due to tolerance) and are associated with a variety of side effects.[24] They are indicated for insomnia symptoms in a short-term period (i.e. no more than three weeks), as long-term therapies are less effective (probably due to tolerance) and related to a wide range of side effects.[34]

*Non-benzodiazepine hypnotics (Z-drugs-zolpidem, zopiclone):* These medications selectively bind to the benzodiazepine (BZD) allosteric binding site on GABAA receptors. A systematic review of four studies on zolpidem in older people found improvements in sleep latency, nocturnal awakenings, and sleep duration compared to placebo. Rebound insomnia is a risk with abrupt discontinuation of Z-drugs, so tapering is suggested. To reduce the risk of tolerance and dependence, intermittent dosing has been successfully tested, with alternative nights or three times per week.[35]

*Melatonin:* Endogenous nocturnal melatonin production decreases with age, with peak excretion being roughly half that of younger patients. Melatonin has infrequent side effects and can deliver mild relief for up to two months. According to a meta-analysis, exogenous melatonin decreased sleep onset latency modestly and provided some benefit to those encountering disturbances to their endogenous circadian rhythms. There is little proof to support long-term melatonin use; at the same time, there have been very few side effects reported up to 6 months. Headaches, irritability, dizziness, nausea, and vomiting are among the less common side effects.[35]

Melatonin is sold over the counter but is not FDA-approved because it is a dietary supplement, and the FDA does not regulate supplements. Nonetheless, the American

Academy of Family Physicians (AAFP) recommends melatonin as the first-line pharmacologic treatment for insomnia. In 2005, the FDA approved ramelteon, a melatonin receptor agonist, for the treatment of insomnia. Melatonin and ramelteon are both mildly effective at reducing sleep latency, particularly in patients with delayed sleep phases (where sleep and wake times are shifted later).[36]

*Antidepressants*

***Tricyclic antidepressants (TCAS):*** TCAS (amitriptyline, nortriptyline, desipramine, clomipramine, imipramine, trimipramine, and doxepin) have pro serotonergic, noradrenergic, dopaminergic, and sodium-channel blocking effects that may explain their efficacy in pain and depression, as well as anticholinergic and antihistaminic effects that cause sedation. All TCAs have been shown to be equally effective in treating neuropathic pain; however, they are not all equal in promoting sleep. Desipramine and imipramine, for example, are less sedative and may cause sleep disturbances. In contrast, amitriptyline, nortriptyline, trimipramine, and doxepin may reduce sleep latency, improve sleep efficiency, and increase total sleep time. TCAs may cause adverse effects such as orthostatic hypotension, dry mouth and eyes, constipation, and cardiac conduction delays due to their anti-$\alpha$-adrenergic and anticholinergic effects. Furthermore, TCAs may prolong the QT interval, increasing the risk of serious cardiac arrhythmias. The risk of cardiac-related adverse effects, such as orthostatic hypotension, increases with age.[36]

***Doxepin:*** At low doses (<10 mg), doxepin acts as a sedating tricyclic antidepressant and a selective histamine H1 receptor antagonist. It is the only TCA approved by the FDA for the treatment of insomnia, with a hypnotic dose of 1 mg to 6 mg versus 150 mg to 300 mg when used as an antidepressant.[36] A recent meta-analysis of six low-dose (3–6 mg) doxepin studies, three of which were conducted in older subjects, found a small to moderate positive effect on sleep maintenance insomnia, with decreased wake after sleep onset and increased sleep efficiency and duration, with a weighted mean total sleep time difference of 23.9 minutes (95% CI 12.0–35.7). Doxepin at moderate to high doses is associated with more frequent side effects and rebound insomnia. Doxepin is also not recommended in the presence of comorbid moderate-severe sleep apnea.[35]

***Mirtazapine:*** An antidepressant with sedative properties caused by the antagonism of type 1 histaminergic and serotonin type 2 receptors. At doses ranging from 15 to 30 mg, it improves sleep latency, total sleep time, and sleep efficiency while decreasing the frequency of night awakenings. It has been demonstrated to improve sleep, pain, appetite, and mood in cancer patients. Mirtazapine has also been shown in several studies to be effective in treating pain caused by recurrent headaches and postherpetic neuralgia.[36]

***Suvorexant:*** A dual orexin receptor antagonist. Orexins are neuropeptides that aid in sleep regulation. In a controlled trial involving 59% of patients over the age of 65, those taking high-dose suvorexant (30 mg for people over 65 and 40 mg for younger people) had improved sleep onset (by 18 minutes) and total sleep time (by 39 minutes) compared to placebo. Higher doses produce more side effects, such as somnolence, fatigue, dry mouth, dyspepsia, and peripheral edema. Severe side effects are uncommon but can include sleepwalking, sleep paralysis, and hallucinations. Suvorexant has a long half-life, and residual effects, such as somnolence, may last the next day, especially at higher doses. Suvorexant has not been proven safe in patients with comorbid sleep apnea or severe chronic obstructive pulmonary disease, so it should be used with caution in these patients. It is available in India, but it is not widely distributed yet.[36]

*GABA receptor antagonists gabapentinoids (gabapentin and pregabalin):* GABA analogues such as gabapentin and pregabalin are frequently used to treat CP conditions accompanied by insomnia. Self-reported sleep outcomes in multiple studies of patients with neuropathic pain and fibromyalgia show positive effects on sleep latency, wakefulness after sleep onset, and deep sleep. Both medications have antidepressant and anxiety-relieving properties. A recent study found that pregabalin was more effective than amitriptyline at improving sleep in diabetic neuropathy patients. Common side effects include dizziness, next-day sedation, gastrointestinal symptoms, and peripheral edema.[36]

However, until now, sleep-promoting pharmacotherapy research has not revealed any consistent augmentation in coexisting chronic pain.

### 2. Targeting Inflammation

Immune dysregulation is involved in a variety of pain disorders and can be precipitated or exacerbated by sleep deprivation. Sleep disturbances are associated with elevated levels of CRP, IL-1, IL-6, and TNF-α. IL-6 has been shown to reduce REM sleep and increase wakefulness in patients, while IL-1 and TNF-α promote spontaneous sleep and sleep rebound after sleep deprivation. Stevens, et al. found that after initiating biological therapy with vedolizumab or anti-TNF agents, IBD patients' sleep and mood quality improved significantly.[37] Karatas, et al. found that anti-TNF-α therapy improved sleep quality but did not improve polysomnography. They concluded that polysomnography parameters may be more closely related to disease pathogenesis than disease activity in ankylosing spondylitis patients.[38] Therefore, immunotherapy may not only improve disease activity but also improve sleep, and cytokine therapy's beneficial effect on sleep in chronic inflammatory diseases may be independent of its effect on disease activity.

### 3. Targeting Postoperative Pain

The goal of postoperative pain management is to alleviate the negative effects of acute postsurgical pain and assist the patient in smoothly returning to normal function. Poor sleep and sleep deprivation have also been linked to increased postoperative pain. Inadequate acute pain management has a variety of negative effects on patient health, including decreased ability to perform daily activities, impaired sleep, low mood, and an increased risk of developing a chronic pain syndrome.[39] There are several external factors that can influence postoperative sleep. Previous research has shown that pain causes the greatest reduction in sleep duration because it is more likely to last throughout the night.[5] Multimodal analgesia, which includes nonsteroidal anti-inflammatory drugs (NSAIDs), paracetamol, and opioids, remains the cornerstone of acute postoperative pain management. A systematic review of 27 randomized controlled trials ($n$ = 1,494) found that patients who received higher intraoperative opioid doses had greater postoperative pain intensity and consumed more morphine 24 hours after surgery, but there were no significant differences in nausea, vomiting, or drowsiness.[40] Patients who were taking opiates prior to surgery are more likely to experience uncontrolled pain as well as opioid-related adverse events and opioid induced hyperalgesia.[41] Studies show that opioids increase wakefulness and the number of sleep-waking state shifts while decreasing total sleep time, sleep efficiency, delta sleep, and rapid eye movement (REM) sleep. Other studies on postoperative patients have also found a reduction in slow-wave sleep with opioid administration.[42] Hence, an individualized acute pain management plan, preferably opioid sparing using a multimodal approach, regional and/or neuraxial anesthetic techniques, and nonpharmacologic therapies (e.g. physical therapy, transcutaneous electrical nerve stimulation, etc.) are necessary to reduce patient suffering, hospital length of stay, thereby aiding in earlier mobilization, ability to perform activities of daily living, and improve patient satisfaction.

## MEDICATIONS WHICH DISTURB SLEEP

Certain medications used for the management of several diseases disturb sleep, thereby potentially augmenting pain and sleep (Table 13.2).

Some analgesics (particularly opioids; see above) have sleep-disturbing or altering effects, as do other classes of drugs such as psychotropic medications (e.g. antidepressants), cardiovascular drugs (e.g. beta-blocking agents), and corticosteroids.[43] Medications that affect neurotransmitters such as norepinephrine, serotonin, acetylcholine, or dopamine are commonly implicated. Antibiotics, antihypertensives, oral contraceptives, and thyroid replacement medications can also cause insomnia in susceptible people.

*Opioid:* Despite providing temporary pain relief, chronic and acute opioid use generally disrupts sleep, as evidenced by decreased slow-wave sleep, REM sleep suppression, and increased awakenings and arousal during sleep. In addition to the well-known risks of dependence and abuse, chronic opioid use increases daytime sedation and the prevalence of breathing disorders, particularly central sleep apnea.[43]

*Antidepressants:* Utilized to treat chronic pain conditions, can have varying effects on sleep depending on the drug class and dosage. Low-dose tricyclic antidepressants,

**Table 13.2: Drugs that potentially affect sleep[31]**

- Antibiotics
- Anticonvulsants
- Antidepressants
- Antihypertensives: α-agonists, β-blockers, centrally acting agents
- Antineoplastic agents
- Caffeine
- Corticotropin (ACTH) and cortisone
- Diuretics
- Ephedrine and pseudoephedrine
- Ethanol
- Levodopa
- Niacin
- Oral contraceptives
- Psychostimulants and amphetamines
- Sedative/hypnotics
- Thyroid preparations

such as amitriptyline and doxepin, promote sleep by increasing slow-wave sleep and sleep continuity, whereas less sedating tricyclic antidepressants, such as imipramine and desipramine, disrupt sleep.

*Beta-blockers:* Insomnia has been reported as a side effect of beta-adrenergic blocking agents such as propranolol and atenolol. These agents also inhibit melatonin production, interfering with its sleep-promoting and circadian phase regulatory properties, which may explain beta-blockers' sleep-disturbing effects.

*Corticosteroids:* Increased endogenous cortisol secretion and/or dysregulation of the diurnal cortisol rhythm have been linked to insomnia and may be the cause of symptoms. According to cross-sectional studies, approximately half of patients exposed to systemic corticosteroids experience sleep disturbances.[43]

## Future Directions

Sleep is a biological necessity, and improving sleep duration and quality can reduce pain intensity in chronic pain patients. The management of chronic pain conditions and sleep disorders must go hand in hand. An assessment of both sleep disturbance and pain in patients with chronic pain, as well as concurrent treatment for both conditions, is required for optimal outcomes. In chronic pain disorders, non-pharmacological methods such as CBT-I are effective in addressing sleep disturbance and may reduce opioid usage.

Given the complicated and interdependent relationship among various organised neurobiological networks, a greater comprehension of potential modulating pathways between pain and sleep is needed. The incorporation of anti-inflammatory and immunomodulating drugs in interventional studies will further our grasp of the process through which interventions influence pain and sleep. Elucidating these mechanisms is critical for developing clinically relevant therapeutic strategies to improve sleep and pain relief in future studies.

The research on chronic pain caused by sleep and its relationship to various chronic pain disorders is still in its early stages. Further understanding of the underlying mechanisms governing the interaction between sleep disorders and chronic pain is critical for establishing more effective pain and sleep management strategies.

The development of objective and validated models for studying sleep and chronic pain, in collaboration with tools such as electrophysiology, brain imaging (e.g. fMRI), and non-invasive brain stimulation techniques, is crucial to personalised management for patients with pain and sleep-related conditions.

Last but not least, clinicians should be aware that many chronic pain conditions, especially cancer pain, are associated with sleep disturbances, and they should encourage patients to improve their sleep habits and educate them on sleep hygiene. Assessment of the multiple dimensions of sleep and basic treatment strategies should be incorporated into pain education and professional training.

## References

1. Gellman MD, Turner JR. Encyclopedia of behavioral medicine. New York: Springer; 2013. (Springer reference).
2. Carskadon M, Dement W. Normal Human Sleep: An Overview. Principles and Practice of Sleep Medicine. MH Kryger (Ed.). WB Saunders Phila. 1989 Jan 1;3–13.

3. Ramar K, Malhotra RK, Carden KA, Martin JL, Abbasi-Feinberg F, Aurora RN, et al. Sleep is essential to health: an American Academy of Sleep Medicine position statement. J Clin Sleep Med. 2021 Oct 15:17(10):2115–9.
4. Worley SL. The Extraordinary Importance of Sleep: The Detrimental Effects of Inadequate Sleep on Health and Public Safety Drive an Explosion of Sleep Research. PT. 2018 Dec;43(12):758–63.
5. Zhao C, Grubbs A, Barber EL. Sleep and gynecological cancer outcomes: opportunities to improve quality of life and survival. Int J Gynecol Cancer. 2022 May 3;32(5):669–675. doi: 10.1136/jgc-2022-003404. PMID: 35331996; PMCID: PMC9064983.
6. Watson NF, Badr MS, Belenky G, Bliwise DI, Buxton OM, Buysse D, et al. Recommended Amount of Sleep for a Healthy Adult: A Joint Consensus Statement of the American Academy of Sleep Medicine and Sleep Research Society. Sleep. 2015 Jun 1;38(6):843–4, doi: 10.5665/sleep.4716. PMID: 26039963; PMCID: PMC4434546.
7. Chokroverty S. Overview of sleep and sleep disorders. Indian J Med Res. 2010 Feb;131(2):126.
8. Husak AJ, Bair MJ. Chronic Pain and Sleep Disturbances: A Pragmatic Review of Their Relationships, Comorbidities, and Treatments. Pain Med. 2020 Jun 1;21(6):1142–52.
9. Büttner-Teleag A, Kim YT, Osel T, Richter K. Sleep Disorders in Cancer-A Systematic Review. Int J Environ Res Public Health. 2021 Nov 7;18(21):11696. doi: 10.3390/ijerph182111696. PMID: 34770209; PMCID: PMC8583058.
10. Mukherjee S, Patel SR, Kales SN, Ayas NT, Strohl KP, Gozal D, et al. An Official American Thoracic Society Statement: The Importance of Healthy Sleep. Recommendations and Future Priorities. Am J Respir Crit Care Med. 2015 Jun 15:191(12):1450–8.
11. Wang RC, Wang SJ, Chang YC, Lin CC. Mood state and quality of sleep in cancer pain patients: a comparison to chronic daily headache. J Pain Symptom Manage. 2007 Jan;33(1):32–9. doi: 10.1016/j.jpainsymman.2006.06.013. PMID: 17196905.
12. Pigeon WR. Diagnosis, prevalence, pathways, consequences & treatment of insomnia. Indian J Med Res. 2010 Feb;131(2):321.
13. Kirsch JL, Robinson ME, McCrae C5, Kacel EL, Wong SS, Patidar S, et al. Associations Among Sleep Latency, Subjective Pain, and Thermal Pain Sensitivity in Gynecologic Cancer. Pain Med. 2020 Jan 1;21(1):5–12. doi: 10.1093/pm/pny236. PMID: 30481329, PMCID: PMC6953342.
14. Krystal AD, Prather AA, Ashbrook LH. The assessment and management of insomnia: An update. World Psychiatry. 2019 Sept 9,18(3):337–52. doi: 10.1002/wps.20674
15. Schrimpf M, Liegl G, Boeckle M, Leitner A, Geisler P, Pieh C. The effect of sleep deprivation on pain perception in healthy subjects: a meta-analysis. Sleep Med. 2015 Nov 1;16(11):1313–20.
16. Liu L, Ancoli-Israel S. Sleep Disturbances in Cancer. Psychiatr Ann. 2008 Sep 1:38(9):627–634. doi: 10.3928/00485713-20080901-01. PMID: 21243092: PMCID: PMC3021374.
17. Gallaway MS, Townsend JS, Shelby D, Puckett MC. Pain Among Cancer Survivors. Prev Chronic Dis. 2020 Jul 9:17:E54, doi: 10.5888/pod17.190367. PMID: 32644924; PMCID: PMC7367076.
18. Fortner BV, Stepanski EJ, Wang SC, Kasprowicz S, Durrence HH. Sleep and quality of life in breast cancer patients. J Pain Symptom Manage. 2002 Nov, 24(5):471–80. doi: 10.1016/s0885-3924(02)00500-6. PMID: 12547047.
19. Fabbri M, Beracci A, Martoni M, Meneo D, Tonetti L, Natale V. Measuring Subjective Sleep Quality: A Review, Int J Environ Res Public Health. 2021 Jan 26,18(3):1082. doi: 10.3390/ijerph 18031082. PMID: 33530453; PMCID: PMC7908437.
20. McCracken LM, Iverson GL. Disrupted sleep patterns and daily functioning in patients with chronic pain. Pain Res Manag. 2002;7(2):75–9.
21. Haythomthwaite JA, Hegel MT, Kerns RD. Development of a sleep diary for chronic pain patients. J Pain Symptom Manage. 1991 Feb;6(2):65–72.
22. Smith MT, Perlis ML, Smith MS, Giles DE, Carmody TP. Sleep quality and presleep arousal in chronic pain. J Behav Med. 2000 Feb;23(1):1–13.
23. Smith MT, Perlis ML, Haythomthwaite JA. Suicidal ideation in outpatients with chronic musculoskeletal pain: an exploratory study of the role of sleep onset insomnia and pain intensity. Clin J Pain. 2004;20(2):111–8.

24. Duo L, Yu X, Hu R, Duan X, Zhou J, Wang K. Sleep disorders in chronic pain and its neurochemical mechanisms a narrative review. Front Psychiatry. 2023,14:1157790.
25. Smith MT, Haythomthwaite JA. How do sleep disturbance and chronic pain inter-relate? Insights from the longitudinal and cognitive-behavioral clinical trials literature. Sleep Med Rev. 2004 Apr:8(2):119–32.
26. Andersen ML, Araujo P, Frange C, Tufik S. Sleep Disturbance and Pain: A Tale of Two Common Problems. Chest. 2018 Nov;154(5):1249–59.
27. Akdeniz Kudubes A, Bektas M, Gerceker GO. The Predictive Power of Pain Characteristics and Sleep Quality on Fatigue in Adolescents With Cancer. J Pediatr Hematol Oncol. 2023 Aug 1:45(6):301–308. doi: 10.1097/MPH.0000000000002707. Epub 2023 Jun 30. PMID: 37494606
28. Finan PH, Goodin BR, Smith MT. The Association of Sleep and Pain: An Update and a Path Forward. J Pain. 2013 Dec 1:14(12):1539–52.
29. Foo H, Mason P. Brainstem modulation of pain during sleep and waking. Sleep Med Rev. 2003 Apr 1;7(2):145–54.
30. Afolalu EF, Ramlee F, Tang NKY. Effects of sleep changes on pain-related health outcomes in the general population: A systematic review of longitudinal studies with exploratory meta-analysis. Sleep Med Rev. 2018 Jun 1:39:82–97.
31. Vitiello MV, McCurry SM, Shortreed SM, Baker LD, Rybarczyk BD, Keefe FJ, et al. Short-term improvement in insomnia symptoms predicts long-term improvements in sleep, pain, and fatigue in older adults with comorbid osteoarthritis and insomnia. Pain. 2014 Aug:155(8):1547–1554. doi: 10.1016/j.pain 2014.04.032. Epub 2014 May 1. PMID: 24793909, PMCID: PMC4104256.
32. McCrae CS, Williams J, Roditi D, Anderson R, Mundt JM, Miller MB, et al. Cognitive behavioral treatments for insomnia and pain in adults with comorbid chronic insomnia and fibromyalgia: clinical outcomes from the SPIN randomized controlled trial. Sleep. 2018 Nov 28:42(3):28y234.
33. Enomoto K, Adachi T, Fujino H, Kugo M, Tatsumi S, Sasaki J. Comparison of the effectiveness of cognitive behavioral therapy for insomnia, cognitive behavioral therapy for pain, and hybrid cognitive behavioral therapy for insomnia and pain in individuals with comorbid insomnia and chronic pain: A systematic review and network meta-analysis. Sleep Med Rev. 2022 Dec;66:101693.
34. Herrero Babiloni A, Beetz G, Bruneau A, Martel MO, Cistulli PA, Nixdorf DR, et al. Multitargeting the sleep-pain interaction with pharmacological approaches: A narrative review with suggestions on new avenues of investigation. Sleep Med Rev. 2021 Oct 1:59:101459.
35. Reynolds AC, Adams RJ. Treatment of sleep disturbance in older adults. J Pharm Pract Res. 2019;49(3):296–304.
36. Cheatle MD, Foster S, Pinkett A, Lesneski M, Qu D, Dhingra L. Assessing and Managing Sleep Disturbance in Patients with Chronic Pain. Anesthesiol Clin. 2016 Jun;34(2):379–93.
37. Stevens BW, Borren NZ, Velonias G, Conway G, Cleland T, Andrews E, et al. Vedolizumab Therapy Is Associated with an Improvement in Sleep Quality and Mood in Inflammatory Bowel Diseases. Dig Dis Sci. 2017 Jan;62(1):197–206.
38. Karatas G, Bal A, Yuceege M, Firat H, Gurcay E, Ardic S, et al. Evaluation of sleep quality in patients with ankylosing spondylitis and efficacy of anti-TNF-α therapy on sleep problems: A polisomnographic study. Int J Rheum Dis. 2018 Jun 1;21(6):1263–9.
39. Hom R. Postoperative pain control [Internet]. US National Library of Medicine, 2024. Available from: https://www.ncbi.nlm.nih.gov/books/NBK544298/
40. Fletcher D, Martinez V. Opioid-induced hyperalgesia in patients after surgery: a systematic review and a meta-analysis. Br J Anaesth. 2014 Jun;112(6):991-1004. doi:10.1093/bja/aeu137. PMID: 24829420.
41. Small C, Laycock H. Acute postoperative pain management. British Journal of Surgery. 2020 Jan; 107(2). doi:10.1002/bjs. 11477
42. Dimsdale JE, Norman D, DeJardin D, Wallace MS. The effect of opioids on sleep architecture. J Clin Sleep Med. 2007 Feb 15,3(1):33-6. PMID: 17557450.
43. Haack M, Simpson N, Sethna N, Kaur S, Mullington J. Sleep deficiency and chronic pain: potential underlying mechanisms and clinical implications. Neuropsychopharmacol Off Publ Am Coll Neuropsychopharmacol. 2020 Jan;45(1):205–16.

Chapter 14

# Pain Management Strategies for Cancer Survivors

• Aparna Chatterjee • Pankaj Singh Rana

## INTRODUCTION

Substantial breakthrough has been achieved in recent decades in cancer therapy. Timely identification, accuracy and less intrusive surgical techniques, along with cytoreductive surgery and more recently the invention of immunotherapy and target specific cancer therapy have transformed the way that cancer is treated. As treatment becomes more intensive, survivor numbers have also increased. Survivors may experience more enduring issues inclusive of pain that will eventually impact their aptitude to perform going forward, quality of life (QoL), and need for medical attention. According to Western literature, approximately 2/3rd patients with cancer live 5 years beyond diagnosis and about 40% of them suffer persistent pain chiefly due to the tumor or cancer treatment.[1,2] India would see 1.57 million cancer cases by 2025, up from 1.46 million cases in 2022.[3] 19.3 million cancer cases were there in 2020 worldwide, according to estimates by the Global Cancer Observatory (GLOBOCAN).[4] Following China and the US, India stood at third place.[5] GLOBOCAN projected that 2.08 million cancer cases would be diagnosed in India by 2040, representing a 57.5% increase from 2020. Overall, the number of cancer survivors has increased due to both advancements in cancer treatment and an increase in the number of patients suffering. However, there is a price to better cancer survival as patients may suffer adverse psychological and physical consequences from both, the diagnosis and treatment. In this chapter, we will explore various aspects related to pain in cancer survivors such as, who can be considered or called a survivor, the cause of pain in survivors, deconditioning and pain, can the WHO ladder be applied in this setting, safety, and validity of long-term opioid therapy (LTOT), guidelines available and their recommendations for survivors.

### Who is a Survivor?

There are variations in the way various organizations interpret the term cancer survivor. According to the National Cancer Institute (NCI), "Survivorship" encompasses the various challenges faced by cancer patients, including emotional, physical, and financial aspects, from diagnosis to the end of life.[6] The National Comprehensive Cancer Network (NCCN) panel also supports the NCI's definition of a cancer survivor.[7] The European Organization for Research and Treatment of Cancer's Survivorship Taskforce[8] defines survivors more narrowly, identifying them as individuals who, with exception of maintenance therapy, have completed primary treatment and do not currently have any active illness.

In summary, cancer survivors are people who have experienced a cancer diagnosis, undergone treatment, and are currently living with or without cancer. The term encompasses a broad spectrum of individuals, including those who are currently in remission, those who have finished their treatment and are regarded as disease-free, and those who may be living with cancer as a chronic condition. Patients with slow-growing tumors, on intermittent treatment, and those with the usually incurable disease but well controlled with systemic therapy and can survive for as long as 10 years or more, are all considered as "Cancer Survivor".

It is important to acknowledge that the understanding of who qualifies as a cancer survivor has developed over time to recognize the diverse experiences of individuals living with cancer. Survivorship includes not only the absence of disease but also the ongoing process of healing and adapting to life after cancer. The term emphasizes resilience, strength, and the ongoing pursuit of a fulfilling and healthy life post-cancer diagnosis and treatment.

## CAUSES OF PAIN IN CANCER SURVIVORS

To fully understand the cause of pain in cancer survivors, it is essential to consider the multidimensional nature of pain and the various factors that may contribute to its development. One factor that can exacerbate distress in cancer survivors is the pathological changes that occur because of the disease and its treatment. These changes may include nerve damage, inflammation, tissue scarring, or the presence of tumors. In some cases, chronic pain that is not related to the illness and its treatment may also be experienced by survivors. Additionally, psychological factors such as stress, anxiety, and depression or social factors such as lack of support or isolation can also contribute to and exacerbate the experience of pain in cancer survivors.[9]

## PATHOPHYSIOLOGY OF PAIN IN CANCER SURVIVORS

Understanding the pathophysiology of pain in cancer survivors is essential for developing appropriate management strategies and elevating cancer patients' quality of living. There are mainly two mechanisms by which cancer pain can occur in cancer survivors (Table 14.1):

*Due to the direct effects of the tumor:* Cancer pain due to tumors usually gets worse as the disease progresses. It can be caused by chemicals secreted by the tumor, acidosis, or direct damage to sensory nerve fibers at the location of the original tumor or its metastases.[10]

But the direct impact of the local tumor and the inflammatory processes that go along with it always produce significant nociceptive mechanisms. In most cases, this is explained by taking into consideration a mixed pathophysiology that includes both nociceptive and neuropathic components.[11] Example of chronic pain syndrome, caused by direct effect to tumor or metastasis includes:

- Cancer induced bone pain as seen in patients with prostate cancer, metastatic breast cancer, and multiple myelomas.

*Due to the effects of various anticancer treatments:* Specific cancer therapies, like chemotherapy and radiation, can occasionally cause pain. The negative effects of these drugs include inflammation, nerve damage, and bone loss, all of which can exacerbate pain.[12] Examples of cancer pain syndrome caused due to effects of anticancer treatments which could persist in a cancer survivor include:

- Cancer-induced bone pain (CIBP)
- Chronic post-surgical pain
- Painful neuropathies
- Post-radiation pain syndrome
- Musculoskeletal pain

**Table 14.1: Chronic pain syndromes in cancer survivors**

| Due to the direct effects of the tumor | Due to the effects of various anticancer treatment |
|---|---|
| Cancer-induced bone pain (CIBP) | *Chronic post-surgical pain (CPSP)*<br>• Postmastectomy syndrome<br>• Post-thoracotomy syndrome<br>• Post-radical neck dissection pain<br>• Post.amputation pain<br>• Postoperative frozen shoulder<br>• Fistula formation<br>• Lymphedema<br>*Painful neuropathies*<br>• Chemotherapy-induced peripheral neuropathy (CIPN)<br>• Monoclonal antibody-related neuropathy<br>• Para-neoplastic neuropathy<br>• Graft versus host disease related neuropathy<br>*Post-radiation pain syndrome*<br>• Brachial or lumbosacral<br>• Plexopathy<br>• Myelopathy<br>• Enteritis or proctitis Lymphedema<br>• Burning perineum syndrome<br>• Osteoradionecrosis<br>• Stroke-like migraine attacks after radiation therapy (SMART) syndrome<br>*Musculoskeletal pain*<br>• Aromatase inhibitor-induced arthralgia (ALA)<br>• Tamoxifen-induced arthralgia |

## Cancer-induced Bone Pain (CIBP)

The term "cancer-induced bone pain" describes the pain that is felt by people whose cancer has metastasized to bones. Tumors such as prostate cancer, metastatic breast cancer and multiple myeloma with prolonged survival have a higher predilection for bone metastasis. It is a constant dull background pain, with intermittent spontaneous flare-ups or movement-related pain. CIBP can be exceedingly crippling for individuals whose life expectancy is already shortened. The mechanisms include the release of growth factors and cytokines by cancer cells, which stimulate the migration and invasion of tumor cells into the bone tissue. Tumor cells release factors such as a parathyroid hormone-related protein that promotes secretion of RANKL by osteoblasts and thus stimulate osteoclast activation, leading to excessive bone resorption and destruction of normal bone structure.[13] These imbalances in the microenvironment with local acidic surroundings and inflammatory mediators further stimulate nerve endings releasing the pain-inducing factors. So, drugs that inhibit osteoclastic cells like bisphosphonates and denosumab are utilized for managing CIBP.

### Chronic Post-surgical Pain (CPSP)

CPSP is a common postoperative complication, which has a major detrimental effect on patients' quality of life and results in financial and health-related burdens. It can develop long after an asymptomatic period. At six to twelve months following surgery, the typical incidence of chronic pain is 20–30%, with a gradual reduction over the course of time.[14,15]

According to the international classification of diseases, eleventh revision (ICD-11),[14] the definition of CPSP includes:

- Pain may appear or become more intense, following surgery or a tissue injury
- Pain that lasts longer than the healing phase, which is three months or more following the trigger event
- Usually, pain is confined to the surgical site or in its territory, or mapped to the nerve's innervation area within this particular location
- Other causes of pain such as infections, cancer, and pre-existing pain problems must be excluded
- More of a neuropathic pain marked by feelings akin to burning, electric shock, and shooting type of sensation
- There is a distinction made between tissue trauma resulting from a regulated medical operation such as surgery and uncontrolled unintentional injury (other traumas)

Among CPSP one of the most frequently encountered postoperative pain syndromes is postmastectomy pain syndrome (PMPS). At Tata Memorial Hospital, an Indian tertiary care cancer centre, its incidence was found to be as high as 35.8% at 6 months following surgery.[16] Even though PMPS historically linked to mastectomy, women who had lumpectomies without lymph node dissection have also reported PMPS.[17] Other CPSP syndromes includes, post-radical neck dissection pain, post-thoracotomy pain, postoperative frozen shoulder, postamputation pain, fistula formation and lymphedema.

### Painful Neuropathies

Cancer treatment can lead to various types of chronic peripheral neuropathies such as chemotherapy-induced peripheral neuropathy (CIPN), monoclonal antibody-related neuropathy, para-neoplastic neuropathy, and Graft versus Host disease related neuropathy. Below is a description of each of these.

#### *Chemotherapy-induced Peripheral Neuropathy (CIPN)*

Chemotherapy agents are cytotoxic not only to the tumor cells but also to the normal tissue including the nervous system. Peripheral nerves stemming from neurons in the dorsal root ganglion lack protection from the blood–brain barrier and are susceptible to injury by chemotherapeutic agents.[18] A "stocking-and-glove" distribution of paresthesia and dysesthesia in the hands and feet is a characteristic of CIPN, which often affects the distal portions of extremities symmetrically.

A variety of chemotherapeutic medications, such as platinum-based (oxaliplatin), plant alkaloids (vincristine), taxanes (paclitaxel), and protease inhibitors (bortezomib) can be neurotoxic. Taxanes induce pain to both hands and feet along with aching sensations. On the other side, platinum-based agents affect hands more than feet, worsen progressively, and develop cold-induced neuropathy. Approximately 30% patients may continue to suffer from CIPN a year, or more, after finishing chemotherapy[19] and hence may continue to distress much after completion of cancer therapy and cure.

#### *Monoclonal Antibody-related Neuropathy*

It is unclear what exactly causes peripheral neuropathy related to monoclonal gammopathy. However, some evidence suggests that monoclonal antibodies such as nivolumab, activate T-cells and produce various inflammatory, autoimmune responses, which leads to myalgia, arthralgia, myositis, and arthritis.[20] In contrast to traditional cancer treatments, the range of toxicities with these immune checkpoint inhibitors (CPIs) is distinct and can affect any organ system, with the gastrointestinal tract, skin, lungs and endocrine glands are the most frequently affected organ systems. And these are known as immune-related adverse events (irAEs).[21]

If there are no contraindications, the first line of treatment for mild-to-moderate rheumatic symptoms should be symptomatic medication, such as non-steroidal anti-inflammatory medications and analgesics. Intra-articular glucocorticoids may be used in case of monoarthritis if other possibilities, such as infection, osteoarthritis have already been ruled out.[22]

#### *Para-neoplastic Peripheral Neuropathy (PPN)*

Paraneoplastic syndrome (PNS) is the consequence of an immunological reaction secondary to the underlying tumor that affects either the central or peripheral nervous system and is not directly associated to coagulopathies, nutritional deficiencies, cancer therapy, or metastases.[23,24] PPN is among the most frequently reported PNS conditions.[25] According to a systematic review and meta-analysis conducted in 2017, the primary cause of PPN (45.7%) was identified as lung cancer, followed by hematological malignancies (16.3%) and malignancies of the gastrointestinal system (12.0%).[26] And the treatment of neuropathic pain does not vary from how pain is managed in cases of paraneoplastic neuropathy.[27]

#### *Graft versus Host Disease Related Neuropathy*

Chronic graft versus host disease (cGVHD) may develop following bone marrow or stem cell transplantation. The management of cGVHD may necessitate immunosuppressive therapy for several years or even decades. The patient's receiving steroids for immunosuppression, might land up in having adverse effects related to it, such as osteoporosis and problems like pain, joint stiffness, etc. cGVHD may also have other painful manifestations like scleroderma, myositis, fasciitis, joint stiffness.[28]

### Post-radiation Pain Syndrome

Radiotherapy is used to treat cancer as well as cancer pain that is amenable to radiation therapy, but radiation itself can also be the cause of pain. Radiation can potentially damage any portion of the nervous system, such as the brain (resulting in radiation encephalopathy), spinal cord (leading to radiation myelopathy), and peripheral nerves (causing radiation neuritis). Radiation-induced damage tends to be permanent and does not diminish with time, and in more severe cases, paralysis or even loss of muscle function may occur. A lancinating and burning feeling that is concentrated in the area where the afflicted nerve structures are distributed characterizes the associated pain, which might manifest for months or even years following therapy.[29]

Even the non-irradiated cells lying adjacent to irradiated cells exhibit effects because of signals received from nearby irradiated cells. This is known as "radiation-induced bystander effects".

Radiation treatment for brain malignancies has been associated with a delayed consequence known as chronic headache syndromes. There are case reports describing "stroke-like migraine attacks after radiation therapy (SMART syndrome)".[30–33] Other post-radiation pain syndromes include brachial plexopathy (breast cancer) or lumbosacral plexopathy (cervix cancer), myelopathy enteritis or proctitis, burning perineum syndrome, and osteoradionecrosis.

Advancement in cancer therapy such as the ability to localize tumors more accurately to direct radiation therapy has improved the ability to spare normal tissues from the harmful effects of radiation exposure. Examples of these techniques and imaging methods include positron emission tomography, CT, MRI, and electronic portal imaging.[33] Intensity-modulated radiotherapy (IMRT), three-dimensional conformal radiotherapy (3DCRT), image-guided radiotherapy (IGT), and particle therapy have advanced planning procedures, precise tumor delineation, and dosage estimation, enabling personalized treatment strategies.[34]

### Musculoskeletal Pain

This type of pain includes aromatase inhibitor-induced arthralgia (AIA); and tamoxifen-induced arthralgia. Aromatase inhibitors (AI) are employed in the management of hormone receptor-positive breast cancers. They inhibit the biosynthesis of estrogen either reversibly (nonsteroidal: anastrozole, letrozole) or irreversibly (steroidal: exemestane). These are associated with adverse effects such as pain in hands, feet, hips, knees, lower back, shoulders, difficulty in sleeping, and early morning stiffness. Pain is severe enough to sometimes discontinue the treatment. The mechanism by which aromatase inhibitors cause arthralgia is not completely known but it is believed that it occurs because of the release of inflammatory markers. Tamoxifen, a hormone therapy drug with anti-estrogen effects can result in arthralgia similar to AIs, but pain severity is not as high as it is with AIs.[35]

## PAIN AND DECONDITIONING: A COMPLEX INTERPLAY

Deconditioning refers to the loss of physical fitness because of prolonged periods of inactivity or reduced physical activity levels. Chronic pain, on the other hand, encompasses a range of persistent painful conditions that can significantly impact an individual's quality of life. Cancer survivors may experience deconditioning, which can even exacerbate non-cancer pain. While these two concepts may seem distinct at first glance, they are intricately connected and can have a profound influence on one another.

When deconditioning occurs, it often leads to a decrease in muscle strength, aerobic capacity, and overall physical fitness. This can subsequently exacerbate the experience of pain and further compromise an individual's capacity to participate in everyday tasks. The resulting cycle of pain and deconditioning sometimes referred to as a pain-deconditioning cycle, can create a vicious loop where pain limits physical activity, leading to further deconditioning, which in turn increases pain levels.

### Mechanisms underlying the Pain-deconditioning Cycle

Several mechanisms contribute to the pain-deconditioning cycle. When individuals experience pain, they may feel inclined to decrease their level of physical activity or even avoid it altogether to avoid exacerbating their pain. This reduction in physical activity can lead to muscle atrophy, decreased joint flexibility, and reduced cardiovascular capacity. Consequently, these physical changes further contribute to the experience of pain.

Additionally, pain can also disrupt sleep patterns, causing fatigue and reducing the energy levels necessary for physical activity. This fatigue can make it even more challenging for individuals to engage in exercise or maintain an active lifestyle. Furthermore, fear of pain and movement, known as kinesiophobia, often develops because of the pain-deconditioning cycle. Kinesiophobia can lead to avoidance of physical activity, perpetuating the deconditioning process and amplifying pain perception.[36,37]

### Breaking the Pain-deconditioning Cycle

Breaking the pain-deconditioning cycle is crucial for managing chronic pain effectively and improving overall physical functioning. Physical therapy, comprising of graded exercise and strength training, can help individuals regain strength, flexibility, and endurance gradually. Additionally, cognitive-behavioral therapy techniques may be employed to address the fear of pain and movement, promoting a positive mindset, and reducing kinesiophobia.

## CAN THE WHO LADDER BE APPLIED IN THE SETTINGS OF PAIN IN CANCER SURVIVORS?

The WHO ladder was proposed in 1986 and provides a framework to guide pain management in cancer patients based on pain intensity. It is till date, considered the standard of care & widely used. This approach categorizes pain intensity into three levels: Mild, moderate, and severe. Opioid analgesics form the basis of pain management based on the WHO ladder. However, pain management in cancer survivors is much more complex. A survivor likely would be trying their best to go back to the normal life which they had before the cancer diagnosis. Thus, while managing their pain, one should take into account and consider the impact of the treatment prescribed on health, physical and mental state, professional aspect, etc. and especially so in those who are now disease free. The WHO ladder is based on opioids and long-term opioid therapy may not be the ideal option for managing pain in a survivor especially those who are disease free.

Managing pain in cancer survivors requires a multidisciplinary team approach. In addition to pharmacological treatments, non-pharmacological interventions can be valuable in managing pain in cancer survivors. These interventions may include physical therapy, cognitive-behavioral therapy, pain education, and relaxation techniques. By addressing physical and psychological aspects of pain, these interventions can improve the overall quality of life for cancer survivors.

## SAFETY AND VALIDITY OF LONG-TERM OPIOID THERAPY (LTOT)

LTOT is not recommended as a first-line therapy for cancer survivors and especially so for those who are disease free. The Agency for Healthcare Research and Quality (AHRQ) published a systematic review in 2020 that found not enough data available to back up the long-term advantages of prescribing opioids to manage chronic pain.[38]

Moreover, there is growing acknowledgment that a common comorbidity among cancer survivors is persistent non-malignant pain.[39] Opioids are classified as the third-line medication in the American Society of Clinical Oncology's (ASCO) guidelines for the management of pain in cancer survivors.[40] For concomitant persistent non-malignant pain, LTOT is not advisable.[41] Among other hazards, LTOT usage has been associated with an increased risk of overdose and opioid abuse.[42] Prescribed opioids also carry dangers not just for patients but also for others and those in close proximity to the patient due to diversion and nonmedical use by people to whom they were not prescribed.

Additionally, opioids can lead to side effects such as constipation, sedation, respiratory depression, and even addiction. Furthermore, there is a risk of developing tolerance to opioids, requiring higher doses over time to achieve the same level of pain relief. This can further increase the likelihood of adverse effects, and dependency and may also interfere with employment. Overdose is most feared with concomitant use of alcohol and benzodiazepines. Even if a patient is started on opioid therapy, should be tapered off slowly to prevent withdrawal.

Validity is another important aspect to consider when assessing the use of long-term opioid therapy in cancer survivors. While opioids can offer substantial pain relief, it is crucial to evaluate whether the benefits outweigh the risks. Alternative pain management approaches, like non-opioid medications and physical therapy, and psychological interventions, should also be considered. Additionally, regular monitoring and assessment of pain levels, functional status, and quality of life are crucial to determining the effectiveness of long-term opioid therapy in cancer survivors. Overall, a comprehensive and individualized approach is necessary to balance the safety and validity of long-term opioid therapy in the management of pain in cancer survivors.

Opioids are only indicated for use in cancer survivors when moderate to severe treatment-related pain persists despite maximally tolerated therapy with non-opioid approaches.[40] Patients receiving opioids should undergo monitoring and gradual tapering whenever possible. Ultimately, the choice to implement long-term opioid therapy in cancer survivors should be based on individual assessment, carefully considering the balance between benefits and risks.

## GUIDELINES AND RECOMMENDATIONS FOR SURVIVORS

There are few available guidelines specific to pain management in cancer survivors. The National Comprehensive Cancer Network (NCCN) does provide recommendations for approaches to screening, prevention, and therapy.[43]

The American Society of Clinical Oncology (ASCO) convened an expert panel that performed a thorough systematic literature search of 63 studies on the management of chronic pain in cancer survivors in 2016.[40] Since there was little high-level evidence, the majority of the recommendations were based on expert consensus. Both ASCO and NCCN recommend a combination of pharmacological and non-pharmacological modalities for managing pain in survivors.

The ASCO essentially covers four elements, which are elaborated upon below.

### 1. Screening and Comprehensive Assessment

- Screening of patient for pain at each encounter and proper documentation at each time.
- Conduct a comprehensive assessment: In-depth discussion, multidimensional nature of pain, comorbid conditions, psychosocial and psychiatric history, prior cancer treatment.
- Recognize the syndromes related to chronic pain that occur with cancer treatment and treatment options.
- Assess and observe for recurrent diseases, second primary malignancy, delayed-onset treatment effects.

### 2. Treatment and Care Options

- The objectives are to assure safety, minimize side effects, increase comfort, and improve function.
- Involve patients, family members, and caregivers in all facets of pain assessment and treatment.
- Ascertain whether more healthcare providers are required to offer individuals with complex needs complete care.
- *Nonpharmacological interventions:* In order to reduce chronic pain and enhance results connected to pain, the physician should refer the patient to other specialists that offer these kinds of interventions
- Pain management and general function can be enhanced by non-pharmacologic interventions such as neurological stimulation therapy, integrative therapy, physical medicine and rehabilitation, integrative therapy, and interventional therapy.
- Physical medicine and rehabilitation include physical therapy (exercises to stretch and strengthen muscles, improve flexibility, and reduce pain), occupational therapy (helps patients regain physical independence), recreational therapy, individualized exercise programs, orthotics, ultrasound, heat/cold.
- Integrative therapies encompass practices such as massage, acupuncture, and music therapy.
- Interventional therapies comprise procedures like nerve blocks, neuraxial infusion (epidural/intrathecal), and vertebroplasty/kyphoplasty.
- Psychological strategies like cognitive behavioral therapy, distraction techniques, mindfulness, relaxation exercises, and guided imagery play a significant role in pain management.
- Neurostimulator therapies, including transcutaneous electrical nerve stimulation (TENS), spinal cord stimulation, peripheral nerve stimulation, and transcranial stimulation, are crucial elements of pain management.

### 3. Pharmacologic Interventions

Medication is often necessary to achieve optimal pain relief in cancer survivors. Analgesics, such as non-steroidal anti-inflammatory drugs (NSAIDs), acetaminophen (paracetamol), or opioids, may be prescribed to manage severe pain.

- NSAIDs and acetaminophen are most effective for nociceptive and chronic non-malignant pain which can be aggravated in survivors.
- Antidepressants, anticonvulsants, and topical agents may also be considered for certain types of pain.
- Duloxetine is currently the only serotonin and norepinephrine reuptake inhibitors (SNRIs) class of antidepressants that is recommended for use in CIPN in doses up to 60 mg daily.[45]
- Anticonvulsants such as gabapentin and pregabalin are useful in managing pain in cancer survivors, along with lamotrigine, and carbamazepine. However, the risk of drowsiness, somnolence, and headache should be kept in mind while prescribing these drugs.
- The routine use of corticosteroids for long-term pain relief in survivors is not recommended due to the significant side effects associated with corticosteroid use.[46]
- Regarding NMDA antagonists such as ketamine and magnesium, some patients may benefit however, long-term effectiveness has not been established.
- Topical analgesics (NSAIDs, local anesthetics, baclofen, amitriptyline, ketamine) can also help manage pain but their use depends upon clinical discretion.
- When it comes to cannabinoids, there is limited evidence supporting the use of medical cannabis as a first-line treatment for survivors. However, some evidence suggests it may be considered as an adjunct or in cases of refractory pain.[47]
- It is important to discuss the benefits and risks of pain medications with the patient and tailor the regimen based on their individual needs.

### 4. Risk Assessment, Mitigation and Universal Precautions with Opioid Use

- Evaluate both the potential risks and benefits when initiating long-term opioid therapy (LTOT) as part of treatment.
- Implement a universal precaution approach to mitigate the risks of abuse, addiction, and adverse outcomes associated with opioid use, including opioid-related fatalities. Caution is necessary while prescribing centrally acting drugs like benzodiazepines
- Educate survivors and families regarding the risks and benefits of LTOT, safe storage, use, and correct disposal of these medications. Address their myths and misconceptions. Sedatives or centrally acting medications, and alcohol should be avoided while on strong opioid therapy.
- Taper opioids when not warranted and in such a way as to avoid abstinence syndrome.

## Conclusion

Pain management in cancer survivors requires a comprehensive and individualized approach. Integrating various strategies, including medication, integrative therapies, psychosocial support, nutritional guidance, and palliative care, can contribute to a more holistic and effective pain management plan. It is essential to involve a multidisciplinary team of healthcare professionals to tailor therapy and interventions to the unique needs of each survivor, promoting their overall well-being and quality of life.

## References


1. Siegel RL, Miller KD, Fuchs HE, Jemal A. Cancer Statistics, 2021. CA Cancer J Clin. 2021 Jan;71(1):7–33.
2. Boland EG, Ahmedzai SH. Persistent pain in cancer survivors. Curr Opin Support Palliat Care. 2017 Sep;11(3):181–90.
3. Sathishkumar K, Chaturvedi M, Das P, Stephen S, Mathur P. Cancer incidence estimates for 2022 and projection for 2025: Result from National Cancer Registry Programme, India. Indian J Med Res. 2022;156(4 & 5):598–607.
4. Sung H, Ferlay J, Siegel RL, Laversanne M, Soerjomataram I, Jemal A, et al. Global Cancer Statistics 2020: GLOBOCAN Estimates of Incidence and Mortality Worldwide for 36 Cancers in 185 Countries. CA Cancer J Clin. 2021 May;71(3):209–49.
5. Ferlay J, Colombet M, Soerjomataram I, Parkin DM, Piñeros M, Znaor A, et al. Cancer statistics for the year 2020: An overview. Int J Cancer. 2021 Apr 5.
6. Definitions | Division of Cancer Control and Population Sciences (DCCPS) [Internet]. [cited 2024 Feb 28]. Available from: https://cancercontrol.cancer.gov/ocs/definitions.
7. Denlinger CS, Carlson RW, Are M, Baker KS, Davis E, Edge SB, et al. Survivorship: introduction and definition. Clinical practice guidelines in oncology. J Natl Compr Canc Netw. 2014 Jan;12(1):34–45.
8. Moser EC, Meunier F. Cancer survivorship: A positive side-effect of more successful cancer treatment. EJC Suppl. 2014 Jun;12(1):1–4.
9. Syrjala KL, Jensen MP, Mendoza ME, Yi JC, Fisher HM, Keefe FJ. Psychological and behavioral approaches to cancer pain management. J Clin Oncol. 2014 Jun 1;32(16):1703–11.
10. Bennett MI, Kaasa S, Barke A, Korwisi B, Rief W, Treede RD, et al. The IASP classification of chronic pain for ICD-11: chronic cancer-related pain. Pain. 2019 Jan;160(1):38–44.
11. Shkodra M, Brunelli C, Zecca E, Formaglio F, Bracchi P, Lo Dico S, et al. Neuropathic pain: clinical classification and assessment in patients with pain due to cancer. Pain. 2021 Mar 1;162(3):866–74.
12. Gupta R, Van de Ven T, Pyati S. Post-Thoracotomy Pain: Current Strategies for Prevention and Treatment. Drugs. 2020 Nov;80(16):1677–84.
13. Zaj czkowska R, Kocot-K pska M, Leppert W, Wordliczek J. Bone Pain in Cancer Patients: Mechanisms and Current Treatment. Int J Mol Sci. 2019 Nov 30;20(23):6047.
14. Schug SA, Lavand'homme P, Barke A, Korwisi B, Rief W, Treede RD, et al. The IASP classification of chronic pain for ICD-11: chronic postsurgical or post-traumatic pain. Pain. 2019 Jan;160(1):45–52.
15. Fletcher D, Pogatzki-Zahn E, Zaslansky R, Meissner W, Pain Out Group. euCPSP: European observational study on chronic post-surgical pain. Eur J Anaesthesiol. 2011 Jun;28(6):461–2.
16. Kakati B, Nair N, Chatterjee A. Post mastectomy pain syndrome at an Indian tertiary cancer centre and its impact on quality of life. Indian J Cancer. 2023;60(2):275–81.
17. Carpenter JS, Andrykowski MA, Sloan P, Cunningham L, Cordova MJ, Studts JL, et al. Postmastectomy/postlumpectomy pain in breast cancer survivors. J Clin Epidemiol. 1998 Dec;51(12):1285–92.
18. Branca JJV, Maresca M, Morucci G, Becatti M, Paternostro F, Gulisano M, et al. Oxaliplatin-induced blood brain barrier loosening: a new point of view on chemotherapy-induced neurotoxicity. Oncotarget. 2018 May 4;9(34):23426–38.
19. Colvin LA. Chemotherapy-induced peripheral neuropathy: where are we now? Pain. 2019 May;160 Suppl 1(Suppl 1):S1–10.
20. Postow MA, Sidlow R, Hellmann MD. Immune-Related Adverse Events Associated with Immune Checkpoint Blockade. N Engl J Med. 2018 Jan 11;378(2):158–68.
21. Kostine M, Finckh A, Bingham CO, Visser K, Leipe J, Schulze-Koops H, et al. EULAR points to consider for the diagnosis and management of rheumatic immune-related adverse events due to cancer immunotherapy with checkpoint inhibitors. Ann Rheum Dis. 2021 Jan;80(1):36–48.
22. Narváez J, Juarez-López P, LLuch J, Narváez JA, Palmero R, García Del Muro X, et al. Rheumatic immune-related adverse events in patients on anti-PD-1 inhibitors: Fasciitis with myositis syndrome as a new complication of immunotherapy. Autoimmun Rev. 2018 Oct;17(10):1040–5.

23. Dalmau JO, Posner JB. Paraneoplastic syndromes affecting the nervous system. Semin Oncol. 1997 Jun;24(3):318–28.
24. Darnell RB. Onconeural antigens and the paraneoplastic neurologic disorders: at the intersection of cancer, immunity, and the brain. Proc Natl Acad Sci U S A. 1996 May 14;93(10):4529–36.
25. Candler PM, Hart PE, Barnett M, Weil R, Rees JH. A follow up study of patients with paraneoplastic neurological disease in the United Kingdom. J Neurol Neurosurg Psychiatry. 2004 Oct 1;75(10):1411–5.
26. Zis P, Paladini A, Piroli A, McHugh PC, Varrassi G, Hadjivassiliou M. Pain as a First Manifestation of Paraneoplastic Neuropathies: A Systematic Review and Meta-Analysis. Pain Ther. 2017 Dec;6(2):143–51.
27. Vadalouca A, Raptis E, Moka E, Zis P, Sykioti P, Siafaka I. Pharmacological treatment of neuropathic cancer pain: a comprehensive review of the current literature. Pain Pract. 2012 Mar;12(3):219–51.
28. Mawardi H, Hashmi SK, Elad S, Aljurf M, Treister N. Chronic graft-versus-host disease: Current management paradigm and future perspectives. Oral Dis. 2019 May;25(4):931–48.
29. Lyne ME, Coyne PJ, Watson AC. Pain management issues for cancer survivors. Cancer Pract. 2002;10 Suppl 1:S27-32.
30. Bartleson JD, Krecke KN, O'Neill BP, Brown PD. Reversible, strokelike migraine attacks in patients with previous radiation therapy. Neuro Oncol. 2003 Apr;5(2):121–7.
31. Pruitt A, Dalmau J, Detre J, Alavi A, Rosenfeld MR. Episodic neurologic dysfunction with migraine and reversible imaging findings after radiation. Neurology. 2006 Aug 22;67(4):676–8.
32. Cordato DJ, Brimage P, Masters LT, Butler P. Post-cranial irradiation syndrome with migraine-like headaches, prolonged and reversible neurological deficits and seizures. J Clin Neurosci. 2006 Jun;13(5):586–90.
33. Partap S, Walker M, Longstreth WT, Spence AM. Prolonged but reversible migraine-like episodes long after cranial irradiation. Neurology. 2006 Apr 11;66(7):1105–7.
34. Koka K, Verma A, Dwarakanath BS, Papineni RVL. Technological Advancements in External Beam Radiation Therapy (EBRT): An Indispensable Tool for Cancer Treatment. Cancer Manag Res. 2022;14:1421–9.
35. Younus J, Kligman L. Management of aromatase inhibitor-induced arthralgia. Curr Oncol. 2010 Feb;17(1):87–90.
36. Ishak NA, Zahari Z, Justine M. Kinesiophobia, Pain, Muscle Functions, and Functional Performances among Older Persons with Low Back Pain. Pain Res Treat. 2017;2017:3489617.
37. Bordeleau M, Vincenot M, Lefevre S, Duport A, Seggio L, Breton T, et al. Treatments for kinesiophobia in people with chronic pain: A scoping review. Front Behav Neurosci. 2022;16:933483.
38. Chou R, Hartung D, Turner J, Blazina I, Chan B, Levander X, et al. Opioid Treatments for Chronic Pain [Internet]. Rockville (MD): Agency for Healthcare Research and Quality (US); 2020 [cited 2024 Feb 28]. (AHRQ Comparative Effectiveness Reviews). Available from: http://www.ncbi.nlm.nih.gov/books/NBK556253/
39. Posternak V, Dunn LB, Dhruva A, Paul SM, Luce J, Mastick J, et al. Differences in demographic, clinical, and symptom characteristics and quality of life outcomes among oncology patients with different types of pain. Pain. 2016 Apr 1;157(4):892–900.
40. Paice JA, Portenoy R, Lacchetti C, Campbell T, Cheville A, Citron M, et al. Management of Chronic Pain in Survivors of Adult Cancers: American Society of Clinical Oncology Clinical Practice Guideline. J Clin Oncol. 2016 Sep 20;34(27):3325–45.
41. Chou R, Turner JA, Devine EB, Hansen RN, Sullivan SD, Blazina I, et al. The effectiveness and risks of long-term opioid therapy for chronic pain: a systematic review for a National Institutes of Health Pathways to Prevention Workshop. Ann Intern Med. 2015 Feb 17;162(4):276–86.
42. Chou R, Deyo R, Devine B, Hansen R, Sullivan S, Jarvik JG, et al. The Effectiveness and Risks of Long-Term Opioid Treatment of Chronic Pain. Evid Rep Technol Assess (Full Rep). 2014 Sep;(218):1–219.

43. Gralow JR, Biermann JS, Farooki A, Fornier MN, Gagel RF, Kumar R, et al. NCCN Task Force Report: Bone Health In Cancer Care. J Natl Compr Canc Netw. 2013 Aug;11 Suppl 3:S1-50; quiz S51.
44. Swarm RA, Paice JA, Anghelescu DL, Are M, Bruce JY, Buga S, et al. Adult Cancer Pain, Version 3.2019, NCCN Clinical Practice Guidelines in Oncology. J Natl Compr Canc Netw. 2019 Aug 1;17(8):977–1007.
45. Hirayama Y, Ishitani K, Sato Y, Iyama S, Takada K, Murase K, et al. Effect of duloxetine in Japanese patients with chemotherapy-induced peripheral neuropathy: a pilot randomized trial. Int J Clin Oncol. 2015 Oct;20(5):866–71.
46. Paulsen Ø, Aass N, Kaasa S, Dale O. Do corticosteroids provide analgesic effects in cancer patients? A systematic literature review. J Pain Symptom Manage. 2013 Jul;46(1):96–105.
47. Lynch ME, Ware MA. Cannabinoids for the Treatment of Chronic Non-Cancer Pain: An Updated Systematic Review of Randomized Controlled Trials. J Neuroimmune Pharmacol. 2015 Jun;10(2):293–301.

Chapter 15

# Psychological Aspects of Cancer Pain

• Savita Goswami • Jayita Deodhar

Pain intensity is defined as a quantification of the severity of pain sensation, while distress associated with pain signifies a level of suffering or discomfort resulting from sensation of pain or the emotional consequences due to severe physical distress. Concurrently, psychosocial distress is a more comprehensive aspect of distress that may or may not be directly connected to pain sensation.[1]

The connection in psychosocial distress and pain is intricate as well as multifaceted.[2] Psychological and emotional distress is a considerable issue for cancer patients undergoing treatment and even for survivors who have completed treatment. Cancer-related uncertainty, the fear of recurrence or progression, symptom burden, and multiple situational demands can elicit emotional turmoil and render individuals physically and mentally vulnerable, ultimately leading to significant distress.[3]

Research on the impact of pain-related distress has commonly assessed it as a comprehensive phenomenon encompassing disturbance in mood, emotional reactions, depression, discomfort, psychosocial issues, depressive feelings, fear, anxiousness, and apprehensions. Studies have consistently demonstrated an association between an increased degree of physical distress and heightened mental health problems.[2]

The relationship between pain perception, its inherent nature, and the resulting suffering due to symptoms such as mood depression, anxiousness, stress, and worry is multifaceted and intricate. The current body of evidence fails to provide a clear and consistent answer regarding whether the perception of pain occurs before or as a result of psychological disorders and the symptoms associated with them.[4]

An Indian prospective study had shown that a lower proportion of patients with no pain reported anxiety (9.2%) compared to patients with severe pain (32.8%), who exhibited significant levels of anxiety. Among patients with no pain, 17.7% experienced depression, while 36.7% of those with severe pain had significant levels of depression. In examining anxiety and depression scores, it was observed that among patients without depression, 6% had anxiety, whereas among those with depression, 44.9% experienced anxiety.[5]

In a recent cross-sectional study, 31.2% of participants presented with significant post-traumatic stress symptoms, and approximately a quarter (25.3%) showed significant psychological distress on the post-traumatic stress symptoms-10 (PTSS-10). Significant symptoms for depression were noted in 13.9% of participants, while anxiety was noted in 15.1% on hospital anxiety depression (HADS) scores.[6]

Persistent pain can lead to the development of negative thought patterns and behaviors that impede daily functioning, exacerbate psychological distress, and prolong the experience of pain. Pain catastrophizing involves magnifying the harmful effects of pain, meditating on the pain, and feeling helpless in dealing with it, has been linked to a host of maladaptive consequences, including among its effects are heightened rates of depression and anxiety, greater impairment and disability resulting from pain, as well as a reduction in overall quality of life.

Patients who tend to exaggerate the severity of their pain often report diminished control over their discomfort, poorer emotional and social functioning, and less favorable effects of medical treatments. Moreover, individuals who catastrophize their pain may impede effective pain management and overall functioning, making it a suitable target for psychological intervention. By addressing catastrophic thoughts related to pain, individuals can experience short-term improvements in their physical and psychological functioning and are more likely to return to work despite persistent pain.[7]

Psychological and physical pain is often addressed through treatments aimed primarily at reducing the somatic symptoms. However, psychological and sociocultural factors can obstruct the management of pain. Psychological factors, including depression, anxiety, and a fear of cancer recurrence or progression, are associated with severe pain in cancer patients. Additionally, when pain is coupled with psychological distress, it can become unrelenting. Moreover, unrecognized psychosocial symptoms such as guilt, grief related to the loss (loss of body part or functioning, alopecia, financial toxicity, etc.) feelings of being dependent, low self-esteem due to change in appearance and body image disturbances, sexual difficulties, lack of pleasure, dissatisfaction with care and socioeconomic factors that cause distress such as family dynamics, relationship conflicts, multiple negative life events, financial constraints, living arrangements, geographical distance from the care center, societal acceptance, stigma, discrimination can exacerbate the severity of pain and excessive use of pain medications.[8,9] Spiritual or existential concerns have the potential to exacerbate the physical and psychological symptoms experienced by cancer patients. Research has uncovered several psychospiritual elements that play a role in the connection between physical distress and depression, including feelings of demoralization, loss of self-respect, guilt, lack of purpose in life, feelings of worthlessness, hopelessness, inability to seek assistance, and insufficient family or social support.[10,11]

## CHALLENGES IN PAIN MANAGEMENT

Insufficient pain management is frequently attributable to a patient's reluctance to disclose their pain and unwillingness to adhere to prescribed treatment. Patients often perceive pain as an inevitable aspect of their cancer diagnosis, while others may hold the belief that acknowledging pain indicates their vulnerability or weakness. The influence of a patient's beliefs and attitudes on their experience and treatment of pain is significant. Cancer patients may refrain from communicating their pain to preserve the perception of being a "good" patient, as they do not want to divert their doctor's attention from treating their cancer or believe that expressing pain signifies disease progression. Patients also express concerns about the potential side effects and fears of addiction and tolerance, and think that resting is the best way to treat pain, as well as unrealistic expectations, misconceptions about pain medications, and varying levels of trust in traditional medicines. Children and geriatric individuals may encounter difficulties in communicating and expressing themselves due to immaturity, cognitive decline, which can lead to altered responses to pain medications and more intricate pain sensations. Inadequate treatment may be attributed to an individual's inability to convey their pain experience to their healthcare provider, inadequate privacy, and socioeconomic difficulties.[12,13]

Healthcare professionals face numerous challenges in providing effective pain management, including excessive workloads, inadequate pain management, poor communication skills, and a lack of training and experience regarding appropriate opioid use and non-pharmacological interventions. Moreover, unintentional biases and time constraints can hinder their ability to provide optimal care. These factors can limit the effectiveness of pain management, which is a critical aspect of patient care.

Effective pain management requires a comprehensive approach that includes a thorough assessment of the patient's pain, medical-psychosocial history, current medications, and the use of appropriate tools for pain assessment. Healthcare professionals must also consider the potential risks and benefits of each treatment option, including opioids and non-pharmacological interventions. It is essential for healthcare providers to be able to communicate effectively with patients and caregivers to be sure that they fully understand their treatment choices and make informed decisions regarding their healthcare.[14]

Patient-reported information about pain, multidimensional distress related to pain, and its impact on quality of life can be evaluated through an interview (verbally), and paper-pencil tests such as The State-Trait Anxiety Inventory (STAI), Hospital Anxiety and Depression Scale total score (HADS-T), Distress Thermometer (DT), Edmonton Symptom Assessment Scale (ESAS), European Organisation for Research and Treatment of Cancer Quality of Life Core Questionnaire (EORTC QLQ-C30), Functional Assessment of Chronic Illness Therapy-Spiritual Well-Being-Expanded (FACIT-Sp-Ex). Visual Analog Scale (VAS) is used for pain assessment commonly and Faces Pain Scale–Revised (FPS-R) is used for young children between 3 and 7 years of age.[15]

## INTERVENTION

Neglecting the sensation of pain is challenging because it serves as a warning sign of physiological imbalance, and paying attention to it can help mitigate its effects.

Non-pharmacological pain management techniques involve the use of methods that do not involve medications, to reduce pain by altering one's thoughts and focusing on different techniques to manage it effectively. These methods are not meant to replace pharmacological treatments but can be used in conjunction with medications to provide a more comprehensive pain management approach. Non-pharmacological techniques are particularly valuable for managing mild to moderate pain.[16]

To alleviate discomfort, various psychological therapies and behavioural pain management techniques can be employed, like talking therapies (psychotherapy), mindfulness exercises, and distraction techniques (Table 15.1). Relaxation exercises like breathing and physical stretching may help in decreasing pain, simple focused deep breathing, sleep hygiene, and yoga such as pranayam, anulom-vilom, yog-asana. Distraction techniques to divert attention from pain can be employed by engaging in activities such as watching television, listening to music, or recounting stories. Moreover, several other approaches can be taken to alleviate patients' discomfort, including

**Table 15.1: Psychological therapies and various techniques for pain management in cancer**

| Relaxation/comforting and distraction techniques | Psychotherapeutic interventions | Therapeutic techniques |
|---|---|---|
| Deep breathing and stretching | Cognitive behavior therapy (CBT) | Psychoeducation, thought reframing<br>Insight-oriented approaches, self management |
| Sleep hygiene | Operant-behavioral therapy | Behavior modification, systematic reinforcement |
| Meditation-dhyana, prayer | Mindfulness-based stress reduction (MBSR)<br>Mindfulness-based interventions (MBI) | Formulation of "nonstriving" response, experiential meditation |
| Aroma therapy | Acceptance and commitment therapy (ACT) | Improving acceptance and emotional regulation |
| Watching TV, playing indoor games | Supportive expressive group therapy | Supportive environment help to confront problems and encourage the expression of emotions |
| Singing, listening to music, storytelling, chanting | Behavior therapy | Self monitoring–structured routine, maintaining diary, lifestyle modifications |
| Light physical exercise | Family/couple therapy | Understanding dynamics—psychoeducation, improving coping, problem solving |
| Expressive art therapy–any art form that enhances expression<br>Art activities (craft, coloring, painting, clay modelling, writing) | Patient and caregiver support groups<br>Parent support group | Allow patients and family caregivers to connect with others, share experience and learn from sharing |
| Massage therapy, heat/cold application | Play therapy for children (toys, mind games, group play therapy, role play, dramatic puppetry, storytelling, animation-cartoon), | Self-expression which offers children the opportunity to communicate, socialise, ventilate emotions like fear, anxiety, sadness helps in psycho-education |
| Companionship | --- | Belongingness, sharing, spending quality time |
| Drama therapy | --- | Role play, psycho drama, role reversal techniques |

companionship, physical exercise, the application of heat or cold, the use of lotions or massage therapy, meditation, music therapy, art therapy, or drama therapy.

Psychotherapy may involve evidence-based interventions such as psychoeducation, mindfulness therapy, supportive psychotherapy, expressive art therapy, group therapy for patient and caregiver support groups.

Operant-behavioral therapy focuses on the process of extinction of maladaptive behavioral responses by altering them to adaptive behavioral responses to pain. This method of therapy modifies behavioral responses by employing reinforcement and punishment contingencies, as well as extinguishing the connections between the fear value of pain and physical actions.

Cognitive-behavioral therapy (CBT) is a therapeutic approach that emphasizes the role of cognitive and behavioral factors in the experience of pain. This approach includes education about pain, pain-related behaviors, and mood, as well as the development of strategies for relaxation, behavioral activation, positive event scheduling, effective communication, and cognitive restructuring of maladaptive thoughts related to pain.

Mindfulness-based stress reduction (MBSR) intervention is a nonjudgmental approach to pain and focuses on separating the biological and psychological aspects of pain. This therapeutic approach enhances learning about "nonstriving" responses to physical distress by improving mindful awareness of the body and through meditative practices.

Acceptance and commitment therapy (ACT) is improving acceptance of emotional reactions and pain, by eliminating inappropriate, maladaptive attempts to control pain through withdrawing and obstructive behavior.

Biofeedback relaxation and progressive muscle relaxation technique (PMRT) give relief from chronic pain by knowing how to control physiological responses to it. It helps patients to release tension and anxiety. Self-monitoring behavioural measures like maintaining a pain diary to monitor pain levels and observe how there is change over time. This technique helps patients develop an understanding of their ability to control and manage pain by using the skills they are practicing.[17–20]

## PAIN MANAGEMENT IN CHILDREN

Cancer treatment is a complex and often invasive process that involves numerous medical procedures, including needle pricks, hospitalizations, and side effects that can cause significant pain. For children, this experience can be particularly traumatic, as they may not fully understand the procedures they are undergoing or have control over them. Moreover, a lack of appropriate explanation and pain management can exacerbate their anxiety and fear. High levels of anxiety can have serious negative impacts on children's health, both physiologically and psychologically. This anxiety can also interfere with their ability to cope with medical treatment, leading to uncooperative behavior and negative emotions toward medical professionals. Anxiety and pain are two major challenges faced by children and adolescents undergoing cancer treatment, and research has shown that increasing anxiety is associated with anticipating more pain and tolerating pain for shorter periods. It is therefore crucial to address both anxiety and pain management to ensure the best possible outcomes for these patients.

Engaging with children and communicating on their level presents a significant challenge. Non-directive play therapy views play as a healing process for a child. Techniques such as storytelling, dramatic puppetry, and doll therapy can be employed, along with indoor games like snake and ladder, X and zero, Ludo, mind games (word games, puzzles, riddles), video games, animations, and pictorial books helps in interaction, distraction and in engaging children. Psychoeducation is also provided to parents to help them learn how to better deal with their children.[21]

Cancer-related chronic pain is a subjective experience; hence, it should be considered a condition rather than a disease that needs management rather than a cure. Evidence-based psychological interventions enhance cognitive, emotional, and behavioural coping; improve self-management and self-efficacy; and help with effective self- and emotional regulation, which minimizes emotional distress while dealing with pain. These benefits are achieved through various behavioural and cognitive techniques such as comforting communication, empathy, therapeutic touch, and unconditional support. Psychological treatment should be considered an important and inevitable part of multidisciplinary care for pain management in cancer patients. Skills that patients acquire through psychological interventions not only empower and enable them to actively manage their illness, but also equip them with valuable life skills that they can utilize in various aspects of their lives.

## References

1. Knotkova H, Crawford Clark W, Mokrejs P, Padour F, Kuhl J. What do ratings on unidimensional pain and emotion scales really mean? A Multidimensional Affect and Pain Survey (MAPS) analysis of cancer patient responses. J Pain Symptom Manage. 2004 Jul;28(1):19–27. doi: 10.1016/j.jpainsymman.2003.11.003. PMID: 15223081.
2. Zaza C, Baine N. Cancer pain and psychosocial factors: a critical review of the literature. J Pain Symptom Manage. 24(5):526–42.
3. Kirkova J, Walsh D, Rybicki L, et al. Symptom frequency and distress in advanced cancer. Palliat Med. 2010;24(3):330–9.
4. Krok J, Baker TA, McMillan SC. Age differences in the presence of pain and psychological distress in younger and older cancer patients. J Hosp PalliatNurs. 2013;15(2):107–13.
5. Arora A, Saini SK, Nautiyal V, Verma SK, Gupta M, Kalra BP, Ahmad M. Cancer Pain, Anxiety, and Depression in Admitted Patients at a Tertiary Care Hospital: A Prospective Observational Study. Indian J Palliat Care. 2019 Oct-Dec;25(4):562–566. doi: 10.4103/IJPC.IJPC_4_19. PMID: 31673213; PMCID: PMC6812432.
6. Unseld M, Zeilinger EL, Fellinger M, Lubowitzki S, Krammer K, Nader IW, et al. Prevalence of pain and its association with symptoms of post-traumatic stress disorder, depression, anxiety and distress in 846 cancer patients: A cross sectional study. Psychooncology. 2021 Apr;30(4):504–510. doi: 10.1002/pon.5595. Epub 2020 Dec 3. PMID: 33210393; PMCID: PMC8049050.
7. Sturgeon JA. Psychological therapies for the management of chronic pain. Psychol Res Behav Manag. 2014 Apr 10;7:115-24. doi: 10.2147/PRBM.S44762. PMID: 24748826; PMCID: PMC3986332.
8. Syrjala KL, Jensen MP, Mendoza ME, Yi JC, Fisher HM, Keefe FJ. Psychological and behavioral approaches to cancer pain management. J Clin Oncol. 2014 Jun 1;32(16):1703–11. doi: 10.1200/JCO.2013.54.4825. Epub 2014 May 5. PMID: 24799497; PMCID: PMC4031190.
9. Karen L Syrjala, et al. Psychological and Behavioral Approaches to Cancer Pain Management. JCO 32, 1703–1711(2014).DOI:10.1200/JCO.2013.54.4825
10. Lee YP, Wu CH, Chiu TY, Chen CY, Morita T, Hung SH, et al. The relationship between pain management and psychospiritual distress in patients with advanced cancer following admission to a palliative care unit. BMC Palliat Care.
11. Delgado-Guay MO, Hui D, Parsons HA, Govan K, De la Cruz M, Thorney S, et al. Spirituality, religiosity, and spiritual pain in advanced cancer patients. J Pain Symptom Manage. 2011;41:986–94 doi: 10.1016/j.jpainsymman.2010.09.017.
12. Ciuc Andrada and Adriana B ban. "Psychological factors and psychosocial interventions for cancer related pain." Romanian Journal of Internal Medicine 55.2 (2017): 63–8.
13. Shute C. The challenges of cancer pain assessment and management. Ulster Med J. 2013 Jan;82(1):40–2. PMID: 23620631; PMCID: PMC3632849.
14. National Institute for Clinical Excellence (NICE) Guidance on cancer services. Improving supportive and palliative care for adults with cancer. 2004. Available from: http://www.nice.org.uk/nicemedia/ live/10893/28816/28816.pdfLast accessed Nov 2012.

15. Mitchell AJ. Short screening tools for cancer-related distress: a review and diagnostic validity meta-analysis. J Natl ComprCancNetw. 2010 Apr;8(4):487–94. doi: 10.6004/jnccn.2010.0035. PMID: 20410338.
16. Mohamed Bayoumi MM, Khonji LMA, Gabr WFM. Are nurses utilizing the non-pharmacological pain management techniques in surgical wards? PLoS One. 2021 Oct 21;16(10):e0258668. doi: 10.1371/journal.pone.0258668. PMID: 34673781; PMCID: PMC8530299.
17. Roditi D, Robinson ME. The role of psychological interventions in the management of patients with chronic pain. Psychol Res Behav Manag. 2011;4:41–9. doi: 10.2147/PRBM.S15375. Epub 2011 May 11. PMID: 22114534; PMCID: PMC3218789.
18. Tsegaye D, Yazew A, Gedfew M, Yilak G, Yalew ZM. Non-Pharmacological Pain Management Practice and Associated Factors Among Nurses Working at Comprehensive Specialized Hospitals. SAGE Open Nurs. 2023 Feb Turk DC, Swanson KS, Tunks ER. Psychological Approaches in the Treatment of Chronic Pain Patients—When Pills, Scalpels, and Needles are Not Enough. The Canadian Journal of Psychiatry. 2008;53(4):213–223. doi:10.1177/070674370805300402
19. Vambheim SM, Kyllo TM, Hegland S, Bystad M. Relaxation techniques as an intervention for chronic pain: A systematic review of randomized controlled trials. Heliyon. 2021 Aug 20;7(8):e07837. doi: 10.1016/j.heliyon.2021.e07837. PMID: 34485731; PMCID: PMC8405991.
20. Williams AC de C, Fisher E, Hearn L, Eccleston C. Psychological therapies for the management of chronic pain (excluding headache) in adults. Cochrane Database of Systematic Reviews 2020, Issue 8. Art. No.: CD007407. DOI: 10.1002/14651858.CD007407.pub4.
21. Scarponi D, Pession A. Play Therapy to Control Pain and Suffering in Pediatric Oncology. Front Pediatr. 2016 Dec 8;4:132. doi: 10.3389/fped.2016.00132. PMID: 28008397; PMCID: PMC5143471.

Section

III

# Perioperative Pain

Chapter 16

# Postoperative Pain

• Virinchi Sanapala • Sumitra Bakshi

## INTRODUCTION

Optimal perioperative analgesia is a vital aspect of anesthesia, representing a key objective for perioperative physicians. Effective pain management enables surgeries to be conducted to the highest standards, minimizing patient discomfort and facilitating swift postoperative recovery for improved outcomes. Regrettably, the prevalence of moderate to severe postoperative pain within the first 24 hours after surgery remains consistently high at approximately 30–35% over the past decade,[1] showing little variation.

While the fundamental surgical principles remain consistent across oncological and non-oncological surgeries, their objectives diverge significantly. In oncological surgery, the primary goal is the complete excision of cancerous tissue with adequate margins and lymph node dissection, necessitating extensive tissue handling, multiple incisions, leading to increased surgical insults and duration of surgery both of which pose the risk of increased severity of postoperative pain in these set of patients. Factors such as preoperative pain, anxiety, opioid use, poor nutrition, and psychological distress further elevate the risk of heightened postoperative discomfort.[1,2] Notably, oncological patients often present with two or more of these factors, highlighting the need for tailored perioperative pain management strategies.

### Pre-emptive and Preventive Analgesia

Injury to peripheral tissues during surgery triggers spinal cord excitation and lowers the pain thresholds of neurons, resulting in increased pain perception during the postoperative phase. This prolonged sensitization of the spinal cord extends the duration of postoperative pain. Preemptive analgesia seeks to mitigate central sensitisation, thereby reducing postoperative pain and promoting quicker return to normal activities, by instituting pain relief before the surgical insult.

The drugs/interventions that have been evaluated initially for preemptive analgesia includes the following:

*NSAIDs:* The diminished synthesis of prostaglandins resulting from oral or parenteral NSAIDs leads to decreased inflammation at the peripheral injury site, ultimately alleviating pain. Preoperative administration of Ketorolac[3] and Celecoxib[4] has been demonstrated to yield superior analgesic effects in the postoperative phase. A single dose of etoricoxib which is more selective inhibitor of COX-2 than COX-1 prior to surgery, showed good analgesic effect in the postoperative period.[5] However, the potential drawback of pre-emptive NSAID usage is the increased risk of bleeding in the perioperative period.

*NMDA antagonists:* The NMDA receptor plays a significant role in central pain processing and neuroplasticity of the spinal cord.[6] Intravenous ketamine has been shown to decrease postoperative opioid needs effectively. When administered as a single IV bolus of 0.5 mg/kg followed by a continuous infusion of 0.25 mg/kg alongside epidural analgesia in major gastrointestinal surgeries,[7] ketamine serves as an adjunct to narcotics and epidural infusion, reducing postoperative pain.[8] A pre-incisional dose of ketamine has been associated with a decreased incidence of wound hyperalgesia in patients undergoing abdominal hysterectomy, although this reduction in secondary hyperalgesia does not necessarily translate to a decrease in postoperative pain or analgesic requirements.[9] Administering ketamine as a pre-incisional single bolus has been linked to reduced postoperative morphine consumption compared to post-closure doses in laparoscopic gynecological surgeries.[10] Epidural ketamine has been found to shorten the time to the first analgesic requirement in the postoperative period, irrespective of whether it was administered prior to or after the surgical incision.[11] Patients who received epidural ketamine also reported less postoperative pain and surgical site sensitivity.[12]

*Steroids:* Glucocorticoids (dexamethasone), known for their anti-inflammatory properties, can reduce tissue damage resulting from surgical procedures. An analgesic effect may necessitate a dose of 0.2 mg/kg,[13] while an 8 mg dose is typically recommended for postoperative pain relief in adults.[14] Additionally, they can delay the need for initial analgesia in surgeries performed under spinal anaesthesia. This carries a minimal risk of hyperglycemia following a single perioperative administration.[15]

*Opioids:* The effectiveness of intrathecal and intravenous opioids in preemptive analgesia has been inconsistent. Incisional pain stemming from hyperalgesia tends to escalate during surgery, often peaking shortly afterward. Administering a pre-incisional injection of 10 mg morphine as an IV bolus during abdominal hysterectomies has demonstrated reductions in VAS scores, postoperative opioid requirements, and secondary hyperalgesia.[16] Interestingly, no significant difference was observed between different morphine doses[17] (10 mg *vs* 20 mg). Early administration of fentanyl has also been linked to a decreased incidence of secondary hyperalgesia in abdominal hysterectomies, albeit without affecting postoperative pain scores or opioid requirements.[9] Some studies have failed to identify a notable difference between pre-incisional and post-incisional opioid administration in terms of postoperative hyperalgesia, opioid requirements, or pain scores.[18] Additionally, larger pre-incisional opioid doses may pose a risk of acute opioid tolerance. Preemptive epidural opioids have demonstrated substantial reductions in postoperative pain scores and analgesic consumption across various procedures such as thoracotomies, lumbar laminectomies, and prostatectomies.[19] Combining epidural opioids with local anaesthetics preemptively in gynecological laparotomies has been associated with decreased postoperative analgesic requirements and secondary hyperalgesia (postoperative morphine).[20] Furthermore, the synergistic effect of combining epidural opioids with ketamine preemptively results in prolonged analgesic action compared to post-incisional administration.

*Gabapentinoids:* Gabapentinoids, i.e. gabapentin and pregabalin mainly act on voltage-gated calcium channels.[21] While they function as anticonvulsants by interacting with these channels, prior meta-analyses have shown that they can enhance postoperative pain relief, albeit with sedative effects. However, recent critical studies have raised concerns about respiratory depression when gabapentinoids are combined with opioids,[22] prompting the FDA to issue a warning in December 2019.[23] Subsequent reviews and advisories have shifted away from widespread use of gabapentinoids. Elderly patients, in particular, are susceptible to these side effects, necessitating dose reduction or avoidance altogether. Nonetheless, for patients exhibiting symptoms indicative of neuropathic pain, such as a burning sensation, gabapentinoids may still offer therapeutic benefits.

*Local anesthetics:* Local anesthetics function by impeding the initiation of action potentials through the blockade of voltage-gated sodium channels, thereby halting afferent input to the spinal cord (neural blockade). They are employed for local infiltration, central neuraxial blockade, and peripheral nerve blocks. Local anaesthetics infiltration in the wound can nullify the axon reflex, thereby curtailing inflammation spread.

Administering local anesthetics for central neuraxial blockade, whether pre-incision or post-incision, has demonstrated comparable efficacy. Some studies showed no difference in postoperative analgesic requirements in patients receiving spinal[24] or epidural bupivacaine[25] irrespective of the time of administration i.e., either prior to or at the end of the surgery in patients undergoing abdominal hysterectomies. In contrast to the previous results, administering 15 ml of epidural bupivacaine before incision in lower abdominal surgeries resulted in a 25% decrease in postoperative morphine consumption through PCA (patient controlled analgesia) and improved McGill pain questionnaire ratings for up to 72 hours post-surgery.[26] The preemptive administration instead of application of epidural bupivacaine also led to increased activity and enhanced function long after discharge in patients undergoing radical prostatectomies.[27]

Pre-emptive analgesia involves administering a single analgesic treatment prior to surgery to prevent central sensitization resulting from the surgical incision, previously considered the sole noxious stimulus during the procedure. However, in prolonged surgeries, factors such as tissue handling and circulating inflammatory mediators also contribute to central and peripheral sensitization, resulting in prolonged pain perception beyond the duration of the pre-surgical analgesic intervention. The impact of tissue damage during surgery can persistently stimulate primary afferent fibers in the postoperative period for days to months. Therefore, the effectiveness and duration of the analgesic intervention become more important than its timing in alleviating postoperative pain. This realization has led to acceptance of a broader concept called preventive analgesia, aimed at controlling pain throughout the perioperative period by implementing a multimodal strategy to mitigate noxious stimuli before, during, and after surgery.[28]

Central sensitization, inhibited during surgery by central neuraxial blockade or peripheral nerve blocks, may reemerge once the blockade wears off due to persistent afferent inputs in the postoperative period likely due to significant tissue injury incurred during the surgery. Continuation of afferent blockade in the postoperative period is equally important as the time point of initiation of the blockade. Late neural blockade can reverse central sensitization and an intense postoperative analgesia prevents it from returning in the postoperative period. Major surgeries which involve intense noxious stimuli warrant a continuous analgesia with adequate afferent blockade during the surgery and even during the postoperative period. Regardless of whether initiated before or after surgery (for colonic surgeries and total knee arthroplasties), patients who received continuous epidural analgesia with bupivacaine and morphine for 48 to 72 hours in the postoperative period exhibited no disparity in analgesic needs or VAS scores.[29]

*Challenges in establishing efficacy of preemptive/preventive analgesia:* Establishing the potential advantage of preemptive treatment is challenging due to the complexities in reconciling inconsistencies among various studies.

Using opioid consumption as a sole measure to gauge the effectiveness of preemptive analgesia is not always optimal. Various patient factors such as anxiety, depression, perception of the surgical process, and overall care can influence opioid usage. Moreover, the intensity of pain and the need for analgesics do not always align. Despite several confounding variables and limitations, total opioid consumption administered via PCA devices has been the most frequently employed method to evaluate preemptive analgesia.

A surgical incision does not just trigger a singular, momentary painful stimulus; instead, it initiates a continuous influx of C fiber and A-delta fiber signals to the spinal cord. Consequently, a single pre-incisional analgesic intervention is unlikely to completely intercept this barrage throughout the postoperative recovery phase, allowing nociceptive impulses to reach the spinal cord and induce central sensitization. Additionally, the inflammatory processes triggered by the surgical incision, whether through directly released mediators or induced gene expression in injured tissues leading to mediator production, also contribute to prolonged central sensitization following surgery. The challenge lies in predicting the duration of this noxious inflammatory state and identifying the individual who is likely to develop chronic post-surgical pain. Surgical technique, patient factors, and other variables play crucial roles in altering the pain pathway, complicating comparative studies.

The efficacy of preventive analgesia is complicated by several factors. Firstly, the variation between single and continuous interventions used in studies adds complexity to the analysis. Secondly, existing evidence inclusive of reviews and meta-analyses, often fails to investigate each technique individually. Thirdly, many studies incorporate premedications, intraoperative analgesic adjuvants, and other analgesic agents, which can obscure differences between control and experimental groups. Additionally, pain assessment lacks a completely objective standard, relying on self-reported pain scales and opioid consumption, which are influenced by psychological factors. In addition, effectively blocking noxious input to the spinal cord during surgery remains elusive, despite the array of analgesic techniques available. This highlights the importance of adopting multimodal analgesia strategies for all surgical procedures.

## Multimodal Analgesia

Perioperative pain encompasses various subtypes, making it challenging to address effectively with a single analgesic. Postoperative pain can manifest as nociceptive, visceral, neuropathic or mixed, depending on the nature of the surgery. MMA is the use of combination of analgesics or techniques that target different mechanisms or pathways in the nociceptive system.[30]

Utilizing a combination of multiple drugs allows for the administration of lower doses of each individual medication, thereby minimizing the side effects associated with each drug while maintaining overall effectiveness. This approach translates to improved pain relief, enhanced functional recovery, and reduced adverse effects related to opioid usage. The American Society of Anesthesiologists (ASA), the American Pain Society (APS), and the American Society of Regional Anesthesia and Pain Medicine (ASRA) strongly advocate for the adoption of MMA in the management of acute perioperative pain, considering it the standard of care for all surgical patients.[31,32] Furthermore, enhanced recovery after surgery (ERAS) protocols emphasize the importance of opioid sparing MMA techniques.[33]

Given the opioid epidemic and widespread drug shortages, it is crucial to develop a comprehensive MMA protocol structured as a checklist rather than a rigid recipe.[30] This approach aims to standardize the selection of analgesics while maintaining flexibility to adjust individual components based on factors such as patients' medical condition, allergies, medications, and prior pain experience.

The components which form the MMA would be non-opioid analgesics, opioids and regional techniques.

## Non-opioid Analgesics

*a. Paracetamol:* Paracetamol, a drug with decades of clinical use, boasts a well-established safety record when administered at appropriate doses and exhibits a favourable perioperative side effect profile. Its primary adverse effect is severe hepatotoxicity, typically induced by the toxic metabolite N-acetyl-p-benzoquinone imine (NAPQI), resulting from either absolute overdosing or pre-existing liver dysfunction.[34] Given its opioid-sparing effects and minimal contraindications except in cases of severe liver disease, paracetamol is a crucial component in MMA protocols. Studies suggest that co-administration of paracetamol can reduce opioid consumption by up to 20%.[35] Additionally, evidence suggests that combining acetaminophen with an adjuvant nonopioid drugs such as an NSAID or COX-2 inhibitor can enhance postoperative analgesia and further decrease opioid use.[36]

*b. NSAIDs:* NSAIDs act by inhibiting COX and prostaglandin synthesis, thereby reducing inflammation at the peripheral site. Several meta-analyses have underscored the potential of NSAIDs to enhance analgesia and mitigate opioid-induced side effects.[36,37] They are recognized for providing effective pain relief for musculoskeletal pain. Despite the known risk of cardiovascular events associated with NSAIDs, a systematic review demonstrated that the efficacy of combining ibuprofen 400 mg and paracetamol 1000 mg in reducing postoperative pain.[38] The selection of NSAIDs and COX-2 inhibitor medications should be guided by both surgical considerations and patient comorbidities. Concerns regarding increased postoperative bleeding risk with NSAIDs have been addressed in a meta-analysis, which negates the belief that use of ketorolac is associated with increased incidence of perioperative bleeding risk.[39] In cases where gastrointestinal ulcers pose a specific concern, substituting a COX-2 selective inhibitor with a non-selective agent may mitigate this risk.[40] Given these considerations and in the absence of contraindications, prescription of NSAIDs or COX inhibitors in the perioperative phase is safe.

*c. NMDA antagonists:* Ketamine is widely recognized for its opioid-sparing effects[41] during the perioperative period and its potential to reduce long-term opioid use in opioid-tolerant patients,[42] as well as mitigate persistent post-surgical pain (persistent post-surgical pain).[43] Recently, the American Society of Regional Anesthesia and Pain Medicine (ASRA) issued guidelines regarding utilisation of ketamine in acute pain management. A consensus statement[32] from ASRA, AAPM, and ASA emphasized the advantages of sub-anesthetic doses of ketamine in reducing postoperative pain in various surgical scenarios, including thoracic, upper and lower abdominal, and orthopedic surgeries (both limb and spine). Infusion doses ranging from 0.35 to 1 mg/kg of ketamine have been shown to significantly reduce the incidence of psychogenic side effects associated with higher doses.[32,41] However, caution should be exercised, as ketamine should be avoided in pregnancy, diagnosed psychiatric illnesses, and uncontrolled cardiovascular disease, and used with care in patients with liver disease.

*d. Magnesium:* Magnesium has shown notable efficacy in reducing postoperative pain when utilized alongside either opioid or non-opioid analgesics, as opposed to when administered in isolation. Its mechanism of action is believed to involve spinal NMDA receptors. Typically, dosing ranges from 30 to 50 mg/kg as a bolus, with an infusion rate of 8 to 15 mg/kg/hr.[47] At therapeutic doses, magnesium demonstrates a favourable safety profile, with a minimal risk of hypermagnesemia in patients with renal disease.[45]

*e. Alpha-2 agonists:* Alpha-2 agonists offer a range of effects including sedation, analgesia, anxiolysis, and hypnosis, which collectively reduce opioid consumption and enhance postoperative pain management.[46] Their efficacy as analgesics and hypnotics without inducing respiratory depression underscores their importance as integral components of MMA.

***Clonidine:*** Clonidine can be administered via various routes, such as intravenous, transdermal, perineural and neuraxial, demonstrating efficacy in reducing opioid[46] and minimum alveolar concentration (MAC) requirements, and serving as an important additive to local anesthetics in regional blocks.[47] However, the POISE 2 trial revealed an increased risk of hypotension and non-fatal cardiac arrest with routine clonidine administration in non-cardiac surgical patients.[48]

***Dexmedetomidine:*** Dexmedetomidine has been extensively utilized perioperatively, showing promise as an additive to intraoperative analgesics and as an adjunct to neuraxial and regional blocks. It has been associated with a 30% reduction in opioid requirements,[46] pain intensity, and nausea, without impacting recovery times, positioning it as a crucial component in Enhanced Recovery After Surgery (ERAS) protocols for different surgical procedures.[49] Despite its efficacy, hypotension and bradycardia are common side effects. Intravenous administration is typical, with bolus doses ranging from 0.25 to 1 μg/kg over 10 minutes, and infusion rates between 0.2 and 0.6 μg/kg/hr. Adjustments may be necessary based on patient hemodynamic, and diligent monitoring is imperative due to its cardiovascular effects. For analgesic purposes, the initial dose should be reduced to 0.5 μg/kg body weight.

*f. Local anesthetic agents*

***Intravenous administration:*** Lignocaine administered intravenously has demonstrated efficacy in reducing postoperative pain and opioid consumption following abdominal and spine surgeries.[50] Additionally, it has been shown to expedite the return of bowel function post-surgery.[51] However, its use in breast surgeries has not significantly improved postoperative pain, though a reduction in persistent postsurgical pain has been noted.[52] Given its cost-effectiveness, intravenous lignocaine infusion is considered a crucial component of Enhanced Recovery After Surgery (ERAS) protocols for abdominal surgeries where neuraxial blockade is contraindicated.[53]

***Local infiltration:*** Local infiltration of the surgical incision site with a local anesthetic agent has shown some benefits in providing analgesia, albeit with short-lived effects. While it has been attempted in laparoscopic cholecystectomies,[54] the extent of analgesia provided is limited. Conversely, intra-articular infiltrations for orthopedic surgeries have demonstrated significant benefits in pain relief and promoting early postoperative ambulation.[55] Incorporating local infiltration techniques into the overall (MMA) strategy for surgeries can be beneficial.

*g. Regional anesthesia techniques:* Although the trend has shifted towards (MMA), there remains a notable reliance on opioids in specific patient populations, considering the risk profiles of each pharmacological component of MMA. Regional techniques, when added to the MMA regimen, offer significant opioid-sparing effects during the perioperative period compared to other components.

The Enhanced Recovery After Surgery (ERAS) guidelines advocate its implementation whenever possible during the perioperative period. In major abdominal surgeries, the debate over the efficacy of fascial plane blocks versus thoracic epidural analgesia (TEA) has intensified in recent years. A significant dilemma arises regarding the choice between thoracic epidural analgesia (TEA) and fascial plane blocks as reliable analgesic approaches for major abdominal surgeries. The abdomen, with both visceral and somatic innervation, exhibits a complex pain perception mechanism. The contribution of the visceral component to the overall perceived pain varies, influenced by factors such as the extent of resection and tissue handling during surgery. While visceral pain, except in pancreatic surgery,[56] is traditionally considered less severe and of shorter duration, its significance should not be underestimated. Some studies suggest that visceral pain is subjectively more unpleasant than somatic pain.

### Thoracic Epidural Analgesia

Thoracic epidural analgesia (TEA) offers comprehensive pain relief for both somatic and visceral pain components. Compared to opioid-based analgesia, TEA recipients benefit from faster extubation times, shorter ICU and hospital stays, reduced rates of postoperative respiratory failure, decreased mortality, lower incidence of postoperative delirium, superior pain management, and earlier restoration of gastrointestinal function.[57,58] However, TEA comes with a reported failure rate of 31% and potential complications such as spinal hematomas, epidural abscesses, lower limb weakness, radicular pain, dural puncture, and hypotension.[59] Its use may interfere with Enhanced Recovery After Surgery (ERAS) protocols, potentially causing hypotension and lower limb weakness, hindering patient mobility postoperatively. Moreover, urinary retention associated with TEA might prolong the need for urinary catheterization. TEA-induced sympathectomy reduces myocardial oxygen demand, lowering the risk of postoperative myocardial infarction. However, splanchnic vasodilation may improve gut perfusion and motility while reducing preload, necessitating increased vasopressor support and fluid administration. Yet, excessive fluid infusion may result in intestinal edema and subsequent surgical complications.[60]

### Fascial Plane Blocks

Fascial plane blocks, targeting the thoracoabdominal nerves innervating the abdominal wall, necessitate substantial volumes of local anesthetic and precise ultrasound guidance. Commonly employed in abdominal surgeries are erector spinae plane blocks, rectus sheath blocks, transversus abdominis plane blocks, and quadratus lumborum blocks. Despite a reported failure rate of approximately 7%, influenced by factors such as surgical trauma, scarring from prior surgeries, and anatomical nerve variations, these blocks generally demonstrate a lower failure rate than thoracic epidural analgesia (TEA). However, bilateral plane block recipients face an elevated risk of local anesthetic systemic toxicity due to the high volumes.

### Comparison of Various Fascial Plane Blocks with Thoracic Epidural Analgesia (TEA)

The comparison between TEA and fascial plane blocks lacks robust, large-scale randomized controlled trials (RCTs), and existing evidence primarily focuses on short-term outcomes, warranting further research into longer-term and functional effects. As minimally invasive surgical techniques become more prevalent, the population undergoing major open abdominal surgeries will decrease, posing challenges to studying this patient cohort. Here are few comparisons of outcomes between the cohorts.

### Rectus Sheath Block

The rectus sheath block involves administering a local anesthetic between the posterior rectus sheath and the rectus abdominis muscle, providing somatic analgesia for midline and paramedial incisions of the abdominal wall. Comparative studies with TEA have shown similar pain scores in patients undergoing colorectal, urological, gastrointestinal, hepatobiliary, and gynecological surgeries.[61] However, TEA exhibited a superior opioid-sparing effect, albeit with a higher incidence of hypotension and longer time to mobilization. No significant differences were found in the duration of hospital stay or ICU stay.

### Transversus Abdominis Plane (TAP) Block

The TAP block involves administering a local anesthetic in the plane between the internal oblique and transversus abdominis muscles, providing coverage from T10 to L1. A lateral approach improves block coverage, while a subcostal approach targets T6 to T9.[62] Comparative studies with TEA have yielded conflicting results, with no major differences in patient satisfaction scores. Most studies[63] demonstrate comparable pain scores, quality of recovery, patient satisfaction, and duration of hospital stay between TAP and TEA groups, with TEA associated with a higher incidence of hypotension and better opioid sparing. PROSPECT guidelines recommend either subcostal TAP or TEA for open liver surgeries, suggesting comparable analgesic efficacy.[64] Even ERAS guidelines for liver surgeries prefer fascial plane blocks over TEA.[65]

### Quadratus Lumborum Block (QLB)

The QLB involves administering a local anesthetic around the quadratus lumborum muscle using various approaches. QLB has shown superiority over other fascial plane

**Table 16.1: Visceral innervation of solid organs**

| Viscera | Visceral innervation |
|---|---|
| Stomach and pancreas | T5–T9—celiac ganglia<br>Cranial nerve X—vagus nerve |
| Liver | T5–T9—celiac ganglia<br>C3–C5—phrenic ganglia<br>Cranial nerve X—vagus nerve |
| Small and large intestine | T5–T9—celiac ganglia<br>T9–T12—superior mesenteric ganglia<br>L1–L2—inferior mesenteric ganglia<br>Cranial Nerve X—vagus nerve |
| Kidney and ureter | T10–T12—least and lesser thoracic nerves<br>Cranial nerve X–vagus nerve |
| Pelvic viscera | T11–L4 |
| Bladder | S2–S4—pelvic splanchnic nerves<br>L1–L2—upper lumbar splanchnic nerves |

blocks for major abdominal surgeries.[66] Although literature comparing QLB with TEA is limited, some randomized controlled trials have demonstrated QLB to be non-inferior to TEA in patients undergoing open liver and renal surgeries.[67]

### Erector Spinae Plane (ESP) Block

The ESP block entails instilling a local anesthetic in the plane between the erector spinae muscle and the transverse processes, representing a relatively newer approach for abdominal surgeries. ESP provides better analgesia compared to TAP block and exhibits a similar analgesic profile to QLB.[68] In comparison with TEA, ESP has shown slightly superior analgesia in patients undergoing hepatectomies, along with a better opioid-sparing effect in hepato-pancreatobiliary surgeries.[69] Additionally, ESP is associated with a lower incidence of hypotension and reduced colloid usage compared to TEA.

## Acute Pain Services

Acute pain services (APS) have evolved significantly over the past 35 years, transitioning from initially focusing solely on postoperative pain management to providing comprehensive care throughout the perioperative period.[70] These dedicated healthcare personnel-driven services assess, monitor, and treat pain and the side effects of various analgesics on a 24-hour basis.[71] Evidence-based protocols tailored to specific surgeries and local environments are now applied consistently across institutions, promoting quality standards, minimizing care fragmentation, reducing variability, and encouraging patient participation in decision-making. Enhanced Recovery After Surgery (ERAS) pathways, which emphasize multidisciplinary, procedure-specific care using evidence-based practices to reduce postoperative complications and facilitate early recovery, highlight the pivotal role of APS in achieving optimal outcomes.[72] Effective pain management remains a cornerstone, essential for facilitating early mobilization, shortening hospital stays, and ensuring patient satisfaction. APS, when integrated into multimodal rehabilitation pathways, contribute to value by promoting good pain control, reducing opioid consumption, and facilitating rapid return to normal activities. Recognizing pain management as a fundamental human right and ethical principle underscores the importance of APS not merely as revenue generators but as cost-saving entities. Patient-reported outcome measures serve as crucial quality indicators, encompassing factors such as lack of complications, early ambulation, oral feeding, maximized function, satisfaction, and long-term outcomes. A cohesive approach integrating surgical and anesthesia services within hospitals, exemplified by programs like ERAS or perioperative surgical home, ensures patient-centred care with pain management as a central focus throughout the continuum of care, thereby mitigating the socioeconomic burden of chronic postsurgical pain transition.[70]

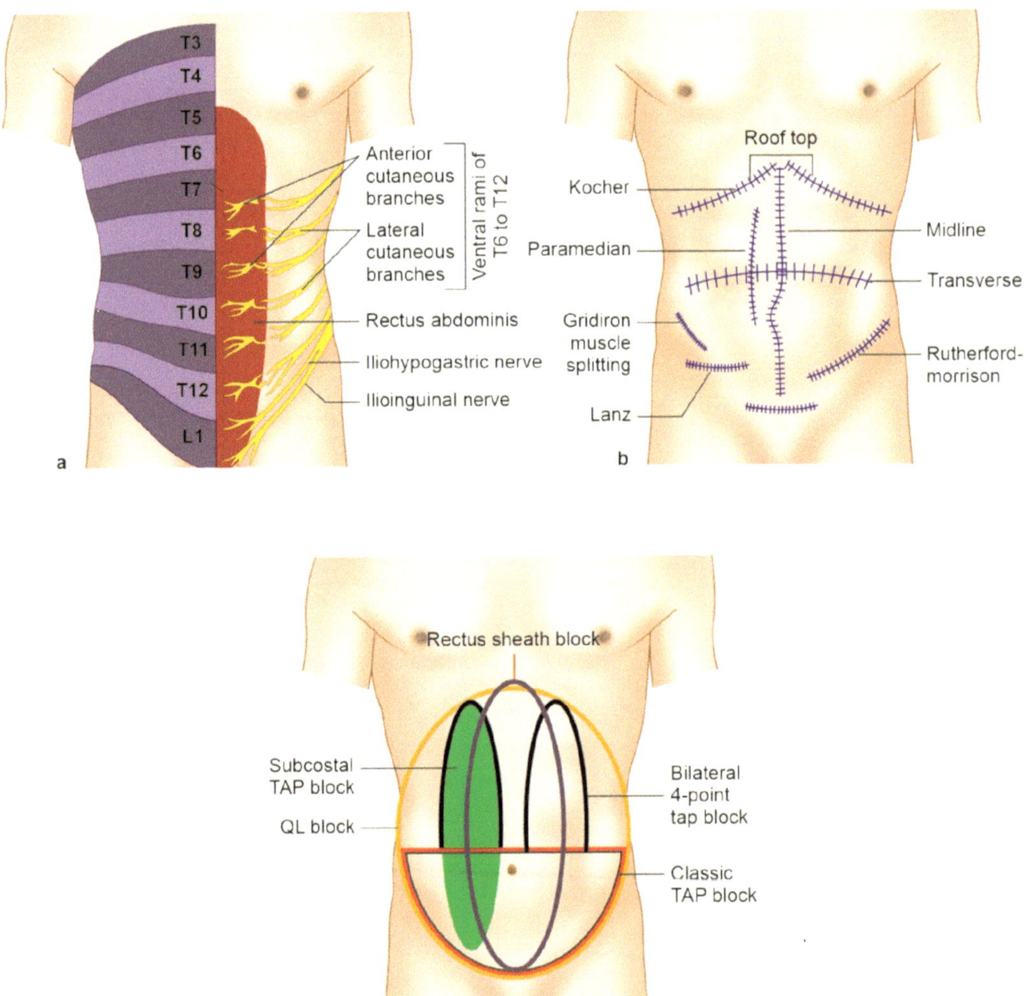


Fig. 16.1: Dermatomal coverage of various fascial plane blocks

## References


1. Park R, Mohiuddin M, Arellano R, Pogatzki-Zahn E, Klar G, Gilron I. Prevalence of postoperative pain after hospital discharge: systematic review and meta-analysis. Pain Rep. 2023 May 8;8(3):e1075.
2. Ip HYV, Abrishami A, Peng PWH, Wong J, Chung F. Predictors of Postoperative Pain and Analgesic Consumption: A Qualitative Systematic Review. Anesthesiology. 2009 Sep 1;111(3):657–77.
3. Norman PH, Daley MD, Lindsey RW. Preemptive analgesic effects of ketorolac in ankle fracture surgery. Anesthesiology. 2001 Apr;94(4):599–603.
4. Senard M, Deflandre EP, Ledoux D, Roediger L, Hubert BM, Radermecker M, et al. Effect of celecoxib combined with thoracic epidural analgesia on pain after thoracotomy. Br J Anaesth. 2010 Aug;105(2):196–200.
5. Clarke R, Derry S, Moore RA. Single dose oral etoricoxib for acute postoperative pain in adults. The Cochrane Database of Systematic Reviews [Internet]. 2014 [cited 2024 Mar 21];2014(5). Available from: https://www.ncbi.nlm.nih.gov/pmc/articles/PMC6485336/
6. Naranjo JoséR, Mellström B, Achaval M, Sassone-Corsit P. Molecular pathways of pain: Fos/Jun-mediated activation of a noncanonical AP-1 site in the prodynorphin gene. Neuron. 1991 Apr 1;6(4):607–17.
7. Lavand'homme P, De Kock M, Waterloos H. Intraoperative epidural analgesia combined with ketamine provides effective preventive analgesia in patients undergoing major digestive surgery. Anesthesiology. 2005 Oct;103(4):813–20.
8. Subramaniam K, Subramaniam B, Steinbrook RA. Ketamine as adjuvant analgesic to opioids: a quantitative and qualitative systematic review. Anesth Analg. 2004 Aug;99(2):482–95, table of contents.
9. Tverskoy M, Oz Y, Isakson A, Finger J, Bradley EL, Kissin I. Preemptive effect of fentanyl and ketamine on postoperative pain and wound hyperalgesia. Anesth Analg. 1994 Feb;78(2):205–9.
10. Kwok RFK, Lim J, Chan MTV, Gin T, Chiu WKY. Preoperative ketamine improves postoperative analgesia after gynecologic laparoscopic surgery. Anesth Analg. 2004 Apr;98(4):1044–9.
11. Wong CS, Lu CC, Cherng CH, Ho ST. Pre-emptive analgesia with ketamine, morphine and epidural lidocaine prior to total knee replacement. Can J Anaesth. 1997 Jan;44(1):31–7.
12. Wilson JA, Nimmo AF, Fleetwood-Walker SM, Colvin LA. A randomised double blind trial of the effect of pre-emptive epidural ketamine on persistent pain after lower limb amputation. Pain. 2008 Mar;135(1–2):108–18.
13. De Oliveira GS, Almeida MD, Benzon HT, McCarthy RJ. Perioperative single dose systemic dexamethasone for postoperative pain: a meta-analysis of randomized controlled trials. Anesthesiology. 2011 Sep;115(3):575–88.
14. Waldron NH, Jones CA, Gan TJ, Allen TK, Habib AS. Impact of perioperative dexamethasone on postoperative analgesia and side-effects: systematic review and meta-analysis. Br J Anaesth. 2013 Feb;110(2):191–200.
15. Herbst RA, Telford OT, Hunting J, Bullock WM, Manning E, Hong BD, et al. The effects of perioperative dexamethasone on glycemic control and postoperative outcomes. Endocr Pract. 2020 Feb;26(2):218–25.
16. Richmond CE, Bromley LM, Woolf CJ. Preoperative morphine pre-empts postoperative pain. Lancet. 1993 Jul 10;342(8863):73–5.
17. Collis R, Brandner B, Bromley LM, Woolf CJ. Is there any clinical advantage of increasing the pre-emptive dose of morphine or combining pre-incisional with postoperative morphine administration? Br J Anaesth. 1995 Apr;74(4):396–9.
18. Mansfield M, Meikle R, Miller C. A trial of pre-emptive analgesia. Influence of timing of peroperative alfentanil on postoperative pain and analgesic requirements. Anaesthesia. 1994 Dec;49(12):1091–3.

19. Katz J, Kavanagh BP, Sandler AN, Nierenberg H, Boylan JF, Friedlander M, et al. Preemptive analgesia. Clinical evidence of neuroplasticity contributing to postoperative pain. Anesthesiology. 1992 Sep;77(3):439–46.
20. Katz J, Cohen L, Schmid R, Chan VWS, Wowk A. Postoperative morphine use and hyperalgesia are reduced by preoperative but not intraoperative epidural analgesia: implications for preemptive analgesia and the prevention of central sensitization. Anesthesiology. 2003 Jun;98(6):1449–60.
21. Tiippana EM, Hamunen K, Kontinen VK, Kalso E. Do surgical patients benefit from perioperative gabapentin/pregabalin? A systematic review of efficacy and safety. Anesth Analg. 2007 Jun;104(6):1545–56, table of contents.
22. Savelloni J, Gunter H, Lee KC, Hsu C, Yi C, Edmonds KP, et al. Risk of respiratory depression with opioids and concomitant gabapentinoids. J Pain Res. 2017;10:2635–41.
23. Kharasch ED, Clark JD, Kheterpal S. Perioperative Gabapentinoids: Deflating the Bubble. Anesthesiology. 2020 Aug;133(2):251–4.
24. Dakin MJ, Osinubi OY, Carli F. Preoperative spinal bupivacaine does not reduce postoperative morphine requirement in women undergoing total abdominal hysterectomy. Reg Anesth. 1996;21(2):99–102.
25. Pryle BJ, Vanner RG, Enriquez N, Reynolds F. Can pre-emptive lumbar epidural blockade reduce postoperative pain following lower abdominal surgery? Anaesthesia. 1993 Feb;48(2):120–3.
26. Katz J, Clairoux M, Kavanagh BP, Roger S, Nierenberg H, Redahan C, et al. Pre-emptive lumbar epidural anaesthesia reduces postoperative pain and patient-controlled morphine consumption after lower abdominal surgery. Pain. 1994 Dec;59(3):395–403.
27. Gottschalk A, Smith DS, Jobes DR, Kennedy SK, Lally SE, Noble VE, et al. Preemptive epidural analgesia and recovery from radical prostatectomy: a randomized controlled trial. JAMA. 1998 Apr 8;279(14):1076–82.
28. Vadivelu N, Mitra S, Schermer E, Kodumudi V, Kaye AD, Urman RD. Preventive analgesia for postoperative pain control: a broader concept. Local Reg Anesth. 2014 May 29;7:17–22.
29. Dahl JB, Hansen BL, Hjortsø NC, Erichsen CJ, Møiniche S, Kehlet H. Influence of timing on the effect of continuous extradural analgesia with bupivacaine and morphine after major abdominal surgery. Br J Anaesth. 1992 Jul;69(1):4–8.
30. Schwenk ES, Mariano ER. Designing the ideal perioperative pain management plan starts with multimodal analgesia. Korean J Anesthesiol. 2018 Oct;71(5):345–52.
31. Guidelines Emphasize Need for Multimodal, Individualized Care for Surgery Patients [Internet]. [cited 2024 Feb 28]. Available from: https://www.asahq.org/about-asa/newsroom/news-releases/2021/09/guidelines-emphasize-need-for-multimodal-individualized-care-for-surgery-patients
32. Schwenk ES, Viscusi ER, Buvanendran A, Hurley RW, Wasan AD, Narouze S, et al. Consensus Guidelines on the Use of Intravenous Ketamine Infusions for Acute Pain Management From the American Society of Regional Anesthesia and Pain Medicine, the American Academy of Pain Medicine, and the American Society of Anesthesiologists. Reg Anesth Pain Med. 2018 Jul;43(5):456–66.
33. Enhanced Recovery After Surgery (ERAS) for gastrointestinal surgery, part 2: consensus statement for anaesthesia practice - PubMed [Internet]. [cited 2023 Jan 11]. Available from: https://pubmed.ncbi.nlm.nih.gov/26514824/
34. Mattia C, Coluzzi F. What anesthesiologists should know about paracetamol (acetaminophen). Minerva Anestesiol. 2009 Nov;75(11):644–53.
35. Remy C, Marret E, Bonnet F. Effects of acetaminophen on morphine side-effects and consumption after major surgery: meta-analysis of randomized controlled trials. Br J Anaesth. 2005 Apr;94(4):505–13.
36. Martinez V, Beloeil H, Marret E, Fletcher D, Ravaud P, Trinquart L. Non-opioid analgesics in adults after major surgery: systematic review with network meta-analysis of randomized trials. Br J Anaesth. 2017 Jan;118(1):22–31.

37. Marret E, Kurdi O, Zufferey P, Bonnet F. Effects of nonsteroidal antiinflammatory drugs on patient-controlled analgesia morphine side effects: meta-analysis of randomized controlled trials. Anesthesiology. 2005 Jun;102(6):1249–60.
38. Derry CJ, Derry S, Moore RA. Single dose oral ibuprofen plus paracetamol (acetaminophen) for acute postoperative pain. Cochrane Database Syst Rev. 2013 Jun 24;2013(6):CD010210.
39. Gobble RM, Hoang HLT, Kachniarz B, Orgill DP. Ketorolac does not increase perioperative bleeding: a meta-analysis of randomized controlled trials. Plast Reconstr Surg. 2014 Mar;133(3):741–55.
40. Rostom A, Muir K, Dubé C, Jolicoeur E, Boucher M, Joyce J, et al. Gastrointestinal safety of cyclooxygenase-2 inhibitors: a Cochrane Collaboration systematic review. Clin Gastroenterol Hepatol. 2007 Jul;5(7):818–28, 828.e1-5; quiz 768.
41. Laskowski K, Stirling A, McKay WP, Lim HJ. A systematic review of intravenous ketamine for postoperative analgesia. Can J Anaesth. 2011 Oct;58(10):911–23.
42. Loftus RW, Yeager MP, Clark JA, Brown JR, Abdu WA, Sengupta DK, et al. Intraoperative ketamine reduces perioperative opiate consumption in opiate-dependent patients with chronic back pain undergoing back surgery. Anesthesiology. 2010 Sep;113(3):639–46.
43. McNicol ED, Schumann R, Haroutounian S. A systematic review and meta-analysis of ketamine for the prevention of persistent post-surgical pain. Acta Anaesthesiol Scand. 2014 Nov;58(10):1199–213.
44. Rodríguez-Rubio L, Nava E, Del Pozo JSG, Jordán J. Influence of the perioperative administration of magnesium sulfate on the total dose of anesthetics during general anesthesia. A systematic review and meta-analysis. J Clin Anesth. 2017 Jun;39:129–38.
45. Bujalska-Zadro ny M, Tatarkiewicz J, Kulik K, Filip M, Naruszewicz M. Magnesium enhances opioid-induced analgesia - What we have learnt in the past decades? Eur J Pharm Sci. 2017 Mar 1;99:113–27.
46. Blaudszun G, Lysakowski C, Elia N, Tramèr MR. Effect of perioperative systemic 2 agonists on postoperative morphine consumption and pain intensity: systematic review and meta-analysis of randomized controlled trials. Anesthesiology. 2012 Jun;116(6):1312–22.
47. Nguyen V, Tiemann D, Park E, Salehi A. Alpha-2 Agonists. Anesthesiol Clin. 2017 Jun;35(2):233–45.
48. Devereaux PJ, Sessler DI, Leslie K, Kurz A, Mrkobrada M, Alonso-Coello P, et al. Clonidine in patients undergoing noncardiac surgery. N Engl J Med. 2014 Apr 17;370(16):1504–13.
49. Kaye AD, Chernobylsky DJ, Thakur P, Siddaiah H, Kaye RJ, Eng LK, et al. Dexmedetomidine in Enhanced Recovery After Surgery (ERAS) Protocols for Postoperative Pain. Curr Pain Headache Rep. 2020;24(5):21.
50. Farag E, Ghobrial M, Sessler DI, Dalton JE, Liu J, Lee JH, et al. Effect of perioperative intravenous lidocaine administration on pain, opioid consumption, and quality of life after complex spine surgery. Anesthesiology. 2013 Oct;119(4):932–40.
51. Weibel S, Jokinen J, Pace NL, Schnabel A, Hollmann MW, Hahnenkamp K, et al. Efficacy and safety of intravenous lidocaine for postoperative analgesia and recovery after surgery: a systematic review with trial sequential analysis. Br J Anaesth. 2016 Jun;116(6):770–83.
52. Chang YC, Liu CL, Liu TP, Yang PS, Chen MJ, Cheng SP. Effect of Perioperative Intravenous Lidocaine Infusion on Acute and Chronic Pain after Breast Surgery: A Meta-Analysis of Randomized Controlled Trials. Pain Pract. 2017 Mar;17(3):336–43.
53. Naik BI, Tsang S, Knisely A, Yerra S, Durieux ME. Retrospective case-control non-inferiority analysis of intravenous lidocaine in a colorectal surgery enhanced recovery program. BMC Anesthesiology. 2017 Jan 31;17(1):16.
54. Loizides S, Gurusamy KS, Nagendran M, Rossi M, Guerrini GP, Davidson BR. Wound infiltration with local anaesthetic agents for laparoscopic cholecystectomy. Cochrane Database Syst Rev. 2014 Mar 12;(3):CD007049.
55. Perlas A, Kirkham KR, Billing R, Tse C, Brull R, Gandhi R, et al. The impact of analgesic modality on early ambulation following total knee arthroplasty. Reg Anesth Pain Med. 2013;38(4):334–9.
56. Analgesia for the Trunk: A Comparison of Epidural, Thoracic Paravertebral and Transversus Abdominis Plane Blocks | IntechOpen [Internet]. [cited 2024 Mar 20]. Available from: https://www.intechopen.com/chapters/46065

57. Epidural pain relief versus systemic opioid-based pain relief for abdominal aortic surgery - Guay, J - 2016 | Cochrane Library [Internet]. [cited 2024 Mar 20]. Available from: https://www.cochranelibrary.com/cdsr/doi/10.1002/14651858.CD005059.pub4/full
58. Epidural local anaesthetics versus opioid-based analgesic regimens for postoperative gastrointestinal paralysis, vomiting and pain after abdominal surgery - Guay, J - 2016 | Cochrane Library [Internet]. [cited 2024 Mar 20]. Available from: https://www.cochranelibrary.com/cdsr/doi/10.1002/14651858.CD001893.pub2/full
59. Ready LB. Acute pain: Lessons learned from 25,000 patients. Regional Anesthesia and Pain Medicine. 1999 Nov 1;24(6):499–505.
60. Chekol WB, Melesse DY, Denu ZA, Tawuye HY. Evidence-based thoracic epidural nerve block: A systematic review. International Journal of Surgery Open [Internet]. 2020 Jan 1 [cited 2024 Aug 27];24:151–5. Available from: https://www.sciencedirect.com/science/article/pii/S2405857220300322
61. Carver A, Wou F, Pawa A. Do Outcomes Differ Between Thoracic Epidurals and Continuous Fascial Plane Blocks in Adults Undergoing Major Abdominal Surgery? Curr Anesthesiol Rep. 2024 Mar 1;14(1):25–41.
62. Furuya T, Kato J, Yamamoto Y, Hirose N, Suzuki T. Comparison of dermatomal sensory block following ultrasound-guided transversus abdominis plane block by the lateral and posterior approaches: A randomized controlled trial. J Anaesthesiol Clin Pharmacol. 2018;34(2):205–10.
63. Perioperative transversus abdominis plane (TAP) blocks for analgesia after abdominal surgery- Osborn, S - 2020 | Cochrane Library [Internet]. [cited 2024 Mar 20]. Available from: https://www.cochranelibrary.com/cdsr/doi/10.1002/14651858.CD007705.pub3/full
64. Pain management after open liver resection: Procedure-Specific Postoperative Pain Management (PROSPECT) recommendations | Regional Anesthesia & Pain Medicine [Internet]. [cited 2024 Mar 20]. Available from: https://rapm.bmj.com/content/46/5/433
65. Joliat GR, Kobayashi K, Hasegawa K, Thomson JE, Padbury R, Scott M, et al. Guidelines for Perioperative Care for Liver Surgery: Enhanced Recovery After Surgery (ERAS) Society Recommendations 2022. World Journal of Surgery. 2023;47(1):11.
66. Ultrasound-guided quadratus lumborum block | JPR [Internet]. [cited 2024 Mar 20]. Available from: https://www.dovepress.com/ultrasound-guided-quadratus-lumborum-block-at-the-lateral-supra-arcuat-peer-reviewed-fulltext-article-JPR
67. Subcostal Anterior Quadratus Lumborum Block Versus Epidural... : Anesthesia & Analgesia [Internet]. [cited 2024 Mar 20]. Available from: https://journals.lww.com/anesthesia-analgesia/fulltext/2021/04000/subcostal_anterior_quadratus_lumborum_block_versus.26.aspx
68. Pawa A, King C, Thang C, White L. Erector spinae plane block: the ultimate 'plan A' block? British Journal of Anaesthesia. 2023 May 1;130(5):497–502.
69. Cureus | Comparison of Continuous Thoracic Epidural With Erector Spinae Block for Postoperative Analgesia in Adult Living Donor Hepatectomy | Article [Internet]. [cited 2024 Mar 20]. Available from: https://www.cureus.com/articles/89711-comparison-of-continuous-thoracic-epidural-with-erector-spinae-block-for-postoperative-analgesia-in-adult-living-donor-hepatectomy#!/
70. Stamer UM, Liguori GA, Rawal N. Thirty-five Years of Acute Pain Services: Where Do We Go From Here? Anesthesia and Analgesia. 2020 Aug;131(2):650.
71. Jain PN, Bakshi SG, Thota RS. Acute pain services in India: A glimpse of the current scenario. J Anaesthesiol Clin Pharmacol. 2015;31(4):554–7.
72. Home-ERAS® Society [Internet]. [cited 2024 Mar 20]. Available from: https://erassociety.org/

Chapter 17

# Controversies in the Use of Opioids in the Postoperative Period

• Pravin Dhakane • Sumitra Bakshi

## INTRODUCTION

The management of pain is paramount in the postoperative period. Opioids have an important role in the management of acute surgical pain due to their potent analgesic properties. However, in recent years, controversies surrounding their usage have increased due to concerns regarding delayed recovery, addiction, misuse, and various other adverse effects.[1] In this chapter, we will cover the controversies surrounding the use of opioids in the postoperative period, exploring both the benefits and risks associated with their administration.

### Routes of Administration

Opioids can be delivered through various routes, each characterized by a distinct onset of action, duration, and potential side effects. Intravenous, oral, neuraxial and transdermal routes are commonly utilized for postoperative pain management.[2]

In the immediate postoperative period, the intravenous route is frequently preferred in the recovery room due to its rapid onset of action.[2] Some of the common opioids administered intravenously, in our country includes fentanyl, morphine, tramadol, butorphanol, nalbuphine and pethidine. Administration of intravenous opioids in monitored areas is essential due to its potential risk of sedation and respiratory depression. Fentanyl a synthetic derivative of morphine, exhibits greater potency and a shorter onset of action (within 60 seconds, with peak action in 2 to 5 minutes) compared to morphine (onset within 1 to 2 minutes, with peak action in 5 to 15 minutes).[2–4] Patient-controlled analgesia (PCA) system is a practical way for intravenous opioid administration, with morphine and fentanyl commonly used in PCA pumps.[2] This approach provides patients with increased autonomy and control over their pain management. However, patients and healthcare staff must undergo training for properly utilizing PCA equipment.[5] Clinical trials comparing intravenous opioid PCA with conventional intravenous "as needed" opioid administration have shown that intravenous PCA provides superior analgesic effects and is preferred by patients based on satisfaction scores.[6]

Once patients resume oral intake in the postoperative period, tramadol and tapentadol may be initiated in the tablet form. It is the preferred route of administration in the postoperative period as it negates the need for an intravenous line, increased patient convenience, and lower cost.[2] These medications can be administered either on a scheduled basis or as needed. The typical oral doses for tramadol and tapentadol range from 50 mg to 100 mg 6–8 hourly, with a maximum of 400 mg within a 24-hour period.[7]

Opioids can also be administered via epidural or intrathecal routes for postoperative analgesia. When opioids are delivered intrathecally or epidurally, they target opioid receptors within the spinal cord, resulting in a more localized effect.[8] Consequently, smaller doses are needed to attain the same level of pain relief as systemic doses, leading to effective pain control with fewer side effects. In epidural analgesia, a catheter is inserted into the epidural space at either the thoracic or lumbar level depending on surgical incision. The addition of opioids with local anesthetics enhances the quality of postoperative epidural analgesia.[2] However, the insertion of epidural catheters presents technical challenges, and despite adequate placement, around 27% of patients experience inadequate analgesia following lumbar insertion and 32% after thoracic insertion.[9] Patients who achieve successful analgesia with continuous epidural infusion may have hypotension, necessitating the administration of additional intravenous fluids. To mitigate such risks, a combination of local anesthetic and opioid can be delivered via a patient-controlled epidural pump, which reduces the required dosage compared to continuous epidural infusion.[10] Administering opioids intrathecally before anesthesia induction offers effective postoperative analgesia for up to 24 hours. This approach proves beneficial when epidural catheter placement is challenging or when difficulties with catheter removal are anticipated in the postoperative period. Among the drugs used, morphine, typically administered at doses ranging from 50 to 500 μg and is most commonly used opioid.[10,11] The duration of analgesia varies based on the type of opioid utilized. Lipophilic opioids like fentanyl generally offer short-term pain control, typically lasting from 1 to 4 hours.[12] In contrast, hydrophilic opioids such as morphine can provide analgesia for up to 24 hours.[5,8,10,13]

Transdermal drug delivery offers a promising, non-invasive approach for the safe and effective administration of opioids. One notable advantage of transdermal opioids is their ability to maintain consistent analgesia without fluctuations in plasma concentration.[14] Conventional transdermal delivery systems depends on passive diffusion to provide effective analgesia. However, the slow absorption process of conventional transdermal patches makes them unsuitable for administering on-demand doses. Therefore, this route is inappropriate with the conventional patches in the postoperative setting, this limitation arises because while pain diminishes over time, fixed-dose transdermal systems continue to deliver medication, potentially leading to respiratory depression and sedation. Advancements in technology have led to the development of an active transdermal fentanyl delivery system utilizing iontophoresis for acute postoperative pain management. The fentanyl HCl iontophoretic transdermal system broadens the scope of transdermal drug delivery to acute pain scenarios, enabling patients to self-administer pre-programmed doses of fentanyl non-invasively. Iontophoresis involves using an electric current to propel ionized drug molecules across the skin and into the systemic circulation. Compared to existing PCA methods, the fentanyl iontophoretic system provides numerous clinical advantages. Its delivery mechanism reduces the risks associated with needle related injuries and infections, while its pre-programmed mechanism reduce the likelihood of dosing errors. Additionally, the system's compact design may facilitate greater patient mobility following surgery.[15] Furthermore, this approach also avoids first-pass drug metabolism by the liver, enhances patient adherence, and offers greater convenience and comfort.[14]

Intramuscular (IM) and subcutaneous (SC) administration in the postoperative period are not recommended due to their painful nature and slower onset of action.[2]

### Benefits

Opioids play a crucial role in managing pain during the postoperative period, offering several benefits to patients recovering from surgery. Firstly, opioids provide effective pain relief, which is essential for ensuring patient comfort and facilitating recovery. By alleviating pain, opioids enable patients to participate better in their physiotherapy and rehabilitation, promoting mobility and preventing complications associated with immobility such as deep vein thrombosis and pneumonia. Moreover, adequate pain control with opioids can enhance patient satisfaction and overall quality of life during the recovery process. Additionally, opioids are versatile medications that can be administered through various routes, allowing the anesthesiologist to use pain management regimens to meet individual patient needs. While opioids are associated with potential adverse effects and risks, when used judiciously and in conjunction with multimodal analgesia approaches, their benefits in managing postoperative pain often outweigh the risks.[16] In situations where non-opioid analgesics such as paracetamol or non-steroidal anti-inflammatory drugs (NSAIDs) are contraindicated or ineffective, opioids offer the best alternative option. Overall, opioids stand as valuable tools in the armamentarium of postoperative pain management, aiding in enhanced patient outcomes and facilitating a smoother recovery process following surgery.[17]

### Adverse Effects

Adverse effects associated with opioids may include respiratory depression, which is more prevalent in patients with obstructive sleep apnea (OSA) and long-standing respiratory diseases. Nausea, vomiting, pruritus, ileus (which may lead to anastomotic leak),[1] constipation, and urinary retention are also potential adverse effects. Additionally, sedation and cognitive impairment may occur, particularly in elderly patients.[18] Mu receptors are primarily located in the brainstem and medial thalamus. Mu 1 receptor activation is responsible for analgesia, while Mu 2 receptor activation causes sedation, vomiting, respiratory depression, pruritus, euphoria, anorexia, and urinary retention. Spinal analgesia results from the activation of delta receptors. Kappa receptors, found in various brain areas and the spinal cord, contribute to analgesia, sedation, psychomimetic effects, miosis, respiratory depression, euphoria, dysphoria, and dyspnea. Opioids, to varying extents, may inhibit N-methyl-D-aspartate (NMDA) receptors, activating descending serotonin and noradrenaline pain pathways from the brainstem. Stimulation of these same NMDA receptors may lead to neuropathic pain and the development of tolerance.[19]

However, it is important to note that the potential adverse effects associated with oral administration are similar to those of the intravenous route. Prolonged opioid use may have risk of opioid dependence and addiction. Epidural or intrathecal routes carry potential risks, including infection (meningitis), sedation, respiratory depression (which is delayed with epidural morphine) and other side effects associated with systemic opioid use. The presence of these adverse effects can result in delayed recovery and an extended duration of hospitalization.[5,8,10,20]

### Opioid Sparing and Opioid Free Analgesia Strategies in Enhanced Recovery Program

Enhanced Recovery After Surgery (ERAS) represents a significant transformation in perioperative care, prioritizing a multidisciplinary and evidence-based approach to enhance patient outcomes and expedite recovery following surgical procedures. ERAS focuses on streamlining the entire surgical journey, encompassing preoperative preparation through postoperative care, aiming to enhance patient recovery while minimizing complications and decreasing duration of hospital stay. The ERAS pathway involves a collaborative effort among surgeons, anesthesiologists, nurses, dieticians, and other healthcare professionals. Preoperatively, patients receive comprehensive education and counselling, emphasizing the importance of active participation in their recovery, adherence to nutritional guidelines, and smoking cessation if applicable. This proactive approach not only empowers patients but also helps to reduce anxiety. Intraoperatively, ERAS protocols prioritize strategies aimed at minimizing surgical stress. This may involve the use of minimally invasive surgical techniques, optimized anesthesia regimens incorporating regional anesthesia and multimodal analgesia, as well as meticulous fluid management and perioperative glycemic control. By reducing the body's stress response to surgery, these interventions help preserve organ function, decrease the risk of postoperative complications, and facilitate early mobilization and return to normal activities.

Postoperatively, the emphasis on early recovery continues with a focus on pain management, nutrition, fluid balance, and mobilization. Early mobilization, encouraged as soon as feasible after surgery, helps to prevent complications such as deep vein thrombosis (DVT) and pneumonia, while also promoting faster recovery.[20,21] Traditionally, opioids have played a significant role in pain management during the postoperative period. However, due to concerns over opioid-related adverse events and the opioid epidemic, there has been a paradigm shift within the protocol of ERAS towards minimizing opioid exposure while ensuring effective pain control.[17] ERAS pathways advocate for the judicious use of opioid-sparing analgesia, supplemented by regional nerve blocks, neuraxial analgesia and non-opioid medications, to minimize pain while minimizing the risk of opioid-related adverse effects and complications.[18]

Nonsteroidal anti-inflammatory drugs (NSAIDs), acetaminophen, gabapentinoids, ketamine and alpha-2 agonists (dexmedetomidine) are the pharmacological agents that can be used in opioid-sparing analgesia strategy within ERAS protocols.[22] Opioid-sparing strategies in ERAS has been associated with a multitude of benefits, including reduced opioid consumption, decreased incidence of opioid-related adverse events, shorter hospital stays, faster recovery of bowel function and ambulation, and improved overall patient satisfaction.[23] Patients with obstructive sleep apnea, chronic obstructive pulmonary disease, and those undergoing bariatric surgery are at high-risk for opioid-related respiratory complications in the postoperative period. Therefore, implementing opioid-sparing and opioid-free analgesia techniques in these patients can aid in early recovery. Moreover, opioid-sparing protocols have the potential to mitigate the risk of chronic opioid use and opioid dependence following surgery.[24]

While opioid-sparing analgesia offers advantages, it has few potential risks associated with non-opioid analgesics. These risks include bradycardia associated with dexmedetomidine. Hepatic damage in vulnerable patients with acetaminophen. There is risk of bleeding, renal impairment, and bronchospasm with NSAIDs. Ketamine use may lead to hallucinations, tachycardia, and addiction. Lidocaine may cause tinnitus, seizures, and cardiac arrest, while gabapentin can induce sedation, and magnesium may result in hypotension.[1]

Opioid-free analgesia (OFA) entails complete avoidance of opioids by using alternative analgesic strategies. These methods include multimodal analgesia, i.e. regional analgesia (peripheral nerve blocks, epidural or intrathecal analgesia, and local infiltration) and nonopioid analgesics. Advantages of opioid free analgesia over opioid sparing analgesia is under review. Additionally, in supra major surgeries, OFA might not be possible in patients where regional analgesia may not sufficiently control pain like in surgeries with multiple incisions, for breakthrough pain episodes or in patients with contraindications to non-opioid analgesics.[18]

Creating a comprehensive preoperative plan to manage conditions such as neuropathic pain and addressing specific psychosocial factors can have a positive impact on both the severity and duration of postoperative pain. It is established that, undertreatment of pain can lead to the development of chronic postsurgical pain (CPSP). Through the implementation of opioid-sparing strategies and multi-modal analgesic pathways, anesthesiologists can enhance surgical outcomes, improve patient comfort, and reduce the potential harm associated with opioids.[1,18]

## Discharge of Patients with Opioid Prescription

Patients generally do not need opioid prescription at discharge. However, many patients with cancer may have been using opioid medications prior to surgery for pain management. Its advisable to gradually taper off these opioids in view of physical dependence and discontinue their use whenever possible following surgery.[16,17,20] Patients with prolonged opioid use may experience opioid tolerance, characterized by a reduced pharmacological response, as well as opioid-induced hyperalgesia, marked by an increase in pain perception. Studies have linked higher opioid doses post-surgery with prolonged hospital stays, elevated 30-day readmission rates, and an overall increase in healthcare costs.[17]

Literature suggests that 49.2% of patients following major onco-surgery need opioids in the early post-discharge period (within 90 days of discharge), while 3.1% of patients need opioid for an extended period after discharge (beyond 90 days after discharge).[25] Discharging patients with opioid prescriptions requires careful attention to ensure the safe and effective pain control while acknowledging the risks associated with opioid usage. This process involves assessment of the patient's pain intensity, medical history, and any potential factors that may increase the risk of harm from the use of opioids. Education has an important role, as patients need to be fully aware of the correct administration of opioids, potential side effects, and the importance of safely storing and disposing these medications.[20] Improper utilization of opioids following discharge from the hospital can elevate the risk of misuse and various patient safety concerns associated with opioids, such as addiction and, in rare cases, overdose-related deaths.[17]

Safe disposal involves returning excess medication to a community or hospital pharmacy to prevent misuse. Patients should be informed about the risks associated with driving or operating machinery while taking opioid medication. It is important to educate patients about the dangers of combining opioids with alcohol or other illicit substances, as this significantly increases the risk of harm. Providing patients with a leaflet or card before discharge can reinforce these important messages. Patients should get access to simple non-opioid analgesics like paracetamol and NSAIDs for reducing the need for opioids.[16] Encouraging patients to keep a record of their opioid and non-opioid analgesics doses, frequency and any associated side effects, can help to optimize their medication.[20]

The hospital discharge documentation must be promptly distributed to all healthcare providers engaged in the patient's treatment, including community pharmacists. This helps to prevent an acute opioid prescription from turning into a repeat prescription unintentionally. Patients should know all the adverse effects associated with opioids, including the risk of addiction. It is important to collaborate with the patient to establish an opioid treatment plan. Renewal of opioid prescriptions for persistent postsurgical pain after discharge should be done only after optimizing analgesic medications to avoid unintentional prolonged use of opioids.[18] Patients should receive guidance regarding medication review after hospital discharge, typically with a prescription for opioids lasting 5 to 7 days. Patients typically should not require long-term opioid medications after surgery. If any individual still needs opioids 90 days post-surgery and is experiencing ongoing pain, a detailed evaluation is warranted. This assessment may involve referring the patient to a chronic pain service to investigate persistent postsurgical pain or, in some cases, to a substance misuse service. It is essential for institutes to have separate protocols for patients being discharged with opioids, and the hospital discharge summary should include the recommended opioid dosage and duration.[16]

### Transitional Pain Service

The concept of the transitional pain service (TPS) emerged from the acknowledgment of insufficient postoperative pain management and the possibility of transitioning to chronic pain after surgery. Its goal is to offer comprehensive, multidisciplinary care to patients during the postoperative period, facilitating the transition from acute to chronic pain management. The services provided by the TPS are classified into three main areas:

1. Introducing and optimizing multimodal analgesia to enhance pain management and support the reduction of opioid usage;
2. Non-pharmacological interventions such as physiotherapy and acupuncture;
3. Psychological interventions delivered by a trained pain psychology team.[26]

This approach is overseen by a team comprised of anesthesiologists, nursing staff, clinical psychologists, palliative care specialists, an exercise physiotherapist, and a patient-care coordinator. The TPS identifies high-risk patients during preoperative clinic visits with the aim of reducing the risk of developing CPSP and postoperative opioid usage.[27] Patients who are not identified during the preoperative visit but meet specific criteria such as preoperative chronic pain, a history of opioid use, a history of substance abuse, severe post-surgical pain, high opioid consumption postoperatively and psychological factors like depression or anxiety can be referred to the TPS.[17,18,27,28]

The transitional pain service (TPS) is essential for several reasons:

1. *Prevention of chronic pain:* TPS facilitates the early identification and intervention of patients who are at risk of developing chronic pain after surgery.
2. *Effective pain management:* By implementing multimodal analgesia in the postoperative period, TPS ensures more effective pain relief.
3. *Enhanced patient satisfaction:* TPS offers continuity of care, education, and support both before and after discharge, empowering patients to actively engage in their recovery. This involvement leads to higher satisfaction levels among patients.

4. *Reduction in healthcare costs:* TPS helps reduce the risk of chronic pain, thereby lowering the utilization of healthcare services, hospital readmissions, and the need for long-term pain management interventions. This results in cost savings for healthcare systems.
5. *Monitoring opioid use:* TPS utilizes a multidisciplinary approach to monitor opioid use postsurgery, with the goal of safely tapering patients off opioids while preserving effective pain management strategies.[26,27]

Incorporating transitional pain services into ERAS protocols could improve both acute and long-term pain management by providing guidelines to prevent CPSP and assisting with the gradual discontinuation of opioid medication.[18] Toronto General Hospital's transitional pain service has identified the patient's opioid dose at the time of discharge as the most significant predictor for opioid-naïve patients' ability to taper off opioids post-surgery. Patients discharged with higher opioid doses are less likely to achieve opioid-free status.[29] Expanding TPS is important for those patients in the intermediate phase when primary physicians have exhausted pain control options but chronic pain specialists have not yet intervened to alleviate pain severity.[27]

Despite the numerous benefits of TPS, limitations hinder its implementation. These limitations include resource constraints (such as staffing shortages and limited funding), a lack of standardized protocols, and limited health literacy among patients.

## Opioid and Cancer Recurrence

In recent years, there has been increased interest and studies regarding the potential role of opioids in cancer recurrence. Opioids are effective analgesic medications and have been an important part of the management of postoperative pain. However, questions have emerged regarding their effect on cancer progression, metastasis and the risk of cancer recurrence.[30]

One proposed mechanism for recurrence and metastasis is the modulation of immune function by opioids, which may affect the body's ability to recognize and eliminate cancer cells. Chronic opioid exposure could potentially suppress immune responses, creating an immunosuppressive (natural killer cells express opioid receptors and undergo apoptosis when exposed with opioid medications) environment to cause tumor growth and recurrence.[30,31] Additionally, opioids may cause angiogenesis—the process of forming new blood vessels which requires for tumor progression, through interactions with angiogenic pathways. Furthermore, opioids might activate cellular signaling pathways which is part of cell proliferation, survival and apoptosis, finally promoting cancer cell survival and metastasis.[32,33] Opioid receptors are overexpressed in several human cancer cells which causes the promotion of tumor growth and metastasis after use of opioids.[14]

Circulating tumor cells (CTCs) are cells released from the primary tumor into the peripheral blood, linked to cancer recurrence and metastasis. Majorities of these CTCs are eliminated through processes such as apoptosis, necrosis, and immune system (mainly by natural killer cells). Similarly, disseminated tumor cells (DTC) refer to the CTCs that have migrated into the bone marrow, often associated with the development of bone metastasis . When immunosuppression occurs due to opioids, CTCs and DTCs may cause unwanted consequence in terms of recurrence and metastasis.[30]

Several studies have indicated a decrease in cancer recurrence, particularly in cases of breast, prostate, and colorectal cancer, where opioid-free anesthesia was adapted.[31] Additionally, comparisons between cancer recurrence rates in surgeries done under general anesthesia with opioids and regional anesthesia have been conducted in several studies. These comparisons have revealed a higher recurrence rate among patients using opioids. However, direct evidence supporting the modification of anesthesia techniques in cancer patients is still inadequate.[14] There exist trials that do not show benefit of regional anesthesia-analgesia when compared with general anesthesia and opioids in the same patient group.[34] This difference in results tells us the complexity of the topic and highlights the need for further research to find out the underlying mechanisms and clarify the impact of opioids on cancer outcome.

## Summary

The controversies surrounding the use of opioids in the postoperative period highlights the need for opioid-sparing strategies. Through the integration of multimodal analgesia, regional anesthesia techniques, non-opioid medications, and alternative therapies, anesthesiologists or pain physicians can customize postoperative pain management plans according to the needs of each patient while minimizing reliance on opioids. Additionally, such strategies not only reduce the risk of opioid-related complications but also contribute to improve patient outcome, reduce hospital stay and promote early recovery. We hope future research on unresolved issues inclusive of cancer recurrence and opioids will answer and resolve the complexities associated with opioid use in modern anesthesia practice.

## References

1. Bohringer C, Astorga C, Liu H. The Benefits of Opioid Free Anesthesia and the Precautions Necessary When Employing It. Transl Perioper Pain Med. 2020;7(1):152–157. PMCID: PMC6844148
2. Puntillo F, Giglio M, Varrassi G. The Routes of Administration for Acute Postoperative Pain Medication. Pain Ther. 2021 Dec;10(2):909–925. PMCID: PMC8586059
3. Yadav S, Ajayababu A, Sinha TP, Bhoi S, Yadav S, Ajayababu A, Sinha TP, Bhoi S. Pain Management in the Emergency Department – Newer Modalities and Current Perspective. Pain Management-From Acute to Chronic and Beyond [Internet]. IntechOpen; 2022 [cited 2024 Mar 3]. Available from: https://www.intechopen.com/chapters/83173
4. Vahedi HSM, Hajebi H, Vahidi E, Nejati A, Saeedi M. Comparison between intravenous morphine versus fentanyl in acute pain relief in drug abusers with acute limb traumatic injury. World J Emerg Med. 2019;10(1):27–32. PMCID: PMC6264977
5. Garimella V, Cellini C. Postoperative pain control. Clin Colon Rectal Surg. 2013 Sep;26(3):191–196. PMCID: PMC3747287
6. Hudcova J, McNicol E, Quah C, Lau J, Carr DB. Patient controlled opioid analgesia versus conventional opioid analgesia for postoperative pain. Cochrane Database Syst Rev. 2006 Oct 18;(4):CD003348. PMID: 17054167
7. Gedela V, Gururaj S. A prospective double blind randomized comparative study of safety and efficacy of Tapentadol versus Tramadol in post-operative orthopaedic patients. International Journal of Basic & Clinical Pharmacology. 2017 Oct 25;6(11):2727–32.
8. DeSousa KA, Chandran R. Intrathecal morphine for postoperative analgesia: Current trends. World Journal of Anesthesiology. Baishideng Publishing Group Inc.; 2014 Nov 27;3(3):191–202.
9. Hermanides J, Hollmann MW, Stevens MF, Lirk P. Failed epidural: causes and management. Br J Anaesth. 2012 Aug;109(2):144–154. PMID: 22735301

10. Borja Mugabure Bujedo MD, Silvia González Santos MD, Amaia Uría Azpiazu MD. A review of epidural and intrathecal opioids used in the management of postoperative pain. Journal of Opioid Management. 2012 May 1;8(3):177–92.
11. Bang YJ, Lee EK, Kim CS, Hahm TS, Jeong H, Cho YJ, Noh JJ, Lee YY, Choi CH, Lee JW, Jeong JS. The Effect of Intrathecal Morphine on Postoperative Opioid Consumption in Patients Undergoing Abdominal Surgery for Gynecologic Malignancy: A Randomized Sham-Controlled Trial. Anesthesia & Analgesia. 2023 Sep;137(3):525.
12. Bernards CM. Recent insights into the pharmacokinetics of spinal opioids and the relevance to opioid selection. Curr Opin Anaesthesiol. 2004 Oct;17(5):441–447. PMID: 17023903
13. Rawal N. Intrathecal opioids for the management of post-operative pain. Best Practice & Research Clinical Anaesthesiology. 2023 Jun 1;37(2):123–32.
14. Gropper MA, Miller RD. Miller's anesthesia [Internet]. Ninth edition. Philadelphia, PA: Elsevier Philadelphia, PA; 2020. Available from: http://www.engineeringvillage.com/controller/servlet/OpenURL?genre=book&isbn=9780323596046>
15. Power I. Fentanyl HCl iontophoretic transdermal system (ITS): clinical application of iontophoretic technology in the management of acute postoperative pain. British Journal of Anaesthesia. 2007 Jan 1;98(1):4–11.
16. Surgery-and-opioids-2021_4.pdf [Internet]. [cited 2024 Feb 29]. Available from: https://fpm.ac.uk/sites/fpm/files/documents/2021-03/surgery-and-opioids-2021_4.pdf
17. Alexander JC, Patel B, Joshi GP. Perioperative use of opioids: Current controversies and concerns. Best Pract Res Clin Anaesthesiol. 2019 Sep;33(3):341–351. PMID: 31785719
18. Echeverria-Villalobos M, Stoicea N, Todeschini AB, Fiorda-Diaz J, Uribe AA, Weaver T, Bergese SD. Enhanced Recovery After Surgery (ERAS): A Perspective Review of Postoperative Pain Management Under ERAS Pathways and Its Role on Opioid Crisis in the United States. Clin J Pain. 2020 Mar;36(3):219–226. PMID: 31868759
19. pdf.pdf [Internet]. [cited 2024 Feb 29]. Available from: https://www.painphysicianjournal.com/current/pdf?article=OTg3&journal=42
20. Srivastava D, Hill S, Carty S, Rockett M, Bastable R, Knaggs R, Lambert D, Levy N, Hughes J, Wilkinson P. Surgery and opioids: evidence-based expert consensus guidelines on the perioperative use of opioids in the United Kingdom. British Journal of Anaesthesia. 2021 Jun;126(6):1208–1216.
21. Altman AD, Helpman L, McGee J, Samouëlian V, Auclair MH, Brar H, Nelson GS. Enhanced recovery after surgery: implementing a new standard of surgical care. CMAJ. 2019 Apr 29;191(17):E469–E475. PMCID: PMC6488471
22. Mauermann E, Ruppen W, Bandschapp O. Different protocols used today to achieve total opioid-free general anesthesia without locoregional blocks. Best Pract Res Clin Anaesthesiol. 2017 Dec;31(4):533–545. PMID: 29739542
23. Carnes KM, Ata A, Cangero T, Mian BM. Impact of Enhanced Recovery after Surgery Protocols on Opioid Prescriptions at Discharge after Major Urological Cancer Surgery. Urology Practice. 2021 Mar;8(2):270–76.
24. Siu EY, Moon TS. Opioid-free and opioid-sparing anesthesia. Int Anesthesiol Clin. 2020;58(2):34–41. PMID: 32004171
25. Clarke H, Soneji N, Ko DT, Yun L, Wijeysundera DN. Rates and risk factors for prolonged opioid use after major surgery: population based cohort study. BMJ. British Medical Journal Publishing Group; 2014 Feb 11;348:g1251. PMID: 24519537
26. Katz J, Weinrib A, Fashler SR, Katznelzon R, Shah BR, Ladak SS, et al. The Toronto General Hospital Transitional Pain Service: development and implementation of a multidisciplinary program to prevent chronic postsurgical pain. Journal of Pain Research. Dove Medical Press; 2015 Oct 12;8:695–702. PMID: 26508886
27. Transitional Pain Services: Closing the Gap Between Acute and Chronic Pain [Internet]. ASRA Pain Medicine. [cited 2024 Feb 29]. Available from: https://www.asra.com/news-publications/

asra-newsletter/newsletter-item/asra-news/2023/02/01/transitional-pain-services-closing-the-gap-between-acute-and-chronic-pain

28. Mikhaeil J, Ayoo K, Clarke H, W sowicz M, Huang A. Review of the Transitional Pain Service as a method of postoperative opioid weaning and a service aimed at minimizing the risk of chronic post-surgical pain. Anaesthesiol Intensive Ther. 2020;52(2):148–153. PMCID: PMC10176534
29. Clarke H, Azargive S, Montbriand J, Nicholls J, Sutherland A, Valeeva L, et al. Opioid weaning and pain management in postsurgical patients at the Toronto General Hospital Transitional Pain Service. Canadian Journal of Pain. Taylor & Francis; 2018 Jan 1;2(1):236–47.
30. Wang K, Qu X, Wang Y, Shen H, Liu Q, Du J. Effect of mu Agonists on Long-Term Survival and Recurrence in Nonsmall Cell Lung Cancer Patients. Medicine (Baltimore). 2015 Aug 21;94(33):e1333. PMCID: PMC4616430
31. Kim R. Anesthetic technique and cancer recurrence in oncologic surgery: unraveling the puzzle. Cancer Metastasis Rev. 2017 Mar;36(1):159–177. PMID: 27866303
32. Opioid-Free Anaesthesia [Internet]. WFSA Resource Library. [cited 2024 Feb 29]. Available from: https://resources.wfsahq.org/atotw/opiod-free-anaesthesia/
33. Nakada T, Ohtsuka T. Impact of opioids on postoperative prognosis in lung cancer. Journal of Thoracic Disease [Internet]. AME Publishing Company; 2023 Oct 31 [cited 2024 Feb 29];15(10). Available from: https://jtd.amegroups.org/article/view/78845
34. Sessler DI, Pei L, Huang Y, Fleischmann E, Marhofer P, Kurz A, et al. Breast Cancer Recurrence Collaboration. Recurrence of breast cancer after regional or general anaesthesia: a randomised controlled trial. Lancet. 2019 Nov 16;394(10211):1807–1815. PMID: 31645288

Chapter 18

# Persistent Post-Surgical Pain

• Gauri R Gangakhedkar

## INTRODUCTION

Tissue trauma that occurs as a result of surgery inevitably results in acute postoperative pain that is expected to resolve over 1–2 weeks, with standard analgesic management.[1] As a result, patients undergoing surgery usually anticipate and accept that there would be discomfort and pain associated with surgery, but also expect that it will subside in due course.

However, of the 310 million major surgeries that are undertaken annually across the world, up to one-third of patients report varying degrees of persistent pain as late as one year after their surgery, namely, persistent post-surgical pain (PPSP).[1,2] This chronic pain can have a significant effect on a patient's quality of life, making it difficult for them to carry out their daily activities, cause limitations in mobility, results in emotional and social distress. It can also lead to depression, anxiety, and sleep disturbances, which can further exacerbate the pain.

Persistence of pain beyond the acute postoperative period, was identified and reported 25 years ago, but our understanding regarding its etiopathogenesis and definitive strategies to prevent occurrence is still limited. This lack of understanding and recognition of its significance, has led to variability in its nomenclature, and a lack of standardization of diagnostic and treatment techniques. Prolonged persistence of postoperative pain has been labelled by various groups as chronic postoperative pain (CPOP), chronic post-surgical pain (CPSP), postoperative chronic pain (POCP), persistent postsurgical pain (PPP) in addition to PPSP. For the purpose of our chapter, we shall refer to the condition as persistent post-surgical pain (PPSP) from here on.[3–6]

## EVOLUTION OF DEFINITION

The definition of PPSP was first proposed in 1999 by Macrae and Davies, and was then further elaborated by Macrae in 2001.[7,8] According to this definition, pain could be labelled as PPSP if it fulfilled the following criteria:

- It must develop after a surgical procedure.
- It should last for at least two months.
- Other causes for the pain should have been excluded.
- The possibility that the pain has occurred due to a pre-existing condition should have also been excluded.

In 2014, another amendment to the definition was proposed by Werner and Kongsgaard, which aligns PPSP as a continuum of pain that occurs after a surgical procedure and takes into consideration the effects that PPSP would have on a patient's life.[9] They suggested, that to be labelled as PPSP, in addition to the original criteria, the pain should either originate after the surgery or increase in intensity, its duration be longer than three months leading to a significant negative impact on the patient's quality of life, and be located either at the surgical site or in the area innervated by a nerve from the surgical field.

The International Association for the Study of Pain (IASP) recognized the burden presented by chronic pain and their collaborative efforts with the World Health Organization led to the successful inclusion of PPSP in the International Code of Diseases (ICD-11) which came into effect in 2022.[10] PPSP is included as one of the seven categories into which chronic pain has been subdivided.[11]

## INCIDENCE

Estimates from epidemiological studies suggest that as 20 to 56% of patients develop PPSP.[5] A study carried out over 11 countries found that moderate to severe PPSP, evaluated 12 months after surgery was as frequent as 11.8% (95% CI, 9.7 to 13.9), while severe pain (numerical rating scale ≥6) was seen in 2.2% (95% CI, 1.2 to 3.3).[12] These numbers cannot be held as absolute, since the specifics of the definitions used to elicit PPSP could vary. For instance, when a study evaluated 'moderate to severe' PPSP, 18% of the patients fit the criteria when only pain in the area of surgery was considered; as opposed to 40% for generalised pain. A further drop to 6% was seen if patients having pre-surgical pain at site of surgery, were excluded from the definition. This variability highlights the need for implementation of uniform criteria for defining PPSP, as is expected to happen after adoption the ICD-11 definition. It is only then that the true global burden of PPSP can be assessed.

## PATHOPHYSIOLOGY AND MECHANISM [5,13–15]

The etiology of PPSP and the biological mechanisms that lead to its development are complex and not yet completely understood. Even for patients undergoing the same surgeries, different pain mechanisms lead to the emergence of diverse pain syndromes. What we understand from animal studies is that the inflammatory reaction resulting from the surgical insult can lead to neuronal excitability due to persistent noxious stimuli. The persistent excitability and triggering leads to maladaptive neuroplasticity which leads to the chronification of pain pathways, which shows an increase in the excitatory mechanism of neurotransmission, and possibly a concurrent reduction in inhibitory mechanisms.

Both central and peripheral sensitisation can be implicated in the development of PPSP (Fig. 18.1). The surgical insult leads to release of inflammatory mediators such as cytokines, prostaglandins, serotonin, histamine, $H^+$ ions, bradykinin, which result in peripheral sensitisation. Nociceptive stimuli also activate the intracellular protein kinase pathway in the dorsal horn of the spinal cord, modify ion channel expression, reception and neurotransmitter density. Amino propanoic acid (AMPA), N-methyl-d-aspartate (NMDA) receptors, substance P, and nitric oxide (NO), are implicated in the increase in

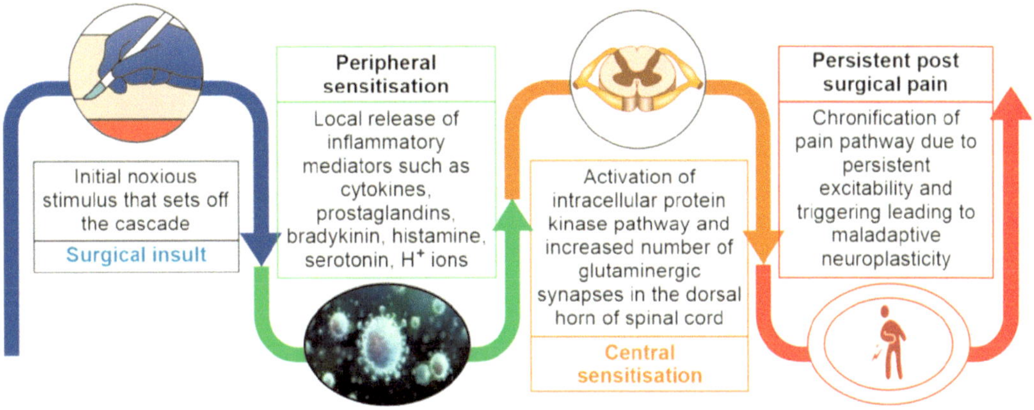


**Fig. 18.1:** Development of persistent post-surgical pain

number of glutaminergic synapses in the dorsal horn of the spinal cord. The increased glutaminergic synapses reinforce transmission of nociceptive stimuli and recruit even non-nociceptive stimuli to the pain pathway, forming the central sensitisation pathway.

## PREDISPOSING FACTORS/RISK FACTORS

Since the pain physicians have understood how detrimental PPSP can be for patients, there has been increased focus on trying to find risk factors to help predict the occurrence of PPSP. Various studies have identified multiple risk factors, and have also led to an understanding that they are not independent, but rather are interconnected, and together, increase the likelihood of occurrence of PPSP in a manner similar to a domino effect. The most commonly identified risk factors include young adults, female gender, presence of preoperative pain particularly that leading to preoperative use of opioids and a psychological profile that makes patients vulnerable to development of PPSP.[16] A classification can also be attempted by identifying the temporal relationship of the pain with the surgery, i.e. preoperative factors, intraoperative factors and post-operative factors.[6] The various risk factors that have been identified are listed in Table 18.1 along with a stratification of level of evidence available to support them.

## CANCER AND CHRONIC POST-SURGICAL PAIN

PPSP is a devastating side effect that can occur in more than 20% of cancer patients undergoing surgery.[17] It has been reported after almost all onco-surgical procedures, with a prevalence being the highest in surgeries requiring thoracotomy (5–65%), amputations (30–85%), and mastectomies (11–57%) as listed in Table 18.2.[18] A higher proportion of patients are seen to undergo a transition from acute pain to PPSP when undergoing oncological procedures as opposed to those undergoing non-oncological procedures, due to the following reasons:[17,19,20]

- The preoperative neoadjuvant therapies can result in central and peripheral sensitisation
- Patients with cancer are more likely to be using opioids in the preoperative period as a consequence of inflammatory mediators released from the tumors or pain secondary to cancer therapy

| Table 18.1: Risk factors for development of PPSP[2,13] | | | |
|---|---|---|---|
| **Patient** | **Anesthesia** | **Surgery** | **Pain** |
| **Young adults**<br>**Comorbidities**<br>**• Disability**<br>**• Addiction**<br>**Lower education**<br>**Smoking**<br>**Psychological factors**<br>**• Fear/anxiety**<br>**• Depression**<br>**• Pain Catastrophising**<br>Female patients<br>Higher BMI<br>Single/ Living alone<br>Unemployed<br>Genetic predisposition | Altered pain processing<br>• Increased pain sensitivity<br>• Reduced endogenous inhibition<br>Use of opioids<br>Use of regional anesthetic techniques | **Longer duration**<br>**Nature of procedure**<br>**Complications**<br>Adjuvant chemotherapy/ radiation<br>Repeated surgery<br>Nerve injury<br>Surgical approach | **Preoperative pain**<br>**• Area of surgery and elsewhere**<br>**• Preoperative opioid use**<br>**Postoperative pain**<br>**• Stronger intensity**<br>**• Duration >5 days**<br>**• Type of pain** |

Risk factors for development of PPSP with more robust evidence are marked in bold

| Table 18.2: Incidence of PPSP at 12 months after surgery[2,6] | |
|---|---|
| **Condition** | **Frequency** |
| Mastectomy | 43–56% |
| Gynecological surgery | 15–40% |
| Thoracotomy | 41.2% |
| Sternotomy | 27% |
| Cholecystectomy | 3–56% |

- Cancer surgeries are inherently long surgeries
- Oncosurgeries can lead to iatrogenic nerve damage
- They require extensive tissue and lymph node dissection to ensure disease clearance
- Effective visualisation, particularly in supra-major surgeries entails a lot of retraction
- The number of surgeries that are undertaken using an open surgical approach is higher
- Drains are used quite frequently
- Cancer surgeries frequently lead to moderate to severe pain in the postoperative period
- Patients with cancer are also likely to undergo multiple surgeries

Since each of the factors mentioned above represent risk factors to the development of PPSP, the cumulative effect often leads to poorer outcomes in cancer patients.

## Prediction of CPSP

Given the exhaustive list of risk factors leading to PPSP, and knowing that risk factors are interdependent, simply identifying risk factors is not enough to predict the likelihood of a patient developing PPSP. Risk prediction models will definitely be more helpful, to ensure that patients are offered appropriate and optimal preventive strategies. Predicting CPSP can allow diversion of adequate resources to the vulnerable patients and allow employment of better resource utilization strategies, particularly in resource limited settings. The validated risk models that are currently in use are modelled for specific surgeries to increase accuracy of prediction. A 6-item predictive scale using only preoperative factors was devised by Montes et al. for patients undergoing hernia repair, hysterectomies (vaginal or abdominal), and thoracotomies.[21] For patients undergoing breast cancer surgeries, a 4-item scale has been developed, that also takes into account pain intensity on postoperative day 7.[22] As a result, the model can only be employed in retrospect. A recent 4-item scale, which was developed by van Driel, et al. can be applied for patients undergoing orthopedic, vascular, trauma, and general surgical procedures.[23] These available prediction models are explained further in Table 18.3. However, even this model includes two postoperative predictors, thus limiting its use in the preoperative period. Building an ideal scale to predict PPSP will be quite a challenge, since scales requiring postoperative factors cannot be implemented in the preoperative period and those including only preoperative factors, will not be able to take into account many of the risk factors for PPSP that develop in the intra-operative or postoperative period.

## Prevention

Development of PPSP can be attributed to such a large number of factors, that it is impossible to pin-point definitive preventive strategies as of now. Due to small

**Table 18.3: Predictive models[21–23]**

| Author (Year) | Montes (2020) | Meretoja (2017) | Van Driel (2022) |
|---|---|---|---|
| Patient population | Thoracotomy | Breast cancer surgery | Orthopedic surgery |
| | Hysterectomy (abdominal/vaginal) | | Vascular surgery |
| | Inguinal hernia repair | | Trauma surgery |
| | | | General surgery |
| Factors | Nature of surgery | Body mass index | Bone surgery |
| | Younger age | Sentinel node dissection/axillary dissection | Preoperative use of steroids |
| | General physical status (SF- 12 score physical) | Pain on postoperative Day 1 | Worst pain score (NRS) on POD 1 |
| | Mental health status (SF- 12 score mental) | Pain on postoperative Day 2 | Presence of pruritus within painful area on POD 1 |
| | Preoperative pain (surgical area) | | Worst pain score (NRS) on POD 14 |
| | Preoperative pain (other area) | | Presence of pruritus within painful area on POD 14 |
| AUC | 0.68–0.69 | 0.70–0.74 | 0.76–0.87 |

volume data and flawed methodology in most of the studies carried out for PPSP, no conclusion could be drawn from a recent meta-analysis too.[24] It is crucial for all practising anesthetists and pain physicians to target identifiable preventive strategies since PPSP provides a window during the acute perioperative period, pre, intra and immediate postoperative period, to intervene and reduce impact of PPSP. The preventive strategies that can be implemented can be broadly categorised as pharmacological and non-pharmacological. They are explained in further detail below.[5,6,25–27]

### A. Pharmacological Strategies

#### 1. *Acetaminophen and NSAIDs*[6,26,27]

Non-steroidal anti-inflammatory drugs (NSAIDs) cause an anti-inflammatory effect, an opioid sparing effect and thus reduce central sensitization and PPSP. NSAIDs are safe, with minimal side effects, However, very limited data is available, and that too is restricted to only a few agents, hence, it is not possible to draw definitive conclusions about their use to prevent PPSP. The same holds true for acetaminophen though it forms an integral part of the current multi-modal acute pain management strategies.

#### 2. *Limiting of use of opioids*[6,26,27]

Though opioids have retained their place as the gold standard for pain relief for moderate to severe perioperative pain, but caution is recommended during their use due to serious side effects and also the risk of developing opioid induced hyperalgesia (OIH), particularly seen with the use of high intraoperative doses of remifentanil.

#### 3. *Multi-modal analgesia*[6,26,27]

Multi-modal anesthesia (MMA) includes use of a combination of agents that possibly have a synergistic effect, use different mechanisms of analgesia and further modulate pain signals at various points of the pain pathway, rather than using a single drug thus effectively reducing PPSP. MMA usually includes NSAIDs, acetaminophen, gabapentinoids and regional anesthesia used together. Pre-clinical studies show good efficacy with use of clinically approved analgesics, and novel pharmacotherapies including a combination of selective Nav1.7 inhibitors. The role of selective voltage-gated sodium channel 1.7 (Nav1.7) inhibitors in chronic pain, generated a lot of interest among pain physicians after patients with loss of Nav1.7 function, showed an insensitivity to pain.[5,28] While the pre-clinical data shows promise, data from clinical studies is awaited.

#### 4. *Gabapentinoids*[6,26,27]

The neuropathic pain component of PPSP can be addressed using that can gabapentinoids such as pregabalin and gabapentin, which reduce pain transmission and central sensitisation by attenuating glutamate release. The widespread use of gabapentinoids has been accentuated by presence of the opioid crisis, but the potential adverse events and inconsistent and conflicting recommendations from pain society guidelines limit their use as a standard protocol.

#### 5. *Anti-depressants*[5,26]

Tricyclic antidepressants and serotonin-norepinephrine reuptake inhibitors are now a part of standard practice to treat chronic pain, since they reduce neuropathic pain and are also help the depression that may be associated with chronic pain. Though their mechanism of action suggests their potential for use, their role in PPSP prevention is still under investigation.

*6. Clonidine*[5,26,27]

The analgesic efficacy of clonidine comes from the selective post-synaptic action in α2-agonist receptors of spinal dorsal horn and hass been used to prevent PPSPIt mimics the action of nor-epinephrine, causes the suppression of excitatory neurotransmitters and, thus, of neuronal excitation in the central nervous system areas which are associated with pain perception. Data from small studies does seem promising but use is limited by its side effects including hypotension, bradycardia and prolongs the effect of peripheral nerve blocks.

*7. Ketamine*[5,26,27]

The analgesic activity of ketamine occurs through antagonism of the N-methyl-d-aspartate (NMDA) receptor,activation of the descending inhibitory monoaminergic system, opioid and cholinergic blockade of sodium channels. Sub-anesthetic doses of ketamine in the perioperative period, have shown to prevent various types of PPSP. A systematic review and meta-analysis done by McNicol et al. showed a statistically significant reduction in the risk of PPSP of 25% and 30%, at 3 and 6 months post-operatively respectively. No significant side effects were noted except for visual disturbances. Another NMDA antagonist Memantine has also been used but relief was not found to persist for long enough to prevent PPSP.

*8. Lignocaine*[26,27]

Local anesthetics reduce pain transmission and central sensitisation by interrupting the sensory information to the spinal cord X. Intravenous lidocaine is increasingly being used for both management of chronic pain, as well as perioperatively reduction of both acute postoperative pain and PPSP. The perioperative use of eutectic mixture of local anesthetic (EMLA) cream has been found to reduce the incidence of chronic pain after a mastectomy.

*9. Steroids*[26,27]

The anti-inflammatory role of steroids is thought to reduce the neuroinflammation that leads to PPSP. Use of steroid in acute pain management is established but little data is available on PPSP prevention. As a result, use of steroids to effectively prevent PPSP cannot be recommended just yet.

### B. Non-pharmacological Strategies

*1. Surgical technique*[6,26]

One risk factor for PPSP is nerve and tissue damage during surgery. Identifying and preserving nerves during surgery can help reduce the development of chronic pain. Minimally invasive surgery may also lead to less persistent pain, but not all studies have been able to show a difference in chronic pain between laparoscopic and open surgery. However, there is still not enough evidence to recommend a definitive surgical technique. Risk can be minimized by avoiding nerve damage and opting for shorter and less invasive surgeries.

*2. Regional anesthesia*[5,6,27]

Regional block techniques have been shown to effectively prevent PPSP in various surgeries by modulating pain signals and neuroplasticity. Thoracic epidural anesthesia has been found to be effective in reducing PPSP in thoracotomy, but thoracic paravertebral block has not been shown to be effective.[29] There is some mention in literature of the use of regional analgesia or local anesthetics in breast cancer surgery to decrease the incidence of PPSP, but the level of evidence is insufficient. Ultrasound-guided fascial plane blocks have shown promise in preventing PPSP, but their precise effects are still unclear. Despite limitations in study methodologies, regional analgesia still remains a promising strategy to prevent PPSP, and its opioid-sparing effect may also contribute to decreasing PPSP.

*3. Psychoeducational support and rehabilitation*[26]

PPSP has a complex etiology that involves biological, psychological, and temporal factors. Focusing only on the perioperative phase may not be adequate and a multidisciplinary approach, which includes non-pharmaceutical therapies, may be more effective. A team should follow-up with at-risk patients not just during the perioperative phase, but also for several weeks after surgery. Operant conditioning and cognitive behavioral therapy (CBT) are also effective for managing chronic pain. Operant conditioning focuses on modifying maladaptive behavior and overt expressions of pain in response to chronic pain, while CBT aims to improve physical and emotional functioning despite the pain. It combines, stress management, goal setting, relaxation, problem-solving, and pacing of activities with positive reinforcement to help patients become desensitized to pain and function.

## Treatment

Several interventions that are commonly employed for acute pain management can also be utilized for the management of PPSP. It is important to first determine the type of pain present when PPSP is suspected, to rule out the possibility of cancer recurrence in cases of cancer surgery or other postoperative complications, like infection. In a manner similar to preventive techniques, treatment techniques can also be divided into pharmacological and non-pharmacological techniques.

## Pharmacological

After a thorough assessment of symptom and their severity, standards analgesics such as paracetamol, NSAIDs, and weak opioids are used in conjunction with adjunct therapy. The use of potent opioids should be avoided during this stage to prevent potential dependency. A large proportion of patients with PPSP present with neuropathic symptoms hence, drugs such as gabapentinoids that are used to treat neuropathic pain, tricyclic anti-depressants and serotonin-norepinephrine reuptake inhibitors form mainstay of therapy.[6] Topical lignocaine, nitroglycerine patches and capsaicin have also been used with some degree of success.[26]

## Non-pharmacological[6,26,30]

Psychological interventions are a significant treatment option for PPSP, as psychological factors have consistently been identified as risk factors for this condition. A systematic review has shown that utilizing cognitive behavioral therapy as a psychological intervention can potentially reduce the severity and disability associated with PPSP.

Pain interventions are usually reserved for those patients that do not respond well to pharmacotherapy. Treatment of sternotomy-induced neuralgia has been successfully attempted using repeated bupivacaine blocks, alcohol blocks or phenol blocks. For lumbar or cervical post-surgery syndrome epidural injections were also seen to provide pain relief . PPSP caused by entrapment of the superficial nerves of the abdominal wall, or trauma to the nerves as a result of surgery, has been treated with local anesthetic-based fascial plane blocks with or without steroid. Botox injections have been used with success for post-thoracotomy pain, abdominal wall pain after ventral hernia repair, and for trigeminal neuropathic pain after dental implants. Mirror therapy, phenol injections or radiofrequency ablation, transcutaneous electrical nerve stimulation, dorsal root entry zone (DREZ) lesioning and motor cord stimulation have all been used to stump and phantom limb pain. Radiofrequency percutaneous partial rhizotomy has been found to be useful in the management of chronic thoracic segmental pain, including post-thoracotomy and post-mastectomy pain. Radiofrequency ablation has also been used for the treatment of chronic ilioinguinal pain following inguinal hernia repair and chronic post-thoracotomy pain, when the DRG or the DREZ have been targeted.

## EFFECTIVE CLINICAL APPROACH TO ADDRESS PPSP[25,26]

PPSP represents a significant challenge to pain physicians given our limited ability to accurately predict, prevent or even treat PPSP. As a result, current recommendations are to implement a variety of strategies at every time-point in order to reduce the incidence of PPSP (Fig. 18.2). The intervention begins in the preoperative period, where the patients who are a high-risk of developing PPSP need to be identified, and multi-disciplinary preventive measures need to be instituted reduce the risk, including psycho-education, choosing the appropriate surgical approach and making a plan for appropriate multi-modal pain management strategies to be employed through the perioperative period. Such patients who have a high risk of developing PPSP and those with pain that does not get controlled with routine institutional analgesic practices, need special attention. A longer postoperative follow-up for longer periods to allow early identification and prompt treatment of patients with PPSP.

## FUTURE DIRECTION OR AVENUES FOR RESEARCH

From the data we have available, it appears that reducing pain sensitization in the postoperative period, is crucial to prevent development of PPSP. Thus, effective utilization of preventive analgesic techniques through the perioperative period, seems

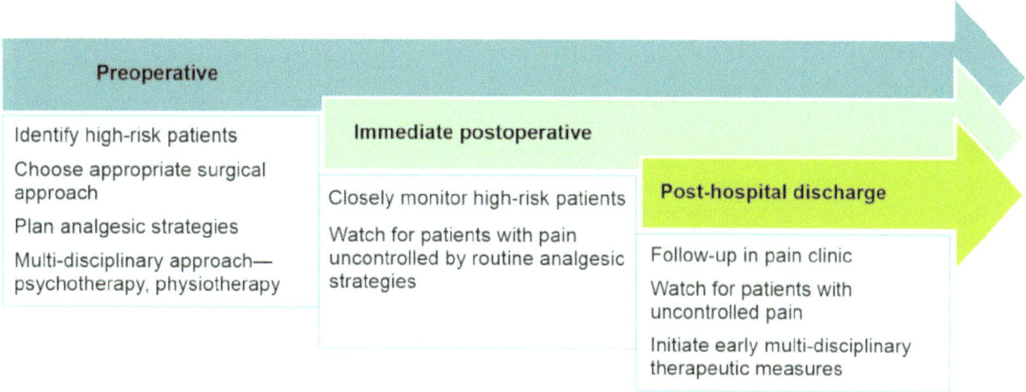


Fig. 18.2: Clinical approach to address PPSP

to hold the key in reducing the incidence of PPSP. The Toronto General Hospital launched the Transitional Pain Service (TPS) in 2014, which is an extremely promising venture in minimizing the risk of occurrence of chronic pain after surgery by providing multidisciplinary pain management. The service operates in three stages: preoperative, immediate postoperative, and outpatient. It includes risk assessment for identifying patients who could potentially develop PPSP, personalized pain management plans that include both, psychological consultations and patient and caregiver education, and follow-up appointments which provide multidisciplinary interventions, including psychological intervention and physiotherapy. TPS has been found to be effective in reducing postoperative pain and opioid use, and can also reduce the severity of chronic pain and associated costs.[31] Unfortunately, the services are available only in a few institutes evaluating their impact on a larger scale still eludes us.

Due to the current lack of standardized protocols, well-designed, large-scale studies that compare various multimodal techniques and follow the patients up for longer periods are necessary to determine the efficacy and thus choose the best agents and techniques for prevention. Research is ongoing to explore the function of other modalities such as the targeting the spinal cord and dorsal root ganglion, use of anti-nerve growth factor and increasing function of endogenous analgesics such as Nav1.7 antagonists.[27] Repurposing of drugs such as minocycline, which have shown attenuation of pain hypersensitivity by inhibition of microglial cell activation, has also shown promise in animal studies.[32]

## Conclusion

The inclusion of PPSP in the ICD-11, only attests to what an important clinical challenge the condition presents to pain physicians. There is an increased focus on preventing PPSP since the biopsychological condition results in a significantly negative effect on the patient's quality of life. Unfortunately, in spite of the current efforts, the evidence on both prevention strategies and pharmacological and non-pharmacological interventions is limited. What remains unequivocally true, is that patients who are at a higher risk of developing PPSP need to be identified. A multidisciplinary holistic approach to address the pain, by use of appropriate pharmacotherapy, pain or surgical interventions and psychological tools has the potential to limit the bio-socio-psychological impact of PPSP.

## References

1. Bruce J, Quinlan J. Chronic Post Surgical Pain. Rev Pain. 2011 Sep;5(3):23–9.
2. Dobson GP. Trauma of major surgery: A global problem that is not going away. Int J Surg. 2020 Sep;81:47–54.
3. Lopes A, Seligman Menezes M, Antonio Moreira de Barros G. Chronic postoperative pain: ubiquitous and scarcely appraised: narrative review. Braz J Anesthesiol. 2021 Nov-Dec; 71(6):649–655.
4. Hofer DM, Lehmann T, Zaslansky R, Harnik M, Meissner W, Stüber F, et al. Rethinking the definition of chronic postsurgical pain: composites of patient-reported pain-related outcomes vs pain intensities alone. Pain. 2022 Dec 1;163(12):2457–2465.
5. Kraychete DC, Sakata RK, Lannes Lde O, Bandeira ID, Sadatsune EJ. Postoperative persistent chronic pain: what do we know about prevention, risk factors, and treatment. Braz J Anesthesiol. 2016 Sep-Oct;66(5):505–12.

6. Fuller AM, Bharde S, Sikandar S. The mechanisms and management of persistent postsurgical pain. Front Pain Res (Lausanne). 2023 Jul 6;4:1154597.
7. Macrae WA, Davies HTO. Chronic postsurgical pain. In: Crombie IK, Linton S, Von Korff M, LeResche L, eds. Epidemiology of Pain. Seattle: IASP Press, 1999;125–42.
8. Macrae WA. Chronic pain after surgery. Br J Anaesth 2001;87:88–98.
9. Werner MU, Kongsgaard UE. I. Defining persistent post-surgical pain: is an update required? Br J Anaesth. 2014 Jul;113(1):1–4.
10. Treede RD, Rief W, Barke A, Aziz Q, Bennett MI, Benoliel R, et al. Chronic pain as a symptom or a disease: the IASP Classification of Chronic Pain for the International Classification of Diseases (ICD-11). Pain. 2019 Jan;160(1):19–27.
11. Schug SA, Lavand'Homme P, Barke A, et al. The IASP classification of chronic pain for ICD-11: chronic postsurgical or post traumatic pain. Pain. 2019;160:45–52.
12. Fletcher D, Stamer UM, Pogatzki-Zahn E, Zaslansky R, Tanase NV, Perruchoud C, et al. Chronic postsurgical pain in Europe: An observational study. Eur J Anaesthesiol. 2015 Oct;32(10):725–34.
13. Rosenberger DC, Pogatzki-Zahn EM. Chronic post-surgical pain – update on incidence, risk factors and preventive treatment options. BJA Educ. 2022 May;22(5):190–196.
14. Gulur P, Nelli A. Persistent postoperative pain: mechanisms and modulators. Curr Opin Anaesthesiol. 2019 Oct;32(5):668–673.
15. Macrae WA. Chronic post-surgical pain: 10 years on. Br Janaesth. 2008;101:77–86.
16. Lopes A, Seligman Menezes M, Antonio Moreira de Barros G. Chronic postoperative pain: ubiquitous and scarcely appraised: narrative review. Braz J Anesthesiol. 2021 Nov-Dec; 71(6):649–655.
17. Glare P, Aubrey K, Gulati A, Lee YC, Moryl N, Overton S. Pharmacologic Management of Persistent Pain in Cancer Survivors. Drugs. 2022 Feb;82(3):275–291.
18. Pellegrino PR, Are M. Pain management in cancer surgery: Global inequities and strategies to address them. J Surg Oncol. 2023 Nov;128(6):1032–1037.
19. Brown M, Farquhar-Smith P. Pain in cancer survivors; filling in the gaps. Br J Anaesth. 2017 Oct 1;119(4):723–736.
20. Humble SR, Varela N, Jayaweera A, Bhaskar A. Chronic postsurgical pain and cancer: the catch of surviving the unsurvivable. Curr Opin Support Palliat Care. 2018 Jun;12(2):118–123.
21. Montes A, Roca G, Cantillo J, Sabate S. Presurgical risk model for chronic postsurgical pain based on 6 clinical predictors: a prospective external validation. Pain 2020; 161: 2611–8.
22. Meretoja TJ, Andersen KG, Bruce J, Haasio L, Sipila R, Scott NW, et al. Clinical prediction model and tool for assessing risk of persistent pain after breast cancer surgery. J Clin Oncol 2017; 35: 1660–7.
23. van Driel MEC, van Dijk JFM, Baart SJ, Meissner W, Huygen FJPM, Rijsdijk M. Development and validation of a multivariable prediction model for early prediction of chronic postsurgical pain in adults: a prospective cohort study. Br J Anaesth 2022; 129:407–15.
24. Carley ME, Chaparro LE, Choinière M, et al. Pharmacotherapy for the prevention of chronic pain after surgery in adults: an updated systematic review and meta-analysis. Anesthesiology 2021; 135: 304e25.
25. Kim BR, Yoon SH, Lee HJ. Practical strategies for the prevention and management of chronic postsurgical pain. Korean J Pain. 2023 Apr 1;36(2):149–162.
26. Thapa P, Euasobhon P. Chronic postsurgical pain: current evidence for prevention and management. Korean J Pain. 2018 Jul;31(3):155–173.
27. Richebé P, Capdevila X, Rivat C. Persistent Postsurgical Pain: Pathophysiology and Preventative Pharmacologic Considerations. Anesthesiology. 2018 Sep;129(3):590–607.
28. Abdel-Magid AF. Nav1.7 Inhibitors: Potential Effective Therapy for the Treatment of Chronic Pain. ACS Med Chem Lett. 2015 Aug 14;6(9):956–7.

29. Na HS, Koo CH, Koo BW, Ryu JH, Jo H, Shin HJ. Effect of the paravertebral block on chronic postsurgical pain after thoracic surgery: a systematic review and meta-analysis of randomized controlled trials. J Cardiothorac Vasc Anesth 2023; 37: 252–60.
30. Nicholls JL, Azam MA, Burns LC, Englesakis M, Sutherland AM, Weinrib AZ, et al. Psychological treatments for the management of postsurgical pain: a systematic review of randomized controlled trials. Patient Relat Outcome Meas 2018; 9: 49–64.
31. Sun EC, Mariano ER, Narouze S, Gabriel RA, Elsharkawy H, Gulur P, et al. Making a business plan for starting a transitional pain service within the US healthcare system. Reg Anesth Pain Med 2021; 46: 727–31.
32. Searle RD, Simpson KH. Chronic post-surgical pain. Continuing Education in Anaesthesia Critical Care &; Pain. 2010 Feb;10(1):12–4.

Chapter 19

# Pain Management in Patients on Opioid Prescriptions

• Chandni Rana • Sumitra Bakshi

## INTRODUCTION

There has been an increase in the availability and rise in opioid consumption for medical reasons in the recent years, due to the ongoing reforms in the regulations related to opioid storage and use.[1] Non-medicinal abuse of opium products is also prevalent and may be under reported in this country, which is also a major exporter of opium. Opioids like Diamorphine (heroin) are often abused in combination with cannabinoids like Tetrahydrocannabinol (THC) and Cannabidiol (CBD). However, despite the indication, prolonged use of opioid leads to alterations in pain pathways. It is important to be aware of these changes and individualize pain treatment of such patients planned for surgery to avoid associated side effects commonly being inadequate pain relief and opioid withdrawal.

A patient is said to be on a chronic pain prescription if he/she is on opioid medications for more than 90 days, which can lead to changes which are clubbed and labelled as opioid use disorder (OUD).[2] Patients who are receiving opioid for more than a year with daily morphine equivalent dose of 120 mg or more (cancer being excluded) are said to be on long term high dose opioid prescription.[3]

OUD includes opioid tolerance, dependence and addiction (details have been covered in Chapter 7). Tolerance is when there is increase in the requirement of the drug for a similar effect. Opioid dependence is the development of physical symptoms/ withdrawal symptoms with abrupt discontinuation of the drug. Opioid addiction is a condition characterized by the continued use of a specific psychoactive substance despite physical, psychological or social harm. In this condition, the person is compelled to take the drug for its effects and to avoid the discomfort of its absence.

## APPLIED PHYSIOLOGY

It is essential to understand OUD with respect to the pain pathway.[4,5] Normally, the detection of a noxious stimuli is by the nociceptors, which are special cells that carry the impulse till the spinal cord via the A delta and C fibers. In the spinal cord, from the dorsal root ganglion, the impulse travels along the spino-thalamic tract reaching the thalamus and then to the somatosensory cortex. Along this transmission, there are inputs from various structures like Peri Aqueductal Gray (PAG) matter, Rostroventral medulla (RVM) in the midbrain. These are termed as the descending pain modulating pathway. These would reduce the neurotransmitter release along the pain pathway and cause anti-nociception. The RVM has on-cells and off-cells. The on-cells are GABAergic (gaba-aminobutyric acid) and off-cells glutaminergic. When a normal pain stimulus travels, the on-cells are activated by GABA and pain is perceived. Activation of off-cells decreases the perception of pain.

There are μ (Mu) opioid receptors in this pathway, which are G protein coupled and have GABAergic neurons. Normally these GABA neurons are tonically active, which would inhibit the PAG and RVM projection in the pain pathway. When μ receptors are stimulated by opioids, they would inhibit the GABA neurons, and enhance the PAG and RVM inhibitory effect on pain. The location of these μ receptors play a role. When the presynaptic μ receptors are stimulated by the opioids, there would be inhibition of voltage gated calcium channels in the presynaptic neuron, leading to decrease in intracellular calcium and hence decrease in the release of GABA at the synapse. When post-synaptic μ receptors are stimulated, there would be influx of potassium, leading to hyperpolarisation of the post-synaptic neuron. At the end, it would decrease the GABA inhibition on the PAG and RVM neurons, and lead to anti-nociception. In addition, μ agonist via the adenylcyclase pathway (reduction in cAMP levels), reduces pain perception.

## OPIOID TOLERANCE

Tolerance to a drug is defined as increased requirement of the drug for a similar response. There is no clear timeline for development of tolerance to opioids. Long-term exposure of opioids at PAG would lead to neuroadaptations and intracellular signaling changes, which would reduce the effect of the opioids and is the basis of development of tolerance. Presence of opioids at PAG for longer duration leads to uncoupling of the μ receptors with the G-protein mediated signaling.[5] This leads to reduction in the inhibition of the calcium channels in the presynaptic neuron. The disinhibition of the GABAergic neurons would be inadequate; hence the pain transmission increases, leading to increase in opioid requirement. Chronic levels of μ agonist causes increase in the level of cAMP and would further increase GABA release.[6] Chronic levels of μ agonist cause upregulation of the Toll like receptors-4 (TLR4) on the astrocytes and glial cells.[4] This upregulation leads to release of excitatory cytokines, which increases the excitatory state of the GABAergic neurons, and contributes to the development of tolerance to opioids.[4]

### Opioid Induced Hyperalgesia (OIH)[7,8]

It is a paradoxical condition where, patients with OUD, develop increased sensitization of pain to a normal/painful stimulus. This hyperalgesia should be suspected when the patient complaints of increased pain, or diffuse allodynia. The molecular mechanism of development of tolerance to opioids and OIH is interlinked, and few hypothesis available to explain the process are as follows:

1. *Central glutaminergic system:* Increase in glutamate causes increase in glial cytokines, and increase activation of N-methyl D-aspartate (NMDA) receptors which play a key role in OIH. If NMDA receptors on the post-synaptic neurons are inhibited, the proportion/incidence of OIH and tolerance reduces. Calcium regulated intracellular protein kinase C is also involved in OIH. There is also a role of NMDA mediated apoptosis of dorsal horn neurons.

2. *Spinal dynorphins:* Prolonged opioid use leads to increased dynorphins levels, which is associated with increased release of cGRP (excitatory neurotransmitter). This develops into a pro-nociceptor state. Cholecystokinin is another excitatory neurotransmitter in medulla, which upregulates the dynorphins in the spinal system, leading to increased nociception.
3. *Descending facilitation:* In normal individual, the descending inhibitory pathway from RVM inhibits pain perception. However, due to repeated activity of opioids at the neuronal level in RVM, it may start stimulating the on cells and cause pain.
4. *Genetics influences:* Study has shown genetic variation in the Catechol O-methyltransferase (COMT) enzyme which would affect the breakdown of neurotransmitter dopamine/adrenaline in the synapses and affect the pain transmission and thus pain modulation.
5. *Decreased reuptake of neurotransmitter and enhanced nociceptive response:* A commonly attributed mechanism. There is a decreased reuptake of neurotransmitter like substance P and glutamate in the primary afferent fibres. With chronic opioid usage, there is increase in the beta-2 adrenergic receptors (β2AR) in spinal pathway. There is an increased responsiveness to the excitatory chemicals like substance P and glutamate. There is an increased sensitivity of the second order neurons to these transmitters after prolonged opioid use, which leads to hyperalgesia.

## GOALS FOR PERIOPERATIVE TREATMENT (OF PATIENTS WITH PRIOR OPIOID USE)

Perioperative pain management of such patients is challenging and require a holistic approach. A brief summary of principles involved includes:

1. Identification of the patients at risk.
2. Adequate preoperative assessment and interdisciplinary discussion involving the surgeon, anesthetist, pain consultant, psychiatrist, nursing staff and the family regarding perioperative pain management, multimodal analgesia, aim of adequate pain relief and possible complications.
3. Clinical examination and optimization
   a. Consideration of comorbid conditions and psychological affect/mood disorders. To get a psychiatrist consultation if required.
   b. Provide with equi-analgesic dosing of baseline opioids to prevent withdrawal.
4. Evaluate and treat OIH
5. Apply additional analgesic treatments for acute pain
   a. Multimodal analgesia: Paracetamol, non-steroidal anti-inflammatory drugs (NSAIDs), ketamine, regional analgesic blocks.
   b. Non-pharmacological therapies—massage, breathing and relaxing exercising, etc.
6. Postoperative assessment and management of pain in the wards via a dedicated pain team
7. Discharge plan: The need to continue the baseline opioids, addition of NSAIDs, paracetamol and gabapentiniods has to be individualized.

Identification of at-risk patient can occur at the surgical out-patient department (OPD) or when the patient comes for the pre-anesthetic evaluation (PAE). Once identified, record all prescription, medicines, route of administration, daily dosing, intake of any additional doses. Elicit history of any physical signs of withdrawal in the past. Patient undergoing a de-addiction program for OUD/substance use disorder (SUD) can also be encountered. For such patients, the history of the duration of addiction, duration of treatment, treatment history, and compliance with the treatment is essential. It is important to note any history of drug craving or drug seeking, relapse, hospital admission with withdrawal, change in social behavior and associated altered mental health.

### Clinical Examination and Optimization

Along with routine physical examination, attention is to be paid to social behavior, inspecting skin for needle marks in SUDs. Optimization of opioid medication in the preoperative period would depend on, when the patient presents to the preanesthetic checkup. If the patient is posted for an elective surgery after 2–3 weeks, non-opioid medications should be added to reduce the requirement of opioids. Paracetamol, NSAIDs, gabapentin/pregabalin, amitriptiline are known to have opioid sparing effect. The tapering of the opioid medications can also be done by an interventional block prior to surgery.

### Providing Equianalgesic Dosing of Ongoing Opioids to Prevent Withdrawal

Majority of the hospitals have a separate designated acute pain service (APS) team lead by a pain consultant. When patients with such opioid requirements come for PAE and get admitted for either elective/emergency surgery, the APS team should be informed and involved. The preoperative changes in the drugs, formulations and route of administration should be done in communication with the APS team.

1. *Oral high dose morphine:* First step is to calculate the daily dose requirement. If adequate days are available, an attempt must be made to reduce the daily requirement of opioid as discussed above. Convert it into the intravenous morphine/fentanyl daily dosing and to be given as basal infusion in the intraoperative and postoperative period.
2. *Opioid agonist (fentanyl) transdermal patches:* If the patient is on transdermal patch-opioid switch should be considered.[9] It is recommended to remove any transdermal patch in the intraoperative period to avoid malfunction of the patch.[9]
3. *Buprenorphine patches/sublingual tablets (buprenorphine maintenance therapy):* There are conflicting recommendations regarding the perioperative buprenorphine treatment. However, consensus and smaller studies have shown good analgesia and lesser incidence of withdrawal when buprenorphine was continued perioperatively.[10,11] If the patient is on lower doses (<70 μg/hr) or <10 mg/day sublingually, by continuing buprenorphine preoperatively, perioperative management of acute pain would not be difficult. If need is to convert from buprenorphine patch to oral morphine, conversion ratio is 1:75.[12] For example: Patient is on 30–35 μg/hr buprenorphine patch (5 mg patch for 7 days), requirement of oral morphine is 35 × 24 × 75 = 60 mg morphine over 24 hr. Its equivalent intravenous morphine can thus be calculated to estimate the daily requirement.
4. *Methadone therapy (methadone maintenance therapy):* Patient is likely to be on methadone (μ agonist) for analgesia (in a previously opioid dependent) or to prevent withdrawal with once daily dosing. It is recommended to continue the methadone dose preoperatively.[11]

5. *Naltrexone:* Naltrexone is a μ receptor antagonist, used during de-addiction either as oral tablets or intramuscular injections. No clear consensus or recommendations exist on the use of naltrexone in the perioperative period. Continuing the naltrexone would block all μ receptors and managing acute pain would become challenging. On the other hand, if discontinued, it would upregulate all the μ receptors and cause hypersensitivity to pain and would need very high doses of short acting μ receptor agonist for acute pain control. It is preferred to manage the pain on non-opioid analgesics and regional analgesia, thus avoiding interference with naltrexone levels and opioid receptors.[13]
6. *Anti-depressants and anxiolytics:* Patients may have concurrent depression/anxiety related/unrelated to cancer and associated pain. These medications have to be continued in the perioperative period.
7. *Cannabinoids:* Recommendations are against sudden tapering/stopping the cannabinoids. Patients should be counselled regarding deaddiction programme and started on the therapy for the same. In case of emergency surgery, last dose of cannabinoid (inhaled/intravenous) should be noted and associated risk about withdrawal and cardiorespiratory complications needs to be explained to the family. Patients on deaddiction treatment would be on naltrexone/dronabinol, which needs to be continued in the perioperative period.[14]

### Evaluation for OIH

It is essential to do a complete pain assessment to elicit altered pain threshold and hyperalgesia. Whenever present, OIH must be treated. The challenge lies in its diagnosis. In patients' with opioid tolerance, increase in the dosage of the opioid, will lead to reduction in pain. Contrary to that, in OIH, the pain would worsen with opioid use. As the main mechanism considered is central sensitization, modulators of NMDA would facilitate in reduction of pain and reversing OIH. Ketamine, dextromethorphan, clonidine and buprenorphine are commonly used.[7] Treatment of OIH would include tapering and reduction of opioids, opioid rotation or starting the patients on non-opioid medications. Methadone has a role in reducing OIH. Advantage of methadone is that it does not have cross tolerance. Buprenorphine being a dynorphin antagonist, partial μ agonist and kappa antagonist, it is the most suitable choice for opioid rotation and analgesia in OIH.[7]

## INTRAOPERATIVE ANALGESIC PLAN

Being on opioids for a long duration may lead to requirement of higher anesthetic depth intraoperatively. Hence when use of muscle relaxants is planned, it is advisable to use appropriate anesthetic depth monitors like Bispectral Index (BIS) to prevent awareness.

Use of regional in addition to systemic multimodal analgesics is the consensus. Regional analgesia includes neuraxial block (epidural, para vertebral), peripheral nerve blocks. Epidural analgesia with local anesthetic without any opioid should be given for the entire duration of surgery. Peripheral nerve blocks including limb blocks and fascial plane blocks with catheters must be considered, details have been covered in Chapter 16. Optimise the use of non-opioid analgesics like paracetamol, NSAIDs, dexmedetomidine, magnesium, ketamine, dexamethasone and lignocaine.

One needs to estimate the daily requirement of opioid, fifty percent of the same is to be given as a basal infusion or in divided doses in the intraoperative and immediate postoperative period (Table 19.1).[15]

*Example 1:* A patient of rectal cancer is on oral morphine 90 mg BD. He has been posted for surgery and need to convert this morphine into intravenous opioids: 90 mg BD is 180 mg oral morphine in 24 hours.

Dose of morphine in 24 hours = 180 mg oral

Dose of morphine in 24 hours IV = 180/3 = 60 mg, half dose (30 mg) needs to be supplemented over 24 hours.

Rate of infusion = 30/24 = 1.25 mg/hr of intravenous morphine.

***Postoperative:*** Managing patients' adequate pain relief without causing anxiety and preventing opioid withdrawal is the real challenge. The patient would need vigilant monitoring by a dedicated team which is generally the APS team. The patients should be monitored in high dependency unit (HDU) with a nurse trained to identify signs of withdrawal or overdosing, refer to Table 19.2.

Continuous epidural analgesia with local anesthetic is recommended in suitable cases. Peripheral nerve block catheters can be inserted for intermittent/continuous local anesthetic administration. The required opioid dose is to be delivered via PCA pump as ongoing basal infusion. The demand dose through the PCA pump would be higher than the dose for an opioid naïve patient. The daily dose calculation would be difficult in patients on illicit drugs/cannabinoids, titrated opioids should be administered via the PCA pump. The advantage of PCA pump is that the patient can control his pain level and receive additional doses of opioid as and when needed. One disadvantage of

**Table 19.1: Equianalgesic doses of opioids and oral morphine equivalents (OME)[16–19]**

| Drug | Parenteral route | Conversion factor to OME | Oral route | Conversion factor to OME |
|---|---|---|---|---|
| | **Intravenous** | | | |
| Morphine | 10 mg IV | 3 | 30 mg | 1 |
| Merperidine | 75 mg IV | 0.4 | 300 mg | 0.1 |
| Pentazocine | 30 mg IV | 1.1 | 50 mg | 0.6 |
| Butorphanol | 2 mg IV | 15 | | |
| Fentanyl | 0.1 mg IV | 300 | | |
| Buprenorphine | 0.3 mg (IV/IM) | 75 | 0.8 mg (S/L) | 38.8 |
| Tramadol | 100 mg | | 150 mg | 0.2 |
| Tapentadol | | | 75 mg | 0.4 |
| | **Transdermal** | | | |
| Buprenorphine | 15 µg/hr* | 75 | | |
| Fentanyl | 12.5 µg/hr# | 2.4 | | |

*This is 30 mg oral morphine equianalgesic dose provided by a 2.5 mg buprenorphine patch—however the least dose commercially available is 5 mg patch. Details of the conversion is explained in the text. (refer paragraph on buprenorphine patch)

#Dose of morphine over 24 hours= 12.5 × 2.4 = 30 mg oral morphine.

**Table 19.2: Cows scale**

| Symptoms | 0 | 1 | 2 | 3 | 4 | 5 |
|---|---|---|---|---|---|---|
| Resting pulse rate (record after sitting/lying for 1 minute) | <80 | 81–100 | 101–120 | - | >120 | - |
| Sweating | No chills/ flushing | Subjective report of chills/ flushing | Flushed/ observable moistness on face | Beads of sweat of face/brows | Sweat streaming of face | - |
| Restlessness | Able to sit still | Reports difficulty in sitting still but able to do it | - | Frequent shifting or extraneous movements of arms/legs | - | Unable to sit still for more than few seconds |
| Pupil size | Normal size for room light | Pupils larger than normal for room light | Pupils moderately dilated | - | - | Pupils so dilated only rim of iris is visible |
| Bones and joint ache (if patient has pain previously, only new component is attributed to withdrawal) | Not present | Mild diffuse discomfort | Patient complaints severe diffuse aching of joints/ muscles | - | Patient is rubbing joints or muscles and is unable to sit still because of discomfort | - |
| Runny nose or tearing (not accounted for by cold symptoms and allergies) | Not present | Nasal stuffiness or usually moist eyes | Nose running or tearing | - | Nose constantly running or tears streaming down the cheeks | - |
| GI upset (over last ½ hour) | No GI symptoms | Stomach cramps | Nausea or loose stools | Vomiting or diarrhea | - | Multiple episodes of diarrhea or vomiting |
| Tremors (observation of outstretched hands) | No tremor | Tremor can be felt but not observed | Slight tremor observable | | Gross tremor or muscle twitching | |

*(Contd...)*

| Table 19.2: Cows scale *(Contd...)* | | | | | | |
|---|---|---|---|---|---|---|
| **Symptoms** | **0** | **1** | **2** | **3** | **4** | **5** |
| Yawning (observation during assessment) | No yawning | Yawning once/twice during assessment | Yawning 3–4 times during assessment | | Yawning several times/ minute | |
| Anxiety/ irritability | None | Patient reports increasing irritability / anxiousness | Patient obvious irritable/ anxious | | Patient so irritable/ anxious that participation in the assessment is difficult | |
| Goose flesh skin | Skin is smooth | | | Piloerection of can be felt or hair standing up on arms | | Prominent piloerection |

PCA in this scenario is the risk of overdosing, hence would need adequate vigilance. Once enteral feeding is established, the daily opioid requirement can be administered orally. Suitable multimodal analgesic needs to be continued in the postoperative period. Gabapentin/pregabalin, if not started preoperatively, should be started in the post-operative period.

## Cows Scale[20]

It is clinical opiate withdrawal scale-used for measuring opiate withdrawal symptoms. For assessment, the 11 items are scored and severity of withdrawal assessed. Mild = 5 to 12, moderate = 13 to 24, moderately severe= 25 to 36 and severe withdrawal >36.

## Discharge

Prior to discharge, the patient needs to be shifted from intravenous to oral opioids. The need of opioids in cancer patients would be reduced after definitive surgery, however, post-surgical pain may persist in some patients. Opioids should not be abruptly reduced, tapering of these drugs by reducing dose weekly or by opioid rotation is preferred. The weaker opioid should be started at 50–75% of equianalgesic dose and eventually tapered. Commonly used preparation include buprenorphine patches/sublingual tablets. Transitional pain service plays a crucial role for pain management in such patients, details covered in Chapter 17.

## Summary

The possibility of encountering patients on opioid treatment for cancer/noncancer pain undergoing surgery is on the increasing trend. Knowledge about the perioperative pain management of such patients becomes important. Detailed preoperative assessment and optimization of analgesics with patient counseling is essential. Interdisciplinary approach involving the surgeon, anesthetist, pain consultant, psychiatrist, nursing staff and the family is recommended for a better perioperative outcome. A thorough knowledge on identification of opioid tolerance, opioid induced hyperalgesia, dependence, withdrawal and its management are of utmost importance. Use of regional and non-opioid analgesics is the line of management with providing daily opioid requirement to prevent sudden withdrawal of the drug. Patient needs to follow-up in the postoperative period for prevention of chronicity of pain and to taper and stop the opioid analgesics.

## References


1. Cleary J, Simha N, Panieri A, et al. Formulary availability and regulatory barriers to accessibility of opioids for cancer pain in India: a report from the Global Opioid Policy Initiative (GOPI). Ann Oncol. 2013;24 Suppl 11:xi33-xi40. doi:10.1093/annonc/mdt501
2. Jackman C. Perioperative Pain Management for the Chronic Pain Patient With Long-Term Opioid Use. Orthop Nurs. 2019;38(2):159–63. doi:10.1097/NOR.0000000000000526
3. Bailey J, Gill S, Poole R. Long-term, high-dose opioid prescription for chronic non-cancer pain in primary care: an observational study. BJGP Open. 2022 Dec 20;6(4):BJGPO.2021.0217. doi: 10.3399/BJGPO.2021.0217. PMID: 35728819; PMCID: PMC9904796.
4. Lueptow LM, Fakira AK and Bobeck EN (2018) The Contribution of the Descending Pain Modulatory Pathway in Opioid Tolerance. Front. Neurosci. 12:886. doi: 10.3389/fnins.2018.00886
5. Mercadante S, Arcuri E, Santoni A. Opioid-induced Tolerance and Hyperalgesia. CNS Drugs 2019;33:943–55. https://doi.org/10.1007/s40263-019-00660-0
6. Khan F, Mehan A. Addressing opioid tolerance and opioid-induced hypersensitivity: Recent developments and future therapeutic strategies. Pharmacol Res Perspect. 2021;9(3):e00789. doi:10.1002/prp2.789
7. Lee M, Silverman SM, Hansen H, Patel VB and Manchikanti L. A comprehensive review of opioid-induced hyperalgesia. Pain physician 2011;14(2):145–61.
8. Akilan Velayudhan, Geoff Bellingham, Patricia Morley-Forster, Opioid-induced hyperalgesia, Continuing Education in Anaesthesia Critical Care & Pain, Volume 14, Issue 3, June 2014, Pages 125–129, https://doi.org/10.1093/bjaceaccp/mkt045
9. Kaye AD, Menard BL, Ehrhardt KP, Gennuso SA, Okereke EC, Tirumala SR, Fox CJ and Cornett EM. Consensus Perioperative Management Best Practices for Patients on Transdermal Fentanyl Patches Undergoing Surgery. Current pain and headache reports, 2019;23(7):50. https://doi.org/10.1007/s11916-019-0780-2
10. Miclescu A. Chronic pain patient and anaesthesia. Romanian journal of anaesthesia and intensive care, 2019;26(1):59–66. https://doi.org/10.2478/rjaic-2019-0009
11. Huxtable CA, Roberts LJ, Somogyi AA, MacIntyre PE. Acute pain management in opioid-tolerant patients: a growing challenge. Anaesth Intensive Care. 2011;39(5):804–823. doi:10.1177/0310057X1103900505
12. Thota RS, Ramanjulu R, Ahmed A, Jain P, Salins N, Bhatnagar S, et al. Indian society for study of pain, cancer pain special interest group guidelines on pharmacological management of cancer pain (Part II). Indian J Palliat Care 2020;26:180–90.
13. Burns SL, Majdak P and Urman RD. Perioperative and Periprocedural anesthetic management of opioid tolerant patients and patients with active and medically treated opioid use disorder. Current opinion in anaesthesiology, 2022 ;35(4), 514–20. https://doi.org/10.1097/ACO.0000000000001157
14. Shah S, Schwenk ES, Sondekoppam RV, et al. ASRA Pain Medicine consensus guidelines on the management of the perioperative patient on cannabis and cannabinoids. Reg Anesth Pain Med. 2023;48(3):97–117. doi:10.1136/rapm-2022-104013
15. Hadi I, Morley-Forster PK, Dain S, Horrill K, Moulin DE. Brief review: perioperative management of the patient with chronic non-cancer pain. Can J Anaesth. 2006;53(12):1190–1199. doi:10.1007/BF03021580

16. Nielsen S, Degenhardt L, Hoban B, Gisev N. A synthesis of oral morphine equivalents (OME) for opioid utilisation studies. Pharmacoepidemiol Drug Saf. 2016;25(6):733–737. doi:10.1002/pds.3945
17. Skaer TL. Dosing considerations with transdermal formulations of fentanyl and buprenorphine for the treatment of cancer pain. J Pain Res. 2014;7:495–503. Published 2014 Aug 19. doi:10.2147/JPR.S36446
18. Gordon DB, Stevenson KK, Griffie J, Muchka S, Rapp C, Ford-Roberts K. Opioid equianalgesic calculations. J Palliat Med. 1999;2(2):209–218. doi:10.1089/jpm.1999.2.209
19. The Royal Australian College of General Practitioners (RACGP). (2019) (n.d.). Approximate potencies of various opioids relative to 10 mg parenteral morphine. Guideline for Prescribing Drugs of Dependence in General Practice. Retrieved August 25, 2024, from https://www.racgp.org.au/getattachment/6099a0ff-4dd6-43c1-891f-7d976fa4d7ee/attachment.aspx?disposition=inline
20. Wesson DR, Ling W. The Clinical Opiate Withdrawal Scale (COWS). J Psychoactive Drugs. 2003;35(2):253–259. doi:10.1080/02791072.2003.10400007

Chapter 20

# Postoperative Pain Management in Children

• Bhakti Trivedi • Akankshya Sarangi

## INTRODUCTION

Perioperative pediatric pain management poses a complex and multifaceted challenge. It requires a tailored strategy that factors in the unique physiological and psychological characteristics of children. Specific challenges can be due to cognitive/emotional/developmental differences, limited communication abilities, and heightened sensitivity to pain.

Appropriate perioperative pain management in this population is a fundamental aspect of their care since it can affect their recovery, well-being, and overall experience during and after surgery. Effective pain alleviation is critical for minimizing discomfort, improving outcomes, and enhancing the entire experience. Communication and collaboration between the anesthetists, surgeon, and the pediatrician is of the utmost importance for good anesthesia and pain management in children.

Herein, we aim to provide a comprehensive overview of perioperative pain management in pediatric patients, covering preoperative assessment, intraoperative strategies, and postoperative pain management. We will discuss the role of multimodal analgesia, regional anesthesia techniques, pharmacological and non-pharmacological interventions in optimizing pain relief and minimizing adverse effects and highlight the importance of a multidisciplinary team approach.

## ETIOLOGY OF PEDIATRIC PAIN

Acute pain in children mainly stem from acute medical illness, procedures, surgeries and trauma. Regardless of the cause of pain, certain factors should always be taken into consideration for successful pain management. These factors include but are not limited to, anticipation of pain, thorough pain assessment, training of the staff involved in caring for these patients, provision of a peaceful environment inclusive of parents/caretakers.[1]

### Pain Assessment

Pain is multi-faceted, having both sensory and an affective dimension to it.[2]

Pediatric pain assessment more often than not, poses a challenge for care providers. The intricacy of pain assessment in this group is usually in discriminating pain from other unpleasant expressions/feelings such as of hunger or fear.[3] The pediatric pain assessment and management should ideally start with screening and identifying patients with potential for developing pain or those in pain. The pain score should be assessed against a pain scale appropriate to their particular age group and their developmental age.

Most commonly used parameters for pediatric pain assessment that are relied upon are as follows:[4]

- *Biological measures:* Any change in heart rate, blood pressure and respiratory rate
- *Observational/behavioral measures:* This includes the child's response towards pain
- *Self-reporting measures:* Relies on the child's account of his experience of pain.

Self-reporting pain measures have been the gold standard of pain assessment in older children who are capable of describing their subjective pain experience.[5]

For this, the faces pain ladder may be employed to assess pediatric pain (Fig. 20.1). This scale consists of a score of 0 to 10, with 0 representing a happy face or no pain at

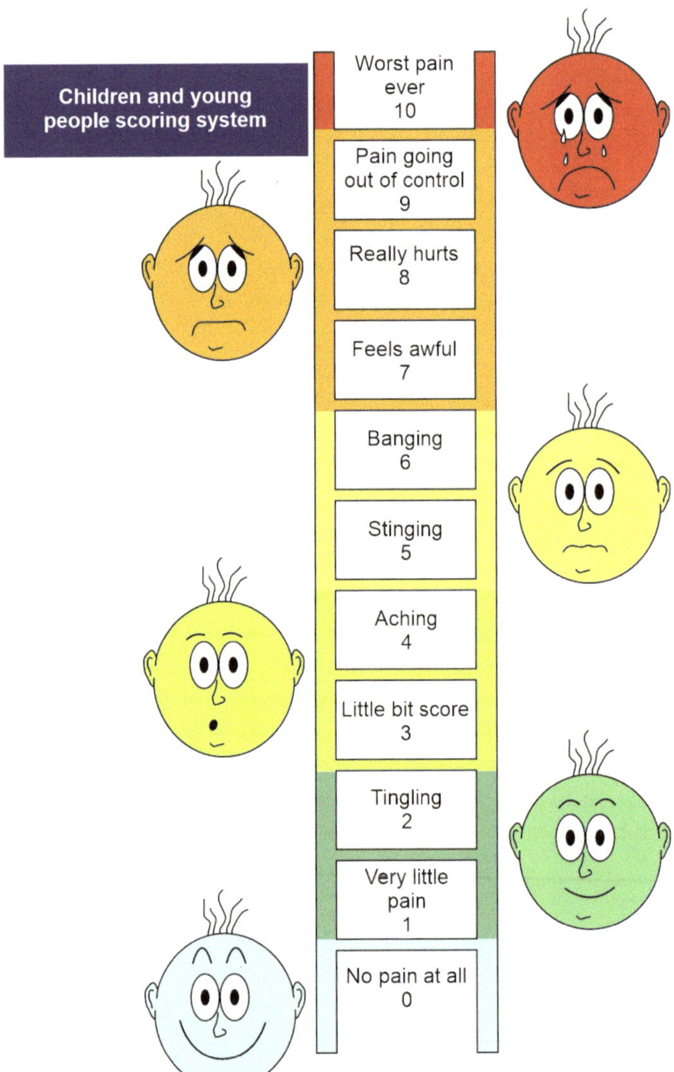
Children and young people scoring system
Worst pain ever 10
Pain going out of control 9
Really hurts 8
Feels awful 7
Banging 6
Stinging 5
Aching 4
Little bit score 3
Tingling 2
Very little pain 1
No pain at all 0

Fig. 20.1: Faces pain ladder[6]

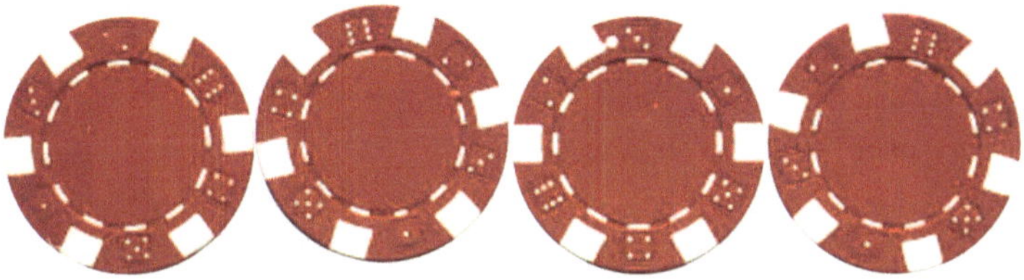

Fig. 20.2: Poker chip pain tool[7,12]

all and 10 corresponding to a crying face or worst pain ever.[6] Similarly another self-reporting pain scale of value is the poker chip pain tool, wherein 4 poker chips are used, with one poker chip referring to little bit of hurt and 4 poker chips quantifying to most hurt possible (Fig. 20.2).[7]

However, in infants and younger children, since self-report measures may not be practical, one has to rely more on behavioral indices like facial expressions, motor responses, crying and even the intricate responses such as changes in the circadian rhythm for pain evaluation.[8] Hence, both observational and self reporting pain scales are routinely used in clinical practice.

Several pain scales are now available to give an objective value to pain (Table 20.1). They may be used to assess the severity of pain, based on the age/intellect of the child.[7–17]

## Management of Perioperative Pain

Effective perioperative pain management is crucial to promote early mobilization, reduce the risk of complications, and improve overall patient satisfaction. An amalgamation of pharmacological and non-pharmacological interventions should be used to provide complete pain relief.

The strategies to decrease perioperative pain in these patients should encompass the idea of blunting the pain response even before it has set in via the use of pre-emptive analgesics as well as the implementation of less invasive surgical techniques.[18]

Involving the next of kin (parents/caretakers) while managing perioperative pain is of utmost importance. Given the dependency of children on their parents/care givers, they are a significant vulnerable section of society, needing special attention.[19]

During surgery, a multimodal approach to pain management is recommended to target both the visceral and somatic pain pathways. Non-opioid analgesics, such as nonsteroidal anti-inflammatory drugs (NSAIDs) and acetaminophen, along with field infiltration of local anesthetic are effective as starting line of treatment for mild to moderate postoperative pain

For major and supramajor surgeries wherever appropriate, regional anesthesia techniques such as epidurals, caudal blocks and/or single shot or continuous peripheral nerve blocks or fascial plane blocks, can provide effective pain relief while reducing the systemic opioid exposure. These techniques can be particularly advantageous for surgeries involving the abdomen, chest, or extremities, particularly beneficial for those undergoing major surgery and at high-risk of opioid-related adverse effects. However, they require close monitoring and expertise to ensure secure and effective administration.

For severe pain, opioids can be used, but their use should be titrated to the lowest effective dose and duration possible. Depending on the age group of the patient, patient-

**Table 20.1: Pediatric pain scales**

| Pain scale acronym | Age group | Score interpretation |
|---|---|---|
| | *Observational scales* | |
| **Premature infant pain profile (PIPP)**<br>Indicators used are gestational age, behavioral state, heart rate, oxygen saturation, brow bulge, eye squeeze and nasolabial furrow | Preterm neonates | Mild: 0–6<br>Moderate: 7–12<br>Severe: 13–15 |
| **CRIES**<br>Components of the scale include crying, oxygen requirement, increase in the vital signs, expressions and sleeplessness | Neonates from 32 weeks of gestational age to 6 months | Mild: 0–3<br>Moderate: 4–6<br>Severe: 7–10 |
| **NIPS (neonatal infant pain scale)**<br>Includes 7 variables – facial expression, cry, breathing pattern, arms, legs, arousal state | Less than 1 year | Mild: 0-2<br>Moderate: 3–4<br>Severe: 5–7 |
| **COMFORT (for critical care setting)**<br>Components include alertness, calmness/agitation, respiratory response, crying, physical movement, muscle tone and facial tension | From birth to 18 years of age | Score of 17–26 indicates adequate pain control and sedation |
| **FLACC**<br>Face, leg, activity, cry, consolability | 2 months–7 years | Mild: 0–3<br>Moderate: 4–6<br>Severe: 7–10 |
| **CHEOPS (Children's Hospital of Eastern Ontario Pain Scale)**<br>Includes 4 parameters: Cry, facial expression, verbal, torso legs | 1 to 12 years | >/5: Consider analgesic<br>>/8: Requires analgesic |
| **MOPS (Modified Objective Pain Scale)**<br>Variables include crying, movement, agitation, posture, verbal | 8 months to 13 years | No pain: 0<br>Mild: 3<br>Moderate: 4–6<br>Severe: 7–10 |
| **EVENDOL (in emergency department)**<br>Consists of components like verbal expression, facial expression, movements, postures and environmental interaction | From birth to 7 years | Score ranges from 0–15<br>Treatment threshold is 4/15 |
| | *Self-reporting scales* | |
| **Wong baker faces** | 3 to 18 years | 0–10; 0 is no hurt and 10 is hurts worst |
| **VAS**<br>Visual Analogue Scale with zero being no pain and 10 being worst pain possible | 3 years to adult | No pain: 0–4 mm<br>Mild: 5–44 mm<br>Moderate: 45–74 mm<br>Severe: 75–100 mm |
| **Poker chip** | 4 to 7 years | One poker chip: Hurts a little bit<br>Two poker chip: Hurts a little more<br>Three poker chip: More yet<br>Four poker chip: Most hurt possible |

controlled analgesia (PCA) devices may be used to allow them to self-administer opioids within predetermined safety limits.

Non-pharmacological interventions, like acupuncture, distraction therapy, physical therapy, massage and music therapy, and psychological interventions, such as cognitive-behavioural therapy and relaxation techniques also play a significant role in reducing anxiety and optimising postoperative pain control. These techniques can help reduce pain intensity, improve functional outcomes, and enhance overall patient satisfaction along with reducing the need for pharmacological interventions.

It is essential to consider the root cause of pain, the onset, location, duration, behavioural and physiological signs as well as the contextual factors.[20] These need to be documented along with the pharmacological and non-pharmacological measures undertaken. The patient should be reassessed at regular intervals and appropriate modifications made.[20]

When commencing pain management, the following non-pharmacological strategies can be adapted as per the age group:[9]

1. *Neonates and infants:* It is important to encourage the parents/next of kin/caretakers to hold and comfort the child, to use both sensory (gentle touch, soft speaking) and comfort techniques (pacifier, swaddling).
2. *1–5 years:* Along with the above, simple and direct communication, demonstration of procedures on a play toy first, use of distraction therapy and offering choices wherever appropriate is essential.
3. *6–12 years:* Should be encouraged to be involved as much as possible in their treatments and the procedures should be explained in a clear, direct and simple language.
4. *Adolescents and older children:* Along with all the above cited techniques, different distraction techniques, gaming, guided imagery and spirituality should be encouraged.

The best way to go about pain management in pediatric population is the pediatric analgesic ladder. It is based or adapted from the World Health Organization (WHO) pain ladder, which was initially framed for adult cancer patients' pain management **(Fig. 20.3)**.

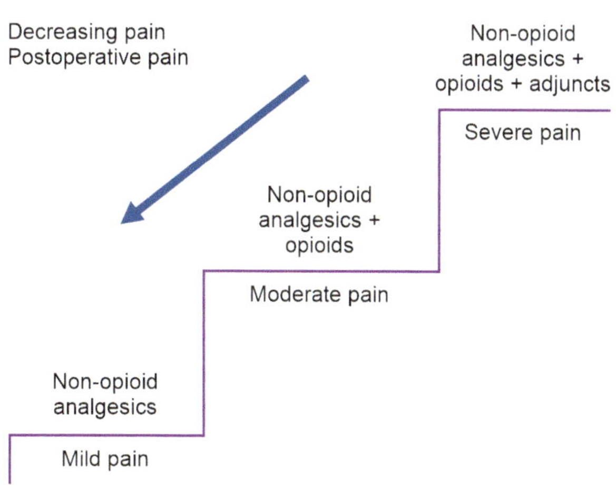


**Fig. 20.3:** Pediatric analgesic ladder (*Adapted from:* WHO Ladder)[21]

Pediatric pain management follows a hierarchical pattern for treatment ranging from mild, moderate to severe. Hence, depending on whether the surgery is superficial/ coelomic/involving neurovascular structures, the quantum of pain may vary and treatment may have to be accelerated immediately postoperative. The pediatric population with moderate to severe pain usually require both non-pharmacological (Fig. 20.4) and pharmacological (Table 20.2) treatment options.[9] Treatment may then be escalated to intravenous routes. However, intravenous route is a safe route and imparts immediate and rapid onset pain relief, but along with being painful, it also requires skill. Hence, it is also necessary to establish the importance of having various analgesic routes in the pediatric population, inclusive of topical, oral, intranasal, perrectal, inhalational/ nebulization (Table 20.3). In certain cases there may be difficulty in securing intravenous access, wherein intranasal routes can be used successfully to deliver analgesia.[22] The

**Table 20.2: Commonly used analgesics**

| Drugs | | Dosages | Notes |
|---|---|---|---|
| Non-opioids/ NSAIDs | Paracetamol or acetaminophen | 10–15 mg/kg, up to 4 times/day Total daily dose not to be exceeded: 100 mg/kg for children; 75 mg/kg for infants; 60 mg/kg for term and preterm neonates older than 32 weeks post-conceptual age; and 40 mg/kg for preterm neonates younger than 32 weeks post-conceptual age | No hematological and gastro-intestinal side effects. Analgesic and antipyretic action, not anti-inflammatory. Very low-risk of liver toxicity if the daily dose of paracetamol does not exceed 90 mg/kg in healthy children |
| | Ibuprofen | For 6 months to 12 years 5–10 mg/kg, every 6–8 hours, maximum 40 mg/kg/day<br>>12 years: 200–400 mg, every 4–6 hours, maximum 1200 mg/day, in severe pain 2400 mg/day | Hematological and gastro-intestinal side effects<br>Anti-inflammatory action |
| | Diclofenac | 1 mg/kg every 8 hours orally, rectally, or intravenously, maximum 2–3 mg/kg/day | Nausea, vomiting, renal toxicity |
| | Naproxen | 5 mg/kg, every 8–12 hours, maximum 1 g/day | Hematological and gastrointestinal side effects<br>Anti-inflammatory action |
| | Ketorolac | 0.5 mg/kg IV, every 6 hours, Not to exceed 5 days | Kidney and liver toxicity<br>Not recommended in less than two years of age |
| | Dextromethorphan | 1 mg/kg, every 6–8 hours | Nausea, drowsiness, confusion |
| | Acetylsalicylic acid | 10–15 mg/kg every 6–8 hours | Reye's syndrome (pre-pubertal children). Gastrointestinal and hematological adverse effects |

*(Contd...)*

**Table 20.2: Commonly used analgesics (*Contd...*)**

| Drugs | | Dosages | Notes |
|---|---|---|---|
| Opiods | Fentanyl | Bolus: 0.5-1 μg/kg 10–15 minutes (with close monitoring)<br>Infusion: 0.5–3 μg/kg/h | Nausea, vomiting, respiratory depression, itching, urinary retention |
| | Morphine | IV: 0.05–0.1 mg/kg every 2–4 hours<br>Oral: 0.5–1 mg/kg every 3–4 hours | Nausea, vomiting, urinary retention |
| | Remifentanil | Bolus: 0.1–0.5 μg/kg every hour<br>Infusion: 0.1-0.25 μg/kg/min | Nausea, vomiting, respiratory depression, itching, urinary retention |
| | Codeine | Oral: 0.5–1 mg/kg every 4 hours<br>However, FDA has issued a warning saying—since codeine carries serious risks, including respiratory depression and even death, which appear to be a greater risk in children younger than 12 years, it should not be used in them | Nausea, vomiting |
| | Hydromorphone | Bolus: 0.015 mg/kg every 2–4 hours<br>Infusion: 0.006 mg/kg/h<br>Oral: 0.06 mg/kg every 3–4 hours | Nausea, vomiting, urinary retention |
| Intravenous analgesia | Patient controlled analgesia (depends on the developmental age and understanding of the concept of the equipment used) | Morphine-most commonly used opioid for pediatric IV-PCA; Bolus dose (usually 0.02 mg/kg) with a lockout period of 5–10 minutes +/- background infusion<br>Along with the IV PCA, a small dose of naloxone infusion (0.25 μg/kg/hour), reduces the opioid related side effects without affecting their analgesic action | Effective pain treatment; allows patients to be in charge of their pain management and provides consistent blood levels of opioids |
| | Parent/nurse controlled analgesia (Pr CA/NCA) | | Although controversial, allows younger or physically/ cognitively impaired children to receive the PCA benefits as the older children<br>A pre-calculated and programmed dosage can be delivered |

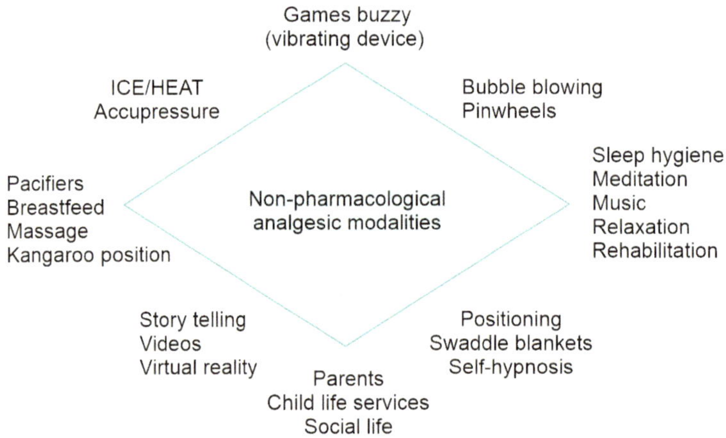


**Fig. 20.4:** Non-pharmacological analgesic modalities[9]

**Table 20.3: Various analgesic modalities and routes**

| *Analgesic modalities and various routes* | |
|---|---|
| **Route** | **Examples** |
| Topical (for prevention and treatment of needle pain) (May also be used in emergency settings as outlined) | EMLA, ethyl chloride, LET |
| | LMX: Lidocaine: For use in >2 years; Onset: 20–30 min, duration ~60 min |
| | EMLA: Lidocaine and prilocaine; Onset: 45–60 min, duration ~120 min |
| | LET: Lidocaine, epinephrine, tetracaine; Onset: 30–45 min, duration varies |
| | Ethyl chloride spray–immediate onset and duration varies according to the application |
| | Pain ease–pentafluoropropane an tetrafluoroethane-immediate onset and Duration ~60 seconds |
| Subcutaneous | Opioids, ketamine |
| Intranasal | Opioids, ketamine, dexmedetomidine |
| Nebulisation | Opioids, ketamine, nitrous oxide |
| Oral (including lollipops) | Acetaminophen, NSAIDs, oral sucrose |
| Intravenous | Acetaminophen, NSAIDs, opioids |
| Per rectal | Acetaminophen, NSAIDs (diclofenac) |

intranasal route along with bypassing the first pass metabolism, provides an easier, more acceptable, faster and a lesser painful way for drug administration.[22] Oral route has a slightly slower onset of action.[23]

While managing pediatric patients in the perioperative period, at every step, analgesia should be considered and administered to avoid development of fear and avoidance of future healthcare. For example: Topical anesthetics are recommended to numb the skin prior to venous cannulation (e.g. EMLA). Various modalities of procedural pain management are available (Table 20.3) to ensure adequate analgesia in the pediatric age group. Some modalities are used more commonly while dealing with chronic pediatric pain like subcutaneous routes, transdermal drug delivery systems and lollipop.

### Multidisciplinary Team Approach

A multidisciplinary team approach is key for effective perioperative pain management in pediatric patients (Fig. 20.5). The team could include pain physicians/anesthesiologists, surgeons, nurses, pharmacists, psychologists, physical therapists and the patients' care givers. Each team member has a unique role in pain assessment, formulating the treatment plan, monitoring the patient's response to therapy, reassessing and making modifications as necessary. Regular communication and collaboration among all the team members involved in patient care are essential to ensure that pain management goals are met and that concerns are addressed promptly.

## ONGOING RESEARCH AND FUTURE DIRECTIONS

Despite progress in perioperative pain treatment, we feel there is still a need for continued research to enhance outcomes in pediatric patients. Areas of focus may include developing new analgesics with least possible side effects, optimising regional anesthesia procedures, implementing creative and dynamic non-pharmacological

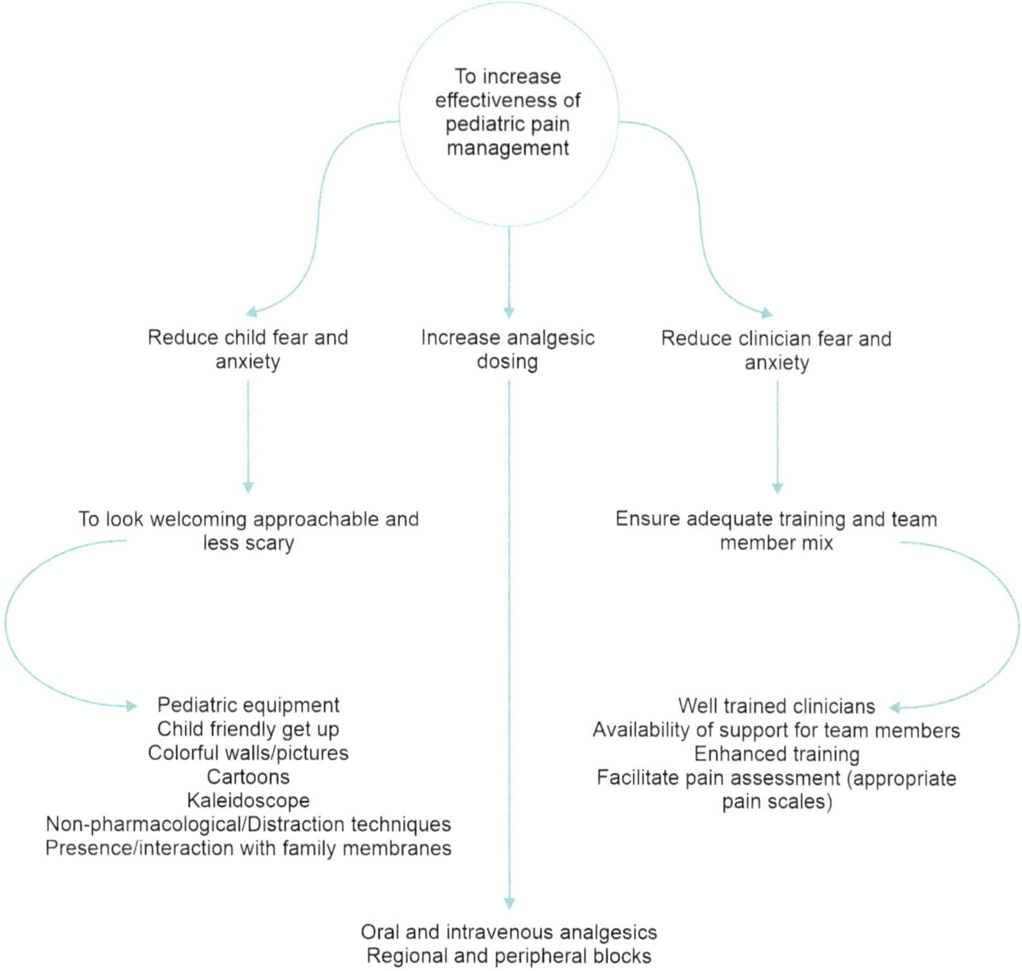


Fig. 20.5: Summarization of pediatric pain management[28]

interventions and making the entire process as comfortable as possible for the children. Also, research on the long-term effects of perioperative pain management, especially that of pharmacological interventions on pediatric patient outcomes and quality of life is required. If not addressed early on, pain in the pediatric population greatly affects their subjective well-being and day to day routine activities including mood, appetite, academic attendance and performance.[29] If not treated, it may also enhance their predisposition to pain later on as they grow up. It is also been seen that in the long run, it may manifest as stress disorder, attention deficit hyperactive disorders, despondency and social uninterest.[29]

## Conclusion

Perioperative pain management in pediatric patients demands that we adapt a comprehensive individualized and tailored approach that incorporates the unique characteristics of each child. A multidisciplinary and multimodal approach, including pharmacological and non-pharmacological interventions is indispensable. By addressing the unique needs of pediatric patients, the care providers can optimize pain management and improve outcomes for children undergoing surgery.

## References


1. Paediatric Pain: Physiology, Assessment and Pharmacology [Internet]. WFSA Resource Library. 2022 [cited 2024 Feb 29]. Available from: https://resources.wfsahq.org/atotw/paediatric-pain-physiology-assessment-and-pharmacology-anaesthesia-tutorial-of-the-week-289/
2. Talbot K, Madden VJ, Jones SL, Moseley GL. The sensory and affective components of pain: are they differentially modifiable dimensions or inseparable aspects of a unitary experience? A systematic review. British Journal of Anaesthesia [Internet]. 2019 Aug 1 [cited 2024 Feb 29];123(2):e263–72. Available from: https://www.ncbi.nlm.nih.gov/pmc/articles/PMC6676053/
3. Rybojad B, Sieniawski D, Paweł Rybojad, Marzena Samardakiewicz, Aftyka A. Pain Evaluation in the Paediatric Emergency Department: Differences in Ratings by Patients, Parents and Nurses. International Journal of Environmental Research and Public Health [Internet]. 2022 Feb 21 [cited 2024 Feb 29];19(4):2489–9. Available from: https://www.ncbi.nlm.nih.gov/pmc/articles/PMC8872586/
4. Lorenzo Di Sarno, Gatto A, Korn D, Pansini V, Curatola A, Ferretti S, et al. Pain management in pediatric age. An update. PubMed [Internet]. 2023 Aug 3 [cited 2024 Feb 29];94(4):e2023174–4. Available from: https://www.ncbi.nlm.nih.gov/pmc/articles/PMC10440769/
5. Pace AK, Melanio Bruceta, Donovan J, Vaida SJ, Eckert JM. An Objective Pain Score for Chronic Pain Clinic Patients. Pain Research & Management [Internet]. 2021 Feb 8 [cited 2024 Feb 29];2021:1–8. Available from: https://www.hindawi.com/journals/prm/2021/6695741/
6. Gandhi M, Thomson C, Lord D, Enoch S. Management of Pain in Children with Burns [Internet]. ResearchGate. Hindawi; 2010 [cited 2024 Mar 1]. Available from: https://www.researchgate.net/publication/47157569_Management_of_Pain_in_Children_with_Burns
7. Carl. Children's Self-Reports of Pain Intensity: Scale Selection, Limitations and Interpretation. Pain Research & Management [Internet]. 2006 Jan 1 [cited 2024 Mar 1];11(3):157–62. Available from: https://www.ncbi.nlm.nih.gov/pmc/articles/PMC2539005/
8. Ganguly A, Bhadesia PJ, Phatak AG, Nimbalkar AS, Nimbalkar SM. Pain profile of premature infants during routine procedures in neonatal intensive care: An observational study. Journal of family medicine and primary care [Internet]. 2020 Jan 1 [cited 2024 Mar 1];9(3):1517–7. Available from: https://www.ncbi.nlm.nih.gov/pmc/articles/PMC7266194/
9. Pediatric Pain [Internet]. Emra.org. 2020 [cited 2024 Mar 1]. Available from: https://www.emra.org/books/pain-management/pediatric-pain

10. Comfort Scale scoring [Internet]. Available from: https://www.georgespicu.org.uk/wp-content/uploads/bsk-pdf-manager/2017/11/Comfort-Score-detail-2017.pdf
11. Uitti JM, Sanna Salanterä, Laine MK, Tähtinen PA, Aino Ruohola. Adaptation of pain scales for parent observation: are pain scales and symptoms useful in detecting pain of young children with the suspicion of acute otitis media? BMC Pediatrics [Internet]. 2018 Dec 1 [cited 2024 Mar 1];18(1). Available from: https://bmcpediatr.biomedcentral.com/articles/10.1186/s12887-018-1361-y/tables/1
12. Zieli ski J, Morawska-Kochman M, Zato ski T. Pain assessment and management in children in the postoperative period: A review of the most commonly used postoperative pain assessment tools, new diagnostic methods and the latest guidelines for postoperative pain therapy in children. Advances in Clinical and Experimental Medicine. 2020 Mar 4;29(3).
13. Canadian Paediatric Society. Best practices in pain assessment and management for children | Canadian Paediatric Society [Internet]. Cps.ca. 2022 [cited 2024 Mar 1]. Available from: https://cps.ca/en/documents/position/pain-assessment-and-management
14. Wong-Baker FACES Foundation. Home - Wong-Baker FACES Foundation [Internet]. Wong-Baker FACES Foundation. 2019 [cited 2024 Mar 1]. Available from: https://wongbakerfaces.org/
15. Jensen MP, Chen C, Brugger AM. Interpretation of visual analog scale ratings and change scores: a reanalysis of two clinical trials of postoperative pain. The Journal of Pain [Internet]. 2003 Sep 1 [cited 2024 Mar 1];4(7):407–14. Available from: https://www.jpain.org/article/S1526-5900(03)00716-8/fulltext
16. Dalia Abdel Latif, Talat MA, Hanaa El Said, Abdelrahman DA. Pain Assessment Scale and Serum Cortisol Level in Children with Cognitive Impairment From Departments of... [Internet]. ResearchGate. unknown; 2021 [cited 2024 Mar 1]. Available from: https://www.researchgate.net/publication/349088486_Pain_Assessment_Scale_and_Serum_Cortisol_Level_in_Children_with_Cognitive_Impairment_From_Departments_of_Pediatrics_1_and_Clinical_Pathology
17. Won Ju Jeong, Woon Young Kim, Man Cook Moon, Duo Jae Min, Yoon Sook Lee, Jae Hwan Kim, et al. The effect of ketamine on the separation anxiety and emergence agitation in children undergoing brief ophthalmic surgery under desflurane general anesthesia. Korean Journal of Anesthesiology [Internet]. 2012 Jan 1 [cited 2024 Mar 1];63(3):203–3. Available from: https://www.ncbi.nlm.nih.gov/pmc/articles/PMC3460147/
18. Escalona-Espinosa A, Maldonado-Sánchez K, Pazos-Alvarado E, Castañeda P, Alcaraz-Ramos R, Aguilar-Romero D, et al. Postoperative Pain in Pediatrics. IntechOpen eBooks [Internet]. 2023 Nov 8 [cited 2024 Mar 1]; Available from: https://www.intechopen.com/chapters/87193
19. For A. Pain in Children: Management—International Association for the Study of Pain (IASP) [Internet]. International Association for the Study of Pain (IASP). 2021 [cited 2024 Mar 1]. Available from: https://www.iasp-pain.org/resources/fact-sheets/pain-in-children-management/
20. Starship.org.nz. gatsby-starship; 2024 [cited 2024 Mar 1]. Available from: https://starship.org.nz/guidelines/paediatric-pain-assessment/
21. Gai N, Naser B, Hanley J, Peliowski A, Hayes J, Aoyama K. A practical guide to acute pain management in children. Journal of Anesthesia [Internet]. 2020 Mar 31 [cited 2024 Mar 1];34(3):421–33. Available from: https://link.springer.com/article/10.1007/s00540-020-02767-x
22. Marcus Glenton Prescott, Ekaterina Iakovleva, Melanie Rae Simpson, Sindre Andre Pedersen, Munblit D, Odd Martin Vallersnes, et al. Intranasal analgesia for acute moderate to severe pain in children – a systematic review and meta-analysis. BMC Pediatrics [Internet]. 2023 Aug 18 [cited 2024 Mar 8];23(1). Available from: https://bmcpediatr.biomedcentral.com/articles/10.1186/s12887-023-04203-x
23. Pansini V, Curatola A, Gatto A, Lazzareschi I, Ruggiero A, Chiaretti A. Intranasal drugs for analgesia and sedation in children admitted to pediatric emergency department: a narrative review. Annals of Translational Medicine [Internet]. 2021 Jan 1 [cited 2024 Mar 8];9(2):189–9. Available from: https://atm.amegroups.org/article/view/51422/html#:~:text=There%20are%20different%20routes%20of,of%20the%20child%20(9).

24. Friedrichsdorf SJ, Liesbet Goubert. Pediatric pain treatment and prevention for hospitalized children. Pain Reports [Internet]. 2020 Jan 1 [cited 2024 Mar 1];5(1):e804–4. Available from: https://journals.lww.com/painrpts/fulltext/2020/02000/pediatric_pain_treatment_and_prevention_for.9.aspx
25. Verghese ST, Hannallah RS. Acute pain management in children. Journal of Pain Research [Internet]. 2010 Jul 1 [cited 2024 Mar 1];105–5. Available from: https://www.ncbi.nlm.nih.gov/pmc/articles/PMC3004641/
26. Pediatriconcall.com. 2024 [cited 2024 Mar 8]. Available from: https://www.pediatriconcall.com/drugs/drugs-a-to-z
27. Mahmoodi AN, Kim PY. Ketorolac [Internet]. Nih.gov. StatPearls Publishing; 2022 [cited 2024 Mar 1]. Available from: https://www.ncbi.nlm.nih.gov/books/NBK545172/
28. Gregory Adam Whitley, Hemingway P, Graham Richard Law, Aloysius Niroshan Siriwardena. Improving ambulance care for children suffering acute pain: a qualitative interview study. BMC Emergency Medicine [Internet]. 2022 Jun 3 [cited 2024 Mar 1];22(1). Available from: https://bmcemergmed.biomedcentral.com/articles/10.1186/s12873-022-00648-y
29. Mathews L. Pain in Children: Neglected, unaddressed and mismanaged. Indian Journal of Palliative Care [Internet]. 2011 Jan 1 [cited 2024 Mar 8];17(4):70–0. Available from: https://www.ncbi.nlm.nih.gov/pmc/articles/PMC3140088/#:~:text=Repeated%20exposure%20to%20pain%20may, patterns%20of%20self%2Ddestructive%20behavior.

# Section IV

# Support Systems and Palliation in Cancer Pain

Chapter 21

# Rehabilitation in Cancer Pain: An Overview

• Anuradha A Daptardar • Ajeeta M Kulkarni

## INTRODUCTION

Rehabilitation of cancer patients includes a multi-disciplinary and biopsychosocial model aiming to reduce the detrimental effects of cancer and its treatment and restore the patients to their maximal function and well-being.[1] Cancer rehabilitation model has four phases, namely preventative, restorative, supportive and palliative (Table 21.1).[2]

In the past, experts have found a combination of pharmacological and non-pharmacological interventions as the best suited method of pain management. Non-pharmacological therapies for pain are an important part of integrative medicine and aim to improve the patient's comfort and quality of life. Physical modalities may be used to improve mobility and alleviate pain. The physical modalities used to control cancer pain may modulate nociception, unload painful structures, or reduce pain caused due to overload of muscles especially post-surgery or due to sarcopenia in late stage.[3] The physical modalities commonly used for cancer pain relief are as follows:

**Table 21.1: Rehabilitation model**

| | |
|---|---|
| Preventative rehabilitation | It is also referred to as prehabilitation or surveillance, which aims at early detection and use of early intervention to delay or reduce the incidence of impairments related to cancer and its treatment |
| Restorative rehabilitation | Aims at full recovery and restoration of functions leading to functional independence |
| Supportive rehabilitation | For patients with permanent disability due to cancer treatment, the focus is on establishing as much functional independence as possible |
| Palliative rehabilitation | It is rehabilitation of cancer patients during terminal stage of disease where the focus is on maximizing comfort and caregiver support |

### Heat and Cold Therapy

Heat application and cold packs for pain relief dates back to ancient times. Mechanisms of action is by causing change in temperature which alters nerve conduction, blood flow and collagen extensibility. Heat therapy causes vasodilatation, results in hyperemia, increases blood circulation and reduces muscle spasm thereby reducing pain. It is more effective in chronic pain by reducing stiffness and relaxing the muscles.[4] Heat therapy is not advocated directly over inflammation and tumor sites. Cold therapy or cryotherapy is usually more beneficial in acute pain. It causes vaso constriction

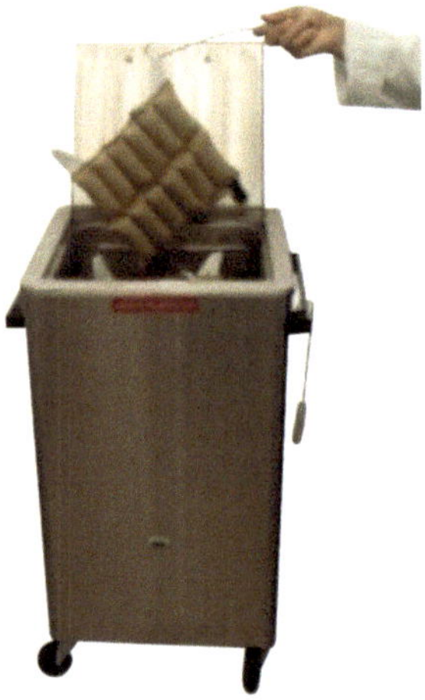

Fig. 21.1: Hot pack

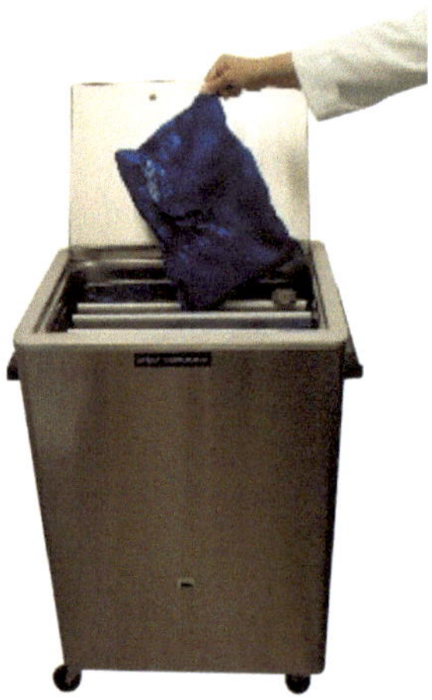

Fig. 21.2: Cold pack

hypothermia, numbing sensation of the tissues and reduces the inflammation and local edema. The duration of application of heat and cold is 10 to 20 minutes. Both heat therapy and cold therapy are more effective when used as adjuncts with exercises and mobilization (Figs 21.1 and 21.2).[5]

### Transcutaneous Electrical Nerve Stimulation (TENS)

TENS is use of high frequency low intensity electrical current delivered through surface electrodes using an inexpensive, portable device. The other type of TENS is the high intensity and low frequency acupuncture type, which is a little uncomfortable and cannot be taken for a long duration. Currently, the TENS is grouped as the burst mode and modulated mode of electrical stimulation. The mechanism of action is based on the pain gate theory, which controls the nociceptive signals by closing the gate of pain transmission and reducing the perception of pain. Duration of use is 10 to 20 minutes. Not advised on tumor site (Fig. 21.3).[6]

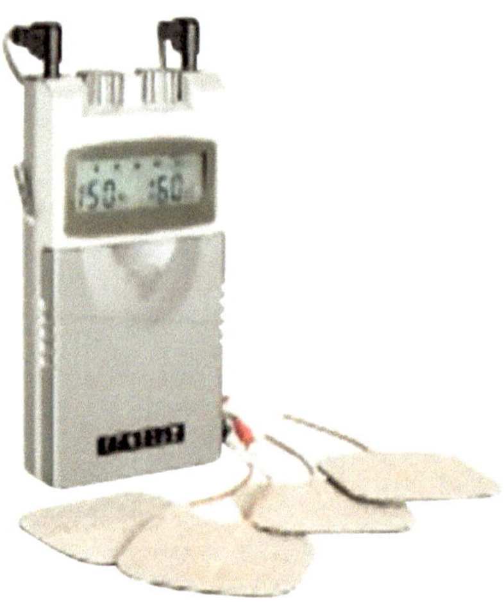

Fig. 21.3: TENS

### Low Level Laser Therapy

Low level laser therapy (LLLT) also known as photobiomodulation (PBM) is application of low intensity light in the wavelength of 650 nm to 1000 nm, intensity of $5W/cm^2$ applied for 30 to 60 seconds at one point for a few times in a week for few weeks. It is used to treat nociceptive and neuropathic pain. LLLT reduces inflammation, lymphedema and helps in tissue repair. The mechanism of action is by promoting a photochemical reaction in the cell, which in turn reduces the conduction velocity and thereby helps in cell proliferation of fibroblasts. Hence, it is effectively used to prevent and reduce oral mucositis and facial lymphedema in patients treated with chemotherapy and radiotherapy for head and neck cancer. It is also known to reduce breast cancer related lymphedema. PBM has also demonstrated moderate pain relief in bone pain due to cancer and cancer treatment. It is safe to administer LLLT in cancer and palliative patients. Care must be taken to protect ones eyes with protective goggles during treatment. LLLT is not to be given on tumor sites.[7]

### Massage Therapy

Massage therapy is a form of manual therapy used by physiotherapists to alleviate pain and increase mobility. It is soft tissue manipulation using hands which affects the muscular and vascular system. In addition to relieving pain, massage therapy also improves circulation, flexibility and reduces stress thereby improving the well-being of patients.[8] The different types of massage techniques are:

1. *Active release technique:* The physiotherapist combines manipulation of soft tissue with movement or stretch to release a tight muscle or tendon.
2. *Trigger point release:* The therapist identifies the painful point and uses her thumb or elbow to give pressure to the painful point to relax the soft tissues and muscles around the point.
3. *Myofascial release:* The physiotherapist releases tight fascia, tendon or muscles by placing her hands on the tight structures and applying slow sustained pressure and stretch to it to relax and realign it.
4. *Soft tissue massage:* The physiotherapist kneads the soft tissues and muscles to break down the muscle knots or adhesions to reduce pain, improve the flexibility and function.[9]
5. *Manual lymphatic drainage (MLD):* MLD is a type of gentle superficial massage to drain the lymph. It is mainly used as a component of complex/complete decongestive therapy (CDT), the gold standard line of management of lymphedema of the arm, leg, breast and head and neck region following cancer treatment. Though its efficacy is questionable, it may be more effective if applied intensively.[10]
6. *Friction massage:* Mainly used to massage and mobilize scar tissues. The physiotherapist uses her fingers to apply pressure on the scar tissue to gently breakdown the adhesions and make the scar more pliable. This massage to be started after the complete healing of the scar.
7. *Percussive massage technique or vibration therapy:* In this technique the physiotherapist cups her hands or uses a massager to percuss the affected area to relieve pain. In addition to improving the flexibility and alleviating pain, percussions delivered to the back or chest can be used in respiratory care to mobilize and clear lung secretions.[11]

The recommended duration of massage is 10–30 minutes for a period of one week or more. A word of caution: All the above massage techniques are contraindicated in infections, over tumor site and on recently irradiated tissues.

### Therapeutic Exercises

They are a combination of physical activity and movement to improve flexibility and function and reduce pain.[12] The different exercise modes are aerobic exercise, resistance exercise, flexibility exercise, balance and co-ordination training.

1. *Aerobic or endurance training:* These normally include low intensity or moderate intensity walking, running, swimming or cycling exercise. The recommended guidelines for aerobic training includes 150 minutes of exercise per week. The aerobic exercises are performed 3–5 times/week for 30 minutes each day. The commonest endurance training exercise is walking.
2. *Strengthening exercises or resistance training (RT):* It is performed against resistance to build up and strengthen the muscles. The resistance used can be in the form of dumbbell, free weights, body weights or resistance bands. It mainly includes isotonic exercises—dynamic movements with constant load, isokinetic exercise—includes a constant velocity with variable load and isometric exercises—static muscle contraction without any change in muscle length. The conventional resistance is calculated as 60–70% of 1 RM (resistance maximum). The frequency is 2–3 times/week. RT includes 8–10 repetitions each of 8–10 exercises targeting major muscle group.[13]
3. *Flexibility exercises:* Slow controlled exercises performed in a gradual manner to improve the range of motion (ROM) of the joints. This can be passive, active assisted or active exercises.
4. *Balance and co-ordination exercises:* Good postural control or balance control helps to prevent injuries and prevents fall. Evidence supports that balance improves with time based or repetition-based programs. A combination of aerobic, resistance and balance exercise is more effective than a single exercise program, as described in a systematic review and meta-analysis published in the journal of physical therapy science in 2021.[14]

Principles of exercise prescription: Based on FITT principle where F—Frequency, number of sessions per week. I—Intensity like low, moderate or vigorous. T—Time for each session. T—Type like aerobic, RT or combination. Increments will be to increase the number of frequency, or time or repetitions or load or resistance. Therapeutic exercise is safe and feasible to administer in cancer population.[13]

Contraindications for exercise in cancer patients[15] (Table 21.2).

### Positioning and Off-loading Painful Structures

Cancer and its treatment have a lot of side effects on the skeletal system. Chemotherapy drugs and steroids affect the bone density making them weak and susceptible to fractures. Radiotherapy to treat cancer locally can make the nearby bones brittle. Cancer induced bone pain (CIBP) is related to the imbalance between the osteoblasts and osteoclasts, leading to bone destruction, inflammation, invasion into the nerve endings in the periosteum, causing severe pain. Non-pharmacological treatment includes TENS, relaxation techniques of the adjacent soft tissues, maintaining range of motion by gradual stretching exercises followed by strengthening. Weight bearing bones have

**Table 21.2: Contraindications for exercise in cancer patients**

| Organ | Parameters | Restrictions |
|---|---|---|
| Hematological | Platelets 20000–50000 | No resistive exercises |
| Platelets | <20000 | No exercises. Limited ambulation |
| Neutrophils | <1000 | Neutropenic precautions |
| Pulmonary | FEV1 or FVC <50% predicted pulse oximetry <90% | Limit aerobic exercises and consider oxygen supplementation |
| Cardiac | HR >80% maximal | Limit aerobic exercises |
| | LVEF <20% | Limit aerobic exercises |
| | Unstable arrhythmias | Exercise only with cardiac monitoring |
| Skeletal | >50% cortical involvement | Non-weight-bearing |
| | 25–50% cortical involvement | Partial weight-bearing |
| | <25% cortical involvement | No high impact activities or sports |
| Gastrointestinal | Uncontrolled emesis or diarrhea | No strenuous activities |

to be protected from impending fractures and can be offloaded by giving some walking aids to enable mobility or by using some orthosis. Positioning and supporting painful structures by appropriate use of pillows or bolsters to reduce the load on them to enable pain free movement.[16]

## Yoga

Yoga is a complementary and alternate therapy for reducing the symptoms of cancer and its treatment and improving the well-being of cancer patients. Evidence supports the feasibility and safe incorporation of yoga in cancer patients.[17] Yoga therapy is a body mind therapy and is a multi-component combination of breathing exercises (*Pranayam*), different stretches and postures for improving flexibility (*Asanas*), meditation and relaxation therapy. It is normally delivered as a group therapy session, for 1 to 3 supervised sessions per week for a period of minimum 4 weeks. After this the sessions are to be continued at home. The benefits of *Yoga* in cancer patients are majorly demonstrated in cancer survivors and the effects are largely seen in physical components like fatigue and sleep, psychological outcomes like anxiety and depression and improvements in overall quality of life (QoL) outcome. Hence Yoga, which is a low cost and safe therapy, having multiple benefits for cancer patients may be recommended as an addition to the standard of care.[18]

## Acupressure/Acupuncture

It is derived from traditional Chinese medicine for healing. It is application of pressure using fingers, thumb or a device or needles for a sustained period of time over certain points of the body called acupoints. Evidence suggests that acupressure and acupuncture is safe and known to relieve cancer pain.[19] The mechanism of action of both acupressure and acupuncture in pain relief is almost the same. The acupoints are stimulated either by pressure or by needles through skin which increases the blood flow and regulates the nerve function by stimulating the peripheral nerves to block the transmission of pain signals and result in autonomous relief of pain.[20]

### Relaxation Techniques

There are various relaxation techniques to alleviate cancer pain. The commonest are meditation, progressive muscle relaxation (PMR), guided imagery, deep breathing exercises, yoga, hypnosis, music therapy, distraction therapy and others. Most of these techniques can be self-practiced except hypnosis. These are body mind exercises that decrease the cortisol levels, relax your body and calm your mind thereby reducing pain perception.[21]

### Benefits of Exercise in the Immediate Postoperative Period

An undesirable by-product of any surgical procedure is the postoperative pain associated with the incisions and the sutures. Postoperative suture pain, especially thoracic and upper abdominal sutures, lead to shallow protective breathing, decreasing the ventilation, eventually leading to pulmonary complications.

Optimization of the patient before surgery is of utmost importance to reduce the postoperative complications. Hence the concept of 'Prehabilitation' has evolved which is a multimodal intervention program to improve the functional capacity, nutritional, physical and psychological wellbeing of patients in preoperative period to prevent or reduce postoperative consequences.[22]

A growing body of evidence has shown that prehabilitation has minimized length of stay, postoperative pain, and postoperative complications. Prehabilitation can be a supervised hospital based program or an unsupervised home based program for a minimum of 4 weeks to 12 weeks. A generic prehabilitation program includes the components of warm-up, flexibility stretching exercises, aerobic and cardiovascular training, resistance training and the functional activities.[23]

The various physiotherapy interventions to improve the postoperative pulmonary function and endurance are as follows:

*Deep breathing exercises:* Deep breathing exercises with segmental and diaphragmatic breathing with sustained maximal inspiration helps in thoracic expansion, thus opening the airways and preventing collapse of alveoli.

*Active cycle of breathing technique (ACBT):* Active cycle of breathing technique (ACBT) are interventions used for gradual increase in inspiratory and expiratory reserve volumes, increase in breath-holding period to improve ventilation and mobilize the secretions, decrease the atelectatic area and prevent collapse of the alveoli. ACBT starts with breathing control where patient breathes through the nose and out through the mouth with pursed lip to create back pressure in airways. Then the chest expansion exercises with 3 seconds breath holding are given followed by huffing or huff coughing. This helps to aerate the small airways and bring more air behind the mucus, if any, which can be easily brought out by huffing and coughing (Fig. 21.4).

Sutures should be guarded with either protective binders or splinting with hand to hold the sutures. Patients are advised to bend forward and hold the sutures before coughing.[24]

A prospective randomized trial concluded that ACBT is effective technique for airway clearance that helps reduce the incidence of postoperative pulmonary complications and other complications like anastomotic leakage and length of stay, after esophagectomy.[25]

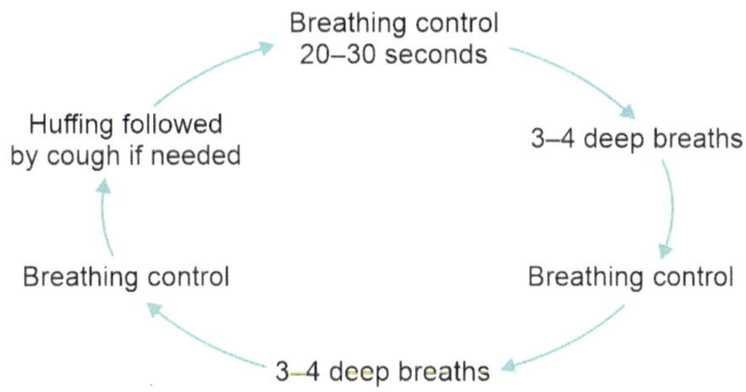


**Fig. 21.4:** ACBT

*Incentive spirometer:* An incentive spirometer is a medical device that helps in sustaining maximal inspiration and indicates the volume of air inhaled into the lungs during inspiration. It is widely used in physiotherapy, encouraging the patient to take slow, deep, prolonged breath allowing the lungs to stretch and opens the alveoli for good ventilation perfusion matching. It also provides a visual feedback, for the patients to check their inspiratory effort, wherein a gender specific targeted volume is set for each patient depending upon their age and height.

The volume based incentive spirometer and the flow based spirometer are the two types of spirometer, of which the volume based spirometer is better.

Flow-oriented incentive spirometers are single balled or three balled spirometers with capacity up to 1200 ml. Volume-based incentive spirometer has one-way valve with capacity up to 5000 ml (Figs 21.5 and 21.6).

Current evidence shows that volume based spirometer improves diaphragmatic function by reducing the work of breathing and pulmonary function more as compared to flow based spirometer.[26]

The lungs are not fully developed in younger children. Positioning and upright posture is of utmost importance to children (Fig. 21.7). Postoperative pain can be reduced

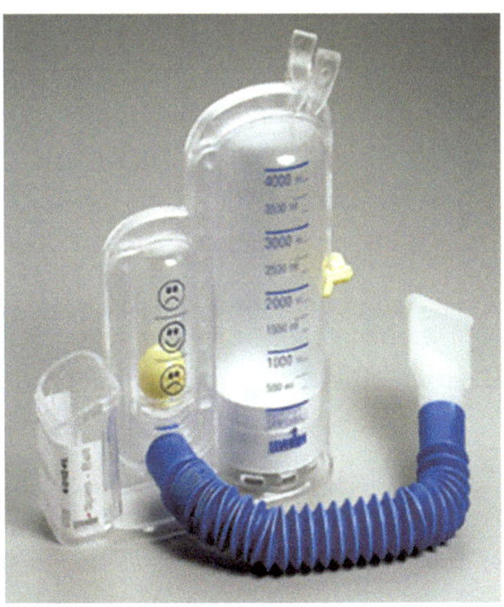

**Fig. 21.5:** Volume based spirometer

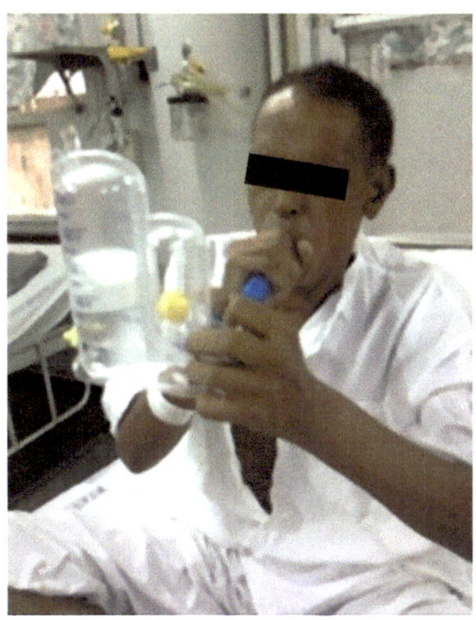

**Fig. 21.6:** Patient performing spirometer exercise

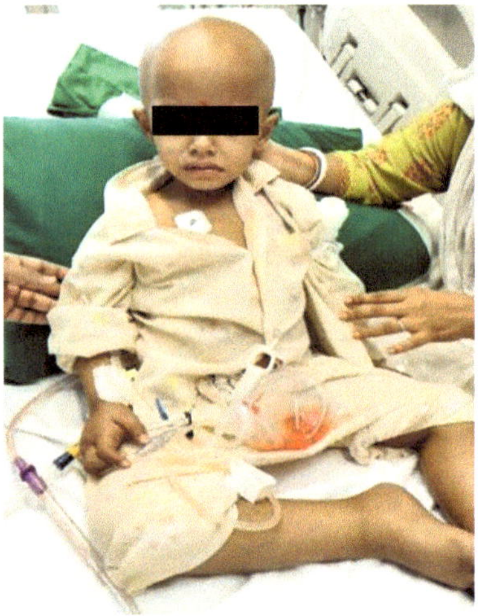

Fig. 21.7: Positioning

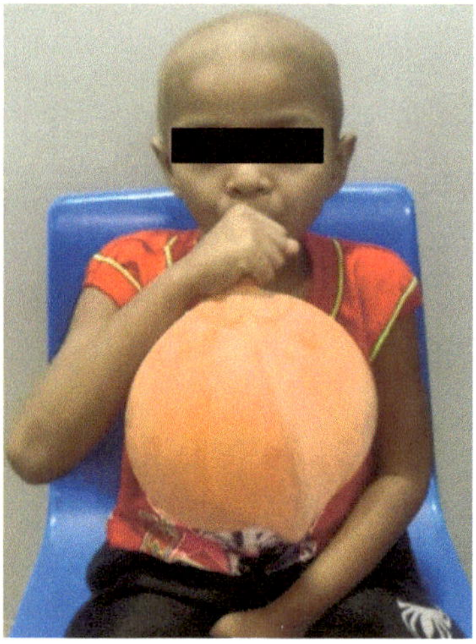

Fig. 21.8: Football balloon bladder

by analgesic and the timing physiotherapy interventions to be adjusted with the timing of medication. Younger children may not be able to perform incentive spirometer, hence a football bladder balloon blowing can be given **(Fig. 21.8)**.

*Inspiratory muscle training:* Various thoracic and upper gastrointestinal surgeries related to cancer are extensive and may lead to respiratory muscles weakness which leads to decreased cough effort and chest compliance thus reducing the physical capacity. Cancer treatment also impacts the respiratory function and physical fitness is reduced in the long run.

Inspiratory muscle training (IMT) is a form of resistance training for the muscles of inspiration, especially the diaphragm to improve its strength and endurance. There is limited evidence regarding the impact of inspiratory muscle training devices on post-operative pulmonary complications (PPC) in cancer patients but there are smaller studies which support the use of inspiratory muscle training in postoperative pulmonary rehabilitation.[27]

A systematic review shows that IMT is effectively improves the pulmonary function in cancer survivors.[28]

Radiation pneumonitis has various symptoms like fever, cough, chest pain, breathlessness and general feeling of discomfort or malaise. During this phase, deep breathing exercises and relaxation techniques help in coping up with the symptoms and reduce pain and breathlessness.

*Exercises for thoracic and shoulder range of motion after thoracotomy:* Patients after thoracotomy usually slouch and sit with protracted shoulders. Postural correction and movements of upper limbs need to be incorporated along with chest expansion exercises. Deep breathing exercises in combination with thoracic movements, shoulder flexion and abduction helps in thoracic expansion.

*Exercises interventions following breast cancers surgeries:* The most common cancer in women with better survival rates is breast cancer; hence, the focus has shifted towards addressing the complications related to breast cancer treatment. Breast cancer surgeries range from lumpectomy to modified radical mastectomy with or without reconstructions. Postoperative nociceptive pain will trigger a protective mechanism subsequently reducing the range of motion at the affected shoulder joint and later elicits the adhesive capsulitis. Cold therapy is an effective non-pharmacological application for relieving postoperative pain and inflammation.[29]

A warm up exercise program which includes active posture correction along with deep breathing and pursed lip breathing, shoulder girdle movements and trunk rotations are to be performed before starting any shoulder exercise. Deep breathing exercises help induce relaxation, reduce pain and relieve the tight structures in the chest.

Shoulder girdle exercises like elevation and shoulder retraction helps in stretching the anterior soft tissues, thus preventing protruded postures and suture scarring. 4–6 weeks after the sutures heal completely; scar massage can be encouraged if the scar become tight and adherent.

The intervention includes shoulder flexion and abduction movements performed in a combination of active assisted ROM, active ROM and stretching exercises (Figs 21.9 and 21.10).[30]

Breast cancer surgery may cause severe long-term morbidity such as impaired range of arm motion, pain, loss of strength, numbness and lymphedema due to axillary lymph node dissection (ALND). Pumping exercises help in improving lymphatic circulation (Fig. 21.11).

Post-mastectomy exercise intervention improves ROM, strength and reduces pain and incidence of lymphedema as is evident according to a trial involving 392 patients conducted at 17 breast cancer centres in England.[31]

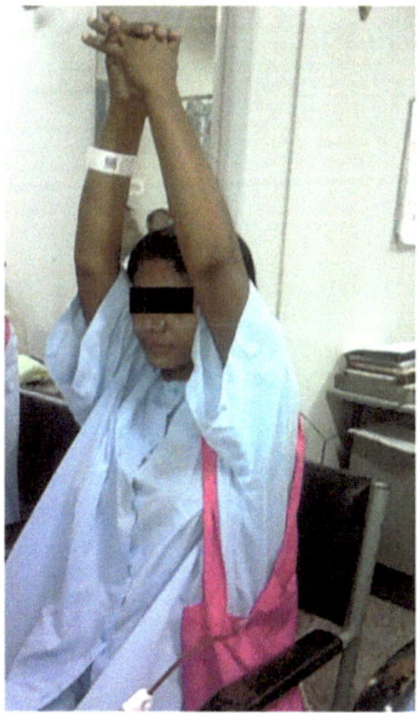

Fig. 21.9: Shoulder flexion

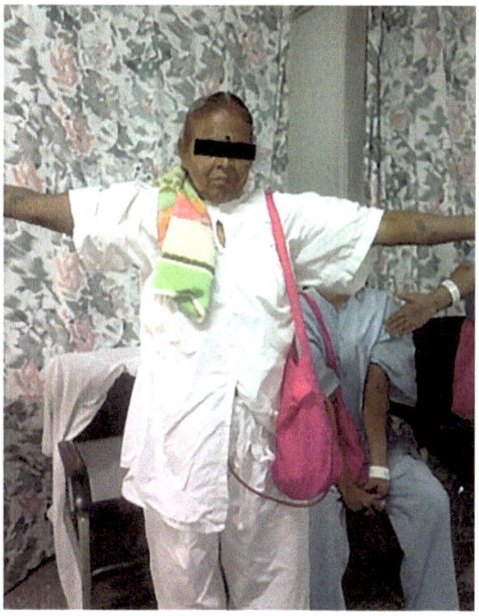

Fig. 21.10: Shoulder abduction

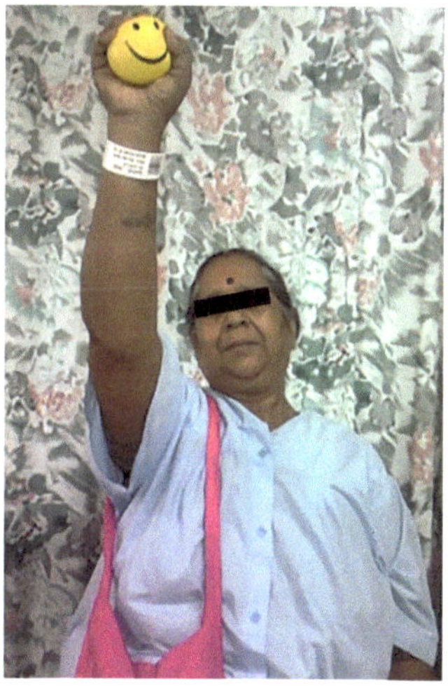

Fig. 21.11: Pumping exercise

## Axillary Web Syndrome (AWS)

Axillary web syndrome (AWS) is a self-limiting condition that can occur as an early or possibly late postoperative complication following ALND. It develops as a fibrotic band or "cords" extending from the axilla into the arm, may cross the cubital fossa, reaching up to the base of thumb. It is clinically associated with pain and restriction of shoulder movement in the affected arm (Fig. 21.12).[32]

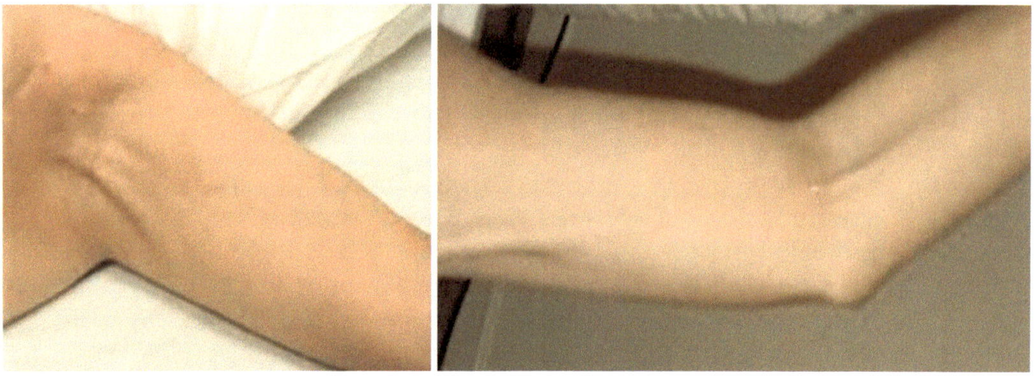

Fig. 21.12: Axillary web syndrome (AWS)

The diagnosis of AWS is based on physical examination with cords either palpable or visible and become more painful and taut during shoulder abduction.[33] Treatment may include pain medicines, physical therapy like soft tissue mobilization, manual lymph drainage (MLD) and stretching. MLD using resorption strokes and arm exercises was found to be more effective in decreasing pain and improving range of shoulder movement both immediately after the intervention and after 3 months.[34] AWS resolves within 3 months but effective clinical intervention shortens its natural course, thus improving the quality of life.

## Postoperative Pain and Movement Restriction after Bone Surgeries

Acute pain immediately following bone surgery is caused by an acute inflammatory reaction, and this pain gradually resolves with resolution of the inflammation. Immediate application of cold packs near incisional site can help in reducing the inflammation and thus reducing the postoperative pain. Major surgeries like internal hemipelvectomy and long bone resections involve a lot of handling of the neurovascular bundle, which indicates persistent neuropathic pain, somatic pain and numbness around the incisional site.[35] Post-surgical exercises should be initiated as early as day 1 in most of the surgeries to minimize the incidence of disuse atrophy and to improve the ROM at the joints. Continuous passive motion (CPM) machine (Fig. 21.13) and pulleys can be used to relax

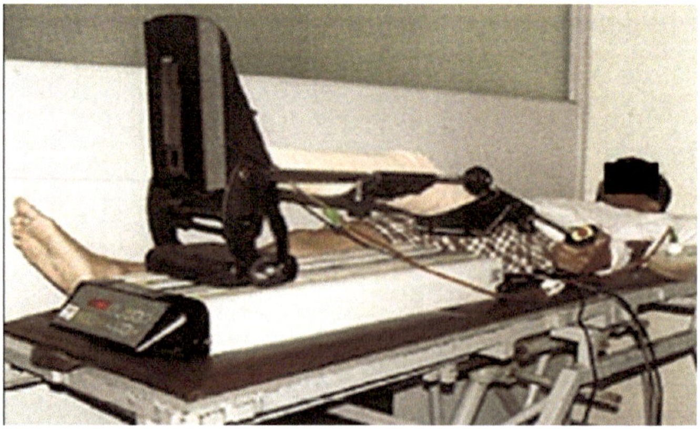

Fig. 21.13: Continuous passive motion (CPM)

the soft tissues, reduce pain and improve joint range. As the mobility increases there is reduction in pain. Postoperative knee range can be improved by patellar mobilization which will reduce pain and increase mobility. If the incisional scar later gets adherent, then scar mobilization can be initiated by deep friction massage and stretching but not immediately on the radiated skin.

### Palliative Care

Physiotherapy in palliative care is still a relatively new concept. This is mainly due to the lack of knowledge and the fear of causing untoward harm during treatment. Perhaps the most valuable contribution skilled physiotherapy has brought to palliative care is the ability to assess accurately a patient's potential for independence. A multimodal person-centred rehabilitation focuses on improving the quality of survival in terminally ill patients, whatever their life expectancy. Timely referral to physiotherapy during palliative care has much to offer in maintaining function, controlling symptoms like pain, weakness, fatigue, etc. and promoting realistic hopes.

### Cancer Survivors

Early diagnosis and better treatment strategies have resulted in an increase in the number of cancer survivor population. Cancer treatment though beneficial, is associated with a lot of adverse effects. Survivors have reported many long-standing problems as a late sequelae to cancer treatment. The commonest issues are cancer-related fatigue, pain, lymphedema, peripheral neuropathy, trismus, shoulder dysfunction, sexual dysfunction and altered sleep.[36] Rehabilitation is an integral part of cancer survivors continuum.

### Cancer Related Fatigue (CRF)

National cancer comprehensive network (NCCN) defines "CRF multidimensional concept of distressing, persistent, subjective sense of physical, emotional, and/or cognitive tiredness or exhaustion related to cancer or cancer treatment, that is, not proportional to recent activity and interferes with usual functioning". CRF is not relieved with rest. 20–30% of cancer survivors experience CRF even after 5 to 10 years post-treatment. Research has established increased inflammatory activity because of cancer treatment as the main cause of CRF.[37] In addition other medical issues like pain, anemia, and psychological factors like anxiety, depression and sleep disturbance are contributing factors to CRF. The management of CRF includes a multidisciplinary approach to combat both physical and psychological needs. Variety of interventions like exercises, yoga, mindfulness, cognitive behavioural therapy (CBT) and acupuncture have demonstrated positive benefits in the management of CRF. Combination of aerobic and resistance exercises along with physical activity is recommended for alleviating CRF.[38]

### Shoulder Dysfunction

Shoulder dysfunction is evident following neck dissection in surgeries of head and neck cancer due to either resection or handling of the spinal accessory nerve which eventually affects the quality of life and return to work. Shoulder dysfunction leads to pain and weakness of the shoulder girdle muscles (Fig. 21.14). Recent systematic review shows the benefits of shoulder exercises after neck dissections and the evidence is most favourable towards progressive resistance exercises and should be considered as the

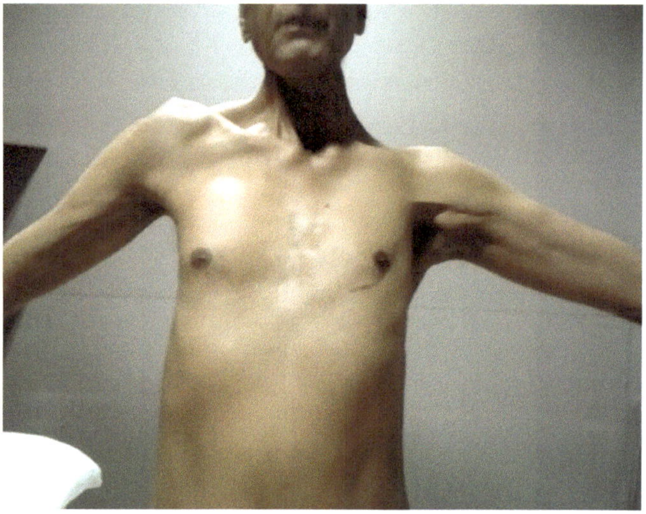

Fig. 21.14: Shoulder dysfunction

standard of care. Progressive resistance exercises can be initiated by resistance bands or weight cuffs or dumbbells starting from as low as half kilograms as per patient's tolerance and gradually increasing the resistance, repetitions or frequency of exercise.[39]

### Trismus

Trismus is reduced mouth opening defined as a maximal interincisal opening (MIO) less than 35 mm in adults. Trismus can be due to a precancerous condition of sub-mucuos fibrosis (SMF) and is also common in post-treatment of head and neck tumors with surgery and/or radiotherapy to the muscles of mastication, temporomandibular joints, oral cavity and the oropharynx. Trismus can become self-limiting, may progress or improve over time, but in most patients trismus remains permanent. Moderate to severe trismus with MIO less than 15–20 mm is usually painful on movement, thus markedly impairing mastication, nutrition, oral hygiene and dental care, thereby affecting patients health and quality of life.[40]

Objective assessment includes measuring the MIO of mouth by either fingers or calliper (Fig. 21.15). Patient Reported Outcome Measures (PROM) like The Gothenburg Trismus Questionnaire (GTQ) and The European Organization for Research and Treatment of Cancer Quality of Life Questionnaire-Core 30 Head and Neck 35-questions (EORTC-QLQ-C30-H&N35) are tools for subjective assessments.

A systematic review with meta-analysis that exercises can lead to improved MIO in patients with trismus following head and neck cancer treatment.[41]

Ice-cream/spatula sticks or wooden tongue depressors can be used to measure and therapeutically increase the MIO by adding number of sticks as per the patient's tolerance (Fig. 21.16).

Various other modalities like jaw stretching devices, low intensity ultrasound therapy, low level laser therapy have been studied in combination with exercises alone, and the additional modalities have proven to give better results in combination with jaw exercises (Fig. 21.17).[42]

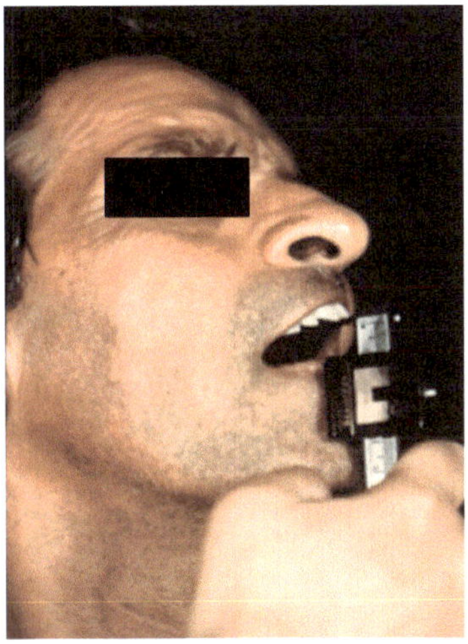

Fig. 21.15: MIO measurement

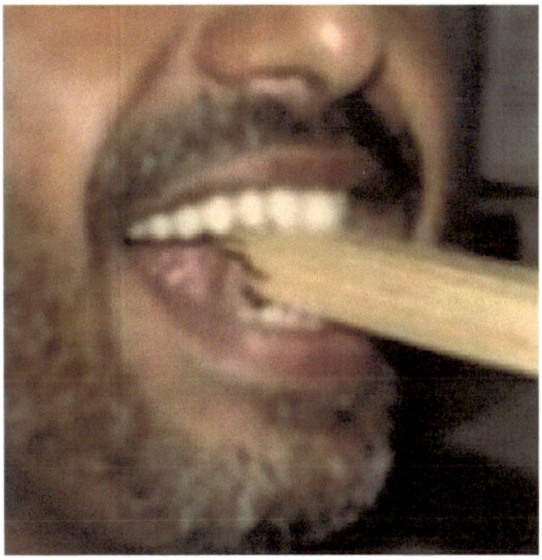

Fig. 21.16: Spatula sticks

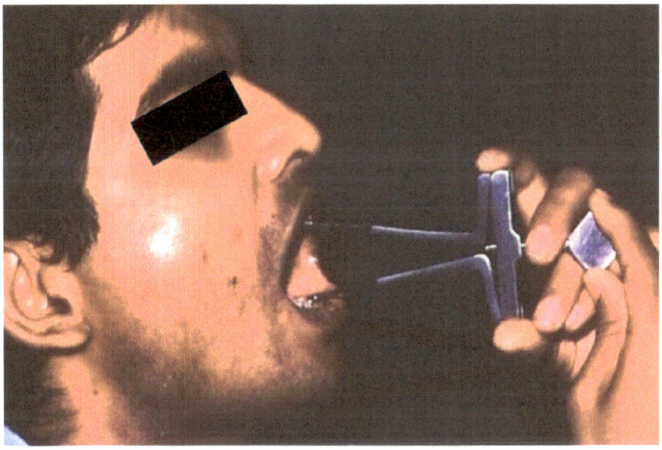

Fig. 21.17: Jaw stretcher key

## Chemotherapy Induced Peripheral Neuropathy (CIPN)

Chemotherapy induced peripheral neuropathy (CIPN) is a pre-dominantly sensory neuropathy that may be accompanied by motor and autonomic changes.

Other non-pharmacological approaches including physical therapy have been explored for CIPN. Exercise was demonstrated to prevent paclitaxel-induced peripheral neuropathy and clinical studies on exercises in CIPN has shown a positive outcome for balance and fitness. A systematic review studied 21 research papers on different non-pharmacological approaches and concluded that only exercise, strength and endurance training along with sensorimotor and balance training show some evidence for the prevention and treatment of CIPN, while data for other treatments like cryotherapy, neurofeedback, ultrasound therapy, low level laser, etc. are very preliminary.[43]

A systematic review on the use of TENS in CIPN shows that it is a safe technique to be administered in cancer patients to relieve different types of pain including the neuropathic pain in CIPN.[44]

Neuropathic pain in children is more associated with the cancer treatment in hematological cancers. Pediatric cancer patients complain of joint pain and refuse to weight bear or walk usually developing tendon Achilles tightness, making weight-bearing further difficult. Weight-bearing activities, obstacle jumping, and balance activities are encouraged.

## Lymphedema

Lymphedema is a late effect of lymph node dissection. Physiotherapy plays an important role in the prevention and management of lymphedema secondary to removal of lymph nodes, especially ALND for upper limbs and groin lymph nodes dissection for lower limbs. Complete decongestive therapy (CDT) which includes skin care, manual lymphatic drainage, multilayer bandaging, compression garments, exercises (active range of motion and progressive resistance exercises) is the gold standard treatment for secondary lymphedema.[45]

CDT in adults is a standard practice but in younger children it becomes more difficult to manage. A pediatric case of neuroblastoma with secondary lymphedema is mentioned in Box 21.1 and Figs 21.18 to 21.20).

**Box 21.1:** Neuroblastoma with lymphedema

| | |
|---|---|
| **Neuroblastoma** | A 10-month-old girl child come with left sided pelvic neuroblastoma with symptoms such as swelling in the abdomen and left leg, colder extremities, difficulty in passing stools and voiding of urine completely |
| **Chemotherapy + surgery** | Child diagnosed at TMH and 2 cycle of neoadjuvant chemotherapy carboplatin+etoposide given with surgical resection of tumor done (95%) along with removal of few lymph nodes |
| **Lymphedema** | Lymphedema developed postoperative day 1, was refereed to physiotherapy department for the same along with difficulty in moving limb, rolling in bed and crawling |

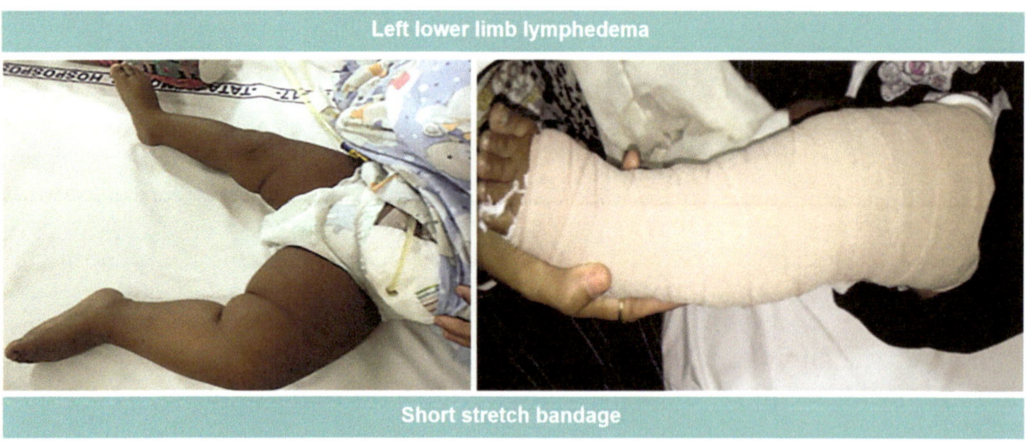


**Fig. 21.18:** Short stretch bandaging functional activities

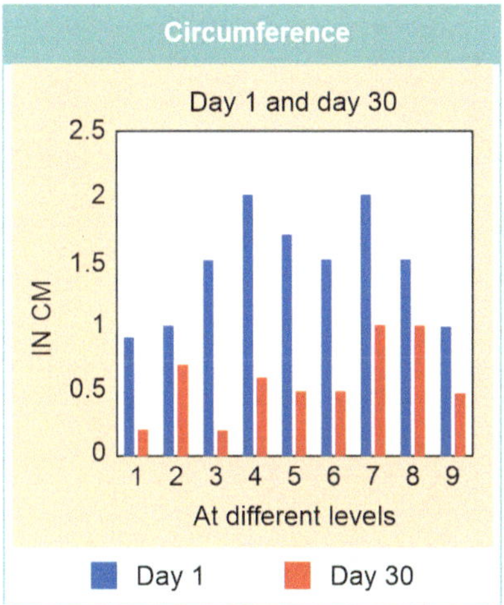


| Gross motor function measured | | | |
|---|---|---|---|
| **Outcome measures:** | **Pre** | **Post** | It assessed gross motor activities in three dimensions |
| Dimension A | 41% | 98% | A: Lying and rolling |
| Dimension B | 30% | 93% | B: Sitting |
| Dimension C | 14% | 83% | C: Crawling and kneeling |
| Gross motor function measure (GMFM) score sheet (GMFM-88 and GMFM-66 scoring) | | | |

**Fig. 21.19:** Assessment

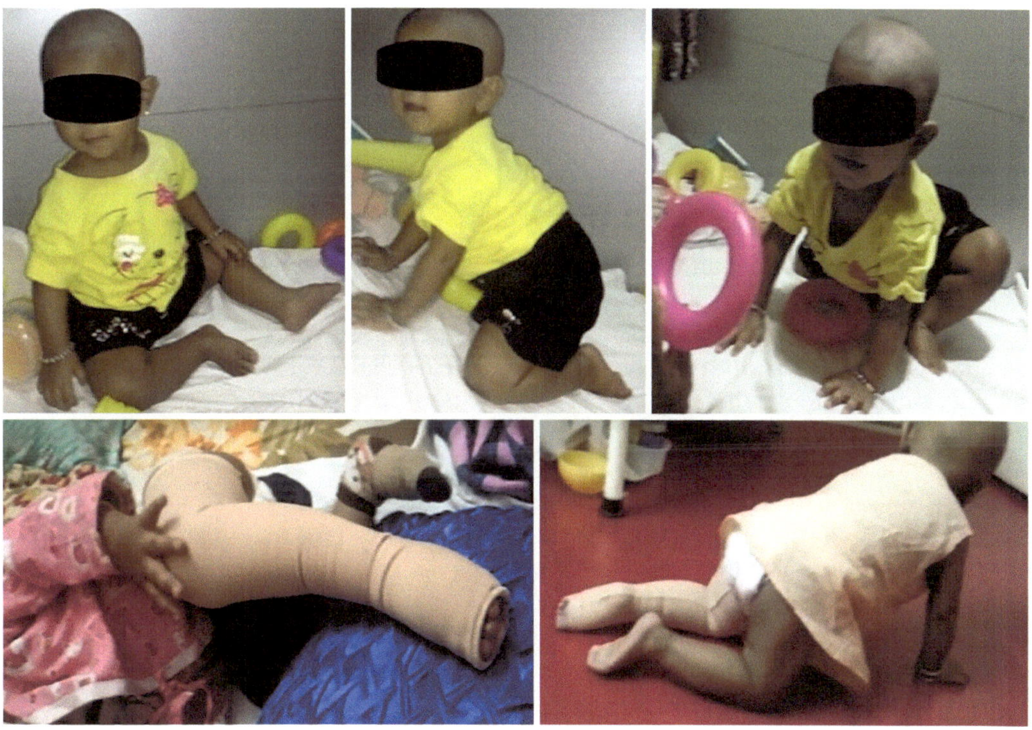

**Fig. 21.20:** Functional activities

## Current Evidence Regarding Virtual Rehabilitation and Tele-rehabilitation

The use of technologies is rapidly increasing in the rehabilitation of patients with cancer. There is evidence showing that virtual reality rehabilitation motivates patients to perform better. Task oriented programs increases patient participation and improves the function as compared to repetitive conventional exercises. Various games can be

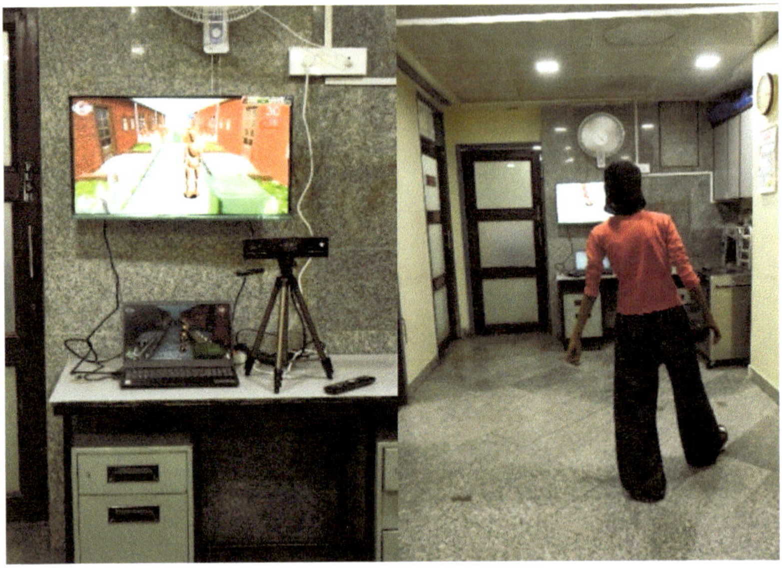

Fig. 21.21: Virtual rehabilitation

combined along with variations in timing and speed which can be targeted to improve patient's range of motion, balance, cognition, pain reduction through distraction and to overcome fear of falls. Virtual reality programs have shown to improve exercise adherence and training intensity resulting in better functional outcome but large trials are needed for best results (Fig. 21.21).[46]

The recent COVID-19 pandemic has led to significant evolution of telemedicine and tele-rehabilitation. Although face to face exercise sessions have an added advantage, tele-rehabilitation can be an alternate way to ensure access to healthcare via affordable technologies like smartphones, tablets or laptop. Tele-rehabilitation services may include the assessment, monitoring of patient's health status, prevention strategies education, consultations and/or interventions through demonstrations which can either be synchronous or asynchronous.

Synchronous tele-rehabilitation is a live, remote exchange of patient information through direct real-time interaction between the patient and the therapist. Asynchronous tele-rehabilitation is a 'store and forward' method wherein patient can share their disease related information which can be viewed later on by the therapist and rehabilitation can be provided through informative videos and demonstrations.[47]

Tele-rehabilitation is the recent, effective means of rehabilitation for the benefit of cancer patients and survivors for their optimal functional improvement.

## Summary

Cancer rehabilitation is a multidisciplinary and biopsychosocial model of physical and rehabilitation medicine, which aims to meet the needs of cancer patients and cancer survivors. Cancer patients are evaluated for physical impairments during and after treatment and if identified, are enrolled in specific rehabilitation program to ensure optimal physical and functional independence. Physiotherapy interventions aim to relieve pain, reduce distress and disability and improve functions, thereby improving the quality of life in cancer patients. Physiotherapy maneuvers like exercises and manual therapy are well tolerated, safe and recommended in cancer patients and cancer survivors. Although there is enough evidence supporting the benefits of rehabilitation in cancer patients, validated prescription guidelines for specific rehabilitation protocols in pain management and physical impairments are scarce and needs investigation.

## References


1. Cheville AL, Mustian K, Winters-Stone K, Zucker DS, Gamble GL, Alfano CM. Cancer Rehabilitation: An Overview of Current Need, Delivery Models, and Levels of Care. Phys. Med. Rehabil. Clin. N. Am. 2017, 28, 1–17.
2. Silver JK, Baima J. Cancer prehabilitation: an opportunity to decrease treatment-relatedmorbidity, increase cancer treatment options, and improve physical and psychologicalhealth outcomes. Am J Phys Med Rehabil 2013; 92:715.
3. Cheville AL, Basford JR. Role of Rehabilitation Medicine and Physical Agents in the Treatment of Cancer-Associated Pain. J ClinOncol 32:1691-1702. 2014 by American Society of Clinical Oncology.
4. Malanga GA, Yan N, Stark J. Mechanisms and efficacy of heat and cold therapies for musculoskeletal injury. Postgrad. Med. 2015, 127, 57–65.
5. Tatiana P. Grazioso, Nabil Djouder. The forgotten art of cold therapeutic properties in cancer: A comprehensive historical guide, iScience. 2023 Jul 21; 26(7): 107010.
6. Hurlow A, Bennett MI, Robb KA, Johnson MI, Simpson KH, xberry SG. Transcutaneous electric nerve stimulation (TENS) for cancer pain in adults. Cochrane Database of Systematic Reviews 2012, Issue 3. Art. No.: CD006276.
7. Howard B Cotler, Roberta T Chow, Michael R Hamblin, James Carroll. The Use of Low Level Laser Therapy (LLLT) For Musculoskeletal Pain MOJ OrthopRheumatol. 2015; 2(5): 00068
8. Crawford C, Boyd C, Paat CF, et al. The impact of massage therapy on function in pain populations—a systematic review and meta-analysis of randomized controlled trials: part I, patients experiencing pain in the general population. Pain Med. 2016;17(7):1353-1375. doi:10.1093/pm/pnw09.
9. Boyd C, Crawford C, Paat CF, Price A, Xenakis L, Zhang W. Evidence for Massage Therapy Working Group. The Impact of Massage Therapy on Function in Pain Populations—A Systematic Review and Meta-Analysis of Randomized Controlled Trials: Part II, Cancer Pain Populations. Pain Med. 2016, 17, 1553–68.
10. Renato G Kasseroller, Erich Brenner. Effectiveness of manual lymphatic drainage in intensive phase I therapy of breast cancer-related lymphedema—a retrospective analysis. Support Care Cancer 2023 Dec 5;32(1):5.
11. Cystic Fibrosis Foundation. Chest physical therapy.
12. Raposo F, Ramos M, Lúcia Cruz A. Effects of exercise on knee osteoarthritis: A systematic review. Musculoskeletal care. 2021 Dec;19(4):399–435.
13. American College of Sports Medicine (ACSM). ACSM guidelinesfor Exercise Testing, 2019.
14. Feng C, Adebero T, DePaul VG, Vafaei A, Norman KE, Auais M. A systematic review and meta-analysis of exercise interventions and use of exercise principles to reduce fear of falling in community-dwelling older adults. Physical Therapy. 2022 Jan;102(1):pzab236.
15. Robert Samuel Mayer, Jessica Engle. Rehabilitation of Individuals with Cancer, AnnRehabil Med 2022;46(2):60-70, pISSN: 2234-0645 • eISSN: 2234-0653
16. Jimenez-Andrade JM, Mantyh WG, Bloom AP, et al. Bone cancer pain. Ann N Y AcadSci 1198:173-181, 2010.
17. Danhauer SCS SJ, Addington EL, Chaoul A, Cohen L. Yoga therapy during cancer treatment The Principles and Practice of Yoga in Health Care ed. East Lothian, UK: Handspring Publishing; 2016.
18. Danhauer SC, Addington EL, Cohen L, Sohl SJ, Van Puymbroeck M, Albinati NK. Yoga for symptom management in oncology: A review of the evidence base and future directions for research. Cancer, 2019;125(12):1979–1989. https://doi.org/10.1002/cncr.31979

19. He YH, Guo XF, Brian HM, Zhang AL, Liu Y, Lu C, et al. Clinical evidence for association of acupuncture and acupressure with improved cancer pain a systematic review and meta-analysis. JAMA Oncol 2020;6(2):271–8. doi: 10.1001/jamaoncol. 2019.5233.
20. Quilt Mai, Xuejing Li, Dan Yang, Xiaoyan Zhang, KePeng, YufangHao. Effects of acupressure on cancer-related pain management: A systematic review and meta-analysis of randomized controlled trials. European Journal of Integrative Medicine. Volume 51, April 2022, 102120.
21. Parás-Bravo P, Alonso-Blanco C, Paz-Zulueta M, Palacios-Ceña D, Sarabia-Cobo CM, Herrero-Montes M, et al. Does Jacobson's relaxation technique reduce consumption of psychotropic and analgesic drugs in cancer patients? A multicenter pre-post intervention study. BMC Complement Altern Med. 2018 May 02;18(1):139.
22. Krishna Moorthy, Laura Halliday. Guide to Enhanced Recovery for Cancer Patients Undergoing Surgery: ERAS and Oesophagectomy. Ann SurgOncol (2022) 29:224–28.
23. Venetia Wynter-Blyth, Krishna Moorthy. Prehabilitation: preparing patients for surgery BMJ 2017;358:j3702
24. Sejal S Shingavi, Atharuddin Kazi, Sambhaji Gunjal, Maria Lamuvel. Effects of active cycle of breathing technique and autogenic drainage in patient with abdominal surgery. International Journal of Applied Research 2017; 3(2): 373-376
25. Zhong J, Zhang S, Li C, Hu Y, Wei W, Liu L, et al. Active cycle of breathing technique may reduce pulmonary complications after esophagectomy: A randomized clinical trial. Thorac Cancer. 2022;13:76–83.
26. Alaparthi GK, Augustine AJ, Anand R, Mahale A. Comparison of diaphragmatic breathing exercise, volume and flow incentive spirometry, on diaphragm excursion and pulmonary function in patients undergoing laparoscopic surgery: a randomized controlled trial. Minimally invasive surgery. 2016 Jan 1;2016.
27. Junghwa Do, et al. The effects of inspiratory muscle training with pulmonary rehabilitation on NSCLC patients during radiation therapy: A pilot clinical study. Thorac Cancer. 2023;14:1567–73.
28. Aida Tórtola-Navarro, et al. Cancer survivor inspiratory muscle training: systematic review and Bayesian meta-analysis. BMJ Supportive & Palliative Care 2023; 13:e561-e569.
29. Selman Emiroglu, et al. Effect of Cold Therapy on Managing Postoperative Pain Following Breast Conserving Surgery. Pain ManagNurs. 2023 Aug; 24(4):452–55.
30. Helen Richmond, et al. Development of an exercise intervention for the prevention of musculoskeletal shoulder problems after breast cancer treatment: the prevention of shoulder problems trial (UK PROSPER). BMC Health Services Research (2018) 18:463
31. Julie Bruce, et al. Exercise to prevent shoulder problems after breast cancer surgery: the PROSPER RCT. Health TechnolAssess . 2022 Feb; 26(15):1–124
32. Konstantinos Dinas, et al. Axillary web syndrome: Incidence, pathogenesis, and management. Current Problems in Cancer 43 (2019)
33. Elan Yang, Xiongwei Li, Xiao Long. Diagnosis and Treatment of Axillary Web Syndrome: An Overview. Chinese Journal of Plastic and Reconstructive Surgery, 2020.
34. María Torres-Lacomba, et al. Manual Lymph Drainage With Progressive Arm Exercises for Axillary Web Syndrome After Breast Cancer Surgery: A Randomized Controlled Trial. Physical Therapy, 2022; 102:1–11.
35. Sumitra Bakshi, et al. Prevalence of chronic pain following resection of pelvic bone tumours: A single centre prospective observational survey. British Journal of Pain 2022, Vol. 16(3) 263–69.
36. Pachman DR, Barton DL, Swetz KM, Loprinzi CL. Troublesome symptoms in cancer survivors: fatigue, insomnia, neuropathy, and pain. J ClinOncol 2012;30(30):3687–96.
37. Bower JE. Cancer-related fatigue–mechanisms, risk factors, and treatments. Nature reviews. Clinical oncology 2014;11(10):597–609.
38. Bei Dong, Yishu Qi, Lu Lin, Tingting Liu, Shaotong Wang, Yueyue Zhang, et al. Orthop Sports PhysTher 2023;53(6):343–352. Epub: 23 March 2023. doi:10.2519/jospt.2023.11251

39. Kleicyane Aguiar, Meireles Almeida, et al. Rehabilitation Interventions for Shoulder Dysfunction in Patients With Head and Neck Cancer: Systematic Review and Meta-Analysis. Physical Therapy 2020, Volume 100 Number 11.
40. Charters E, et al. Trismus therapy devices: A systematic review. Oral Oncology 126 (2022).
41. Chia-Hui Shao, et al. Exercise therapy for cancer treatment-induced trismus in patients with head and neck cancer: A systematic review and meta-analysis of randomized controlled trials. Radiotherapy and Oncology; Volume 151, October 2020, Pages 249–255.
42. Shuzhen Chee, et al. Interventions for Trismus in Head and Neck Cancer Patients: A Systematic Review of Randomized Controlled Trials Integrative Cancer Therapies 2021, Volume 20: 1–12
43. Stefano Tamburin, et al. Rehabilitation, exercise, and related non-pharmacological interventions for chemotherapy-induced peripheral neurotoxicity: Systematic review and evidence-based recommendations Critical Reviews in Oncology / Hematology 171 (2022) 103575.
44. MiroslawaPuskulluoglu, et al. Effects of Transcutaneous Electrical Nerve Stimulation on pain and Chemotherapy induced Peripheral Neuropathy in Cancer patients: A systematic Review. Medicina 2022;58:284.
45. Mitali Naik, Priyanka Nayak, KU Dhanesh Kumar. Effect of Physiotherapy in the Prevention and Relief of Secondary Lymphoedema in Subjects with Postoperative Breast Cancer—A Systematic Review of Randomised Controlled Trials. Journal of Clinical and Diagnostic Research. 2021;15(5).
46. Antonio Melillo, Andrea Chirico, Giuseppe De Pietro, Luigi Gallo, Giuseppe Caggianese, Daniela Barone, et al. Virtual Reality Rehabilitation Systems for Cancer Survivors: A Narrative Review of the Literature. Cancers 2022, 14, 3163.
47. Yu He, Xiaochai Han, Wenchen Zou, Xuemin Liu, Nianyi Sun, Fenghua Zhou. Telerehabilitation programmes for patients with cancer and survivors: a protocol for a systematic review. BMJ Open 2022.

Chapter 22

# Role of Occupational Therapy in Cancer Pain Management

• Manjusha Vagal

## INTRODUCTION

Pain is multifaceted phenomenon that impacts not only the physical components but affects the cognitive, psychological, social, spiritual and behavioural components of an individual.[1] Pain acts as a barrier that prevents an individual from successful participation in the valued and meaningful routine task and roles.

Occupational therapy (OT) plays a multifaceted role in oncology and cancer-related pain management.[2] Occupational therapists are valued members of the interdisciplinary team due to their unique ability to assess the effect of pain on an individuals capacity to participate in purposeful activities.[2] Referral to occupational therapy is prompted when pain interferes with the patient's capacity to participate in meaningful daily activities or tasks.

### Occupational Therapy in Cancer Pain Assessment

Considering the multifactorial etiology of pain its proper assessment is challenging. Pain assessment is multiprofessional, multidimensional and is repeated at regular intervals to guide initial and ongoing treatment. As a multidisciplinary team member an occupational therapist evaluates the factors that influence patients' pain perception and its interference in daily life. Occupational therapists identify the factors that decreases occupational performance, disrupts occupational roles and diminishes quality of life. They objectively assess the occupational performances to determine patients' occupational profile and the value of those occupations.[3] Since pain is recognised as a subjective experience[4] 'self-report' measures represent the predominant form of pain assessments. Occupational therapists follow holistic approach to pain assessment for providing comprehensive care. In occupational therapy the clinical comprehensive cancer pain assessment focuses on finding onset of pain, location(s), intensity, frequency, duration, exacerbating and relieving pain factors, pain treatments (past and current), mood, and occupational performance. Some of the commonly used validated and reliable self-reporting measures are 'Visual analogue scale' (VAS)[5,6] 'Numerical rating scale' (NRS), 'Verbal reporting scale' (VRS), 'Brief pain inventory' (BPI),[7] 'Pain disability index' (PDI),[8] 'Canadian occupational performance measure' (COPM). Patients pain behaviors can be evaluated before, during, and after intervention using alabama pain behavior scale.[9] Activity diaries are highly reliable and valid[10] and often used as an assessment technique and outcome measure for occupational performance.[11] Simple descriptive pain distress scale, faces scale and McGill Pain questionnaire[12] are other measures which can be used to assess and monitor cancer pain. For patients with limited communication skills and cognitive functions different observational scales are used.[13]

Ultrasonography is the preferred method for objectively assessing 'myofascial trigger points' as it effectively distinguishes these points from surrounding normal tissues. However, in routine clinical practice, these trigger points are typically assessed manually using palpation techniques.[14]

Both the 'NRS' and the 'VAS' can be utilized in patients having myofacial pain syndrome (MPS) which is recognized as one of the most important causes of pain in cancer patients with cancer.[15]

Initial pain assessment is intends to find the cause of pain while frequent and regular reassessment guide the ongoing pain management. It is important that the therapist is aware of red flags and possibility of disease progression on reports of new pain.

## Occupational Therapy in Cancer Pain Management

Malignant pain, stemming directly from cancer itself, often demands urgent and potent pain relief due to its severity and progressive nature. Non-malignant pain, on the other hand, can arise from various sources related to cancer treatment or other medical conditions, and it may manifest acutely, sub-acutely or develop into a chronic issue over time.

The World Health Organization (WHO) guidelines recommend a combination of pharmacologic and non-pharmacologic treatments as the standard of care for managing cancer pain. Non-pharmacologic interventions play a significant role as adjuncts to pharmacologic treatment, offering additional means not only for pain relief but also for alleviating mood disturbances, improving patients' participation in life roles and are thus helpful in improving quality of life. Considering, that cancer pain is multifactorial phenomenon having physical, psychological, social and spiritual affectation on person's quality of life, the biopsychosocial model of cure is applied in cancer pain management.[16] In cancer pain management, occupational therapist evaluates and applies evidence based therapeutic methods to help individuals overcome challenges in performing their daily activities.

Occupational therapy plays a crucial role in promoting holistic pain management and improving patients' overall quality of life by addressing the psychosocial and physical aspects of cancer pain. Cancer pain management based on occupational therapy approaches can briefly be divided into psychosocial interventions and physical interventions.

### Psychosocial Interventions

There is robust evidence backing the effectiveness of psychosocial interventions in managing cancer pain.[17] These interventions primarily target altering the perception of pain, mitigating associated fears, and empowering individuals to take charge of their pain. Occupational therapy holds a pivotal role in utilizing psychosocial interventions for cancer pain management. Some commonly used interventions include:

*Education:* Counseling as well as patient and caregiver education forms are crucial components of pain management. Occupational therapists educate patients about pain physiology, non-pharmacological interventions, self-management approach, the importance of adherence to treatment plans and clarify their treatment expectations as it prepares them for active participation in the pain management. Similarly, they teach patients and caregivers technical vocabulary to describe pain symptoms and enhances their ability to communicate effectively with the medical team.[18]

*Active listening:* Patients may harbour various beliefs and fears about cancer related pain like 'cancer pain is inevitable', 'pain might be a sign of disease progression', 'pain complaint might stop treatment'. Active listening is a crucial skill that occupational therapists utilize to understand and address these concerns effectively and provide proper guidance.[18]

*Communication of pain and social skill training:* Communication of pain is an important and critical aspect of pain management. Discrimination and social skill training are important domains in controlling pain language. Discrimination training is directed towards teaching patients. Appreciating their efforts at discussing their pain only with the concerned healthcare professional, and at right time and appropriate place. Social skill training aims at reinforcing patient's behavior which does not revolve around their pain especially in social contacts.

*Relaxation training:* Relaxation training indeed plays a crucial role in helping patients manage pain by enhancing their ability to self-regulate pain perception. Occupational therapists often guide patients through various relaxation techniques like 'progressive muscle relaxation', 'autogenic training', and 'guided mental imagery' to help them manage their pain perception. Each of these methods targets different aspects of relaxation which are tailored as per patient's to the individual needs and preferences. By teaching and practicing these relaxation techniques, occupational therapists empower patients in actively managing their pain and improving their overall well-being. Relaxation training may include the use of biofeedback to facilitate learning to voluntarily control musculoskeletal and vascular responses that precipitate pain experience. According to literature relaxation training has multiple benefits including reduction in anxiety and fatigue, giving patients sense of control over pain.[19,20] Evidence suggests relaxation rehearsal may help in reducing perceived pain intensity, duration and frequency.[21,22]

*Distraction:* Purposeful activities play a crucial role in occupational therapy interventions by addressing physical, functional, and psychosocial goals, including pain management and distraction from pain sensations. It has demonstrated to improve pain tolerance.[23] Distraction activities target increased pain awareness which is usually experienced during the periods of low environmental stimulation and during minimal activity periods. 'Play based' occupational therapy can improve pain, fatigue and anxiety in children admitted for cancer treatment.[24] Balance between work, leisure and social participation is important for distracting attention from pain.

*Coping skills:* Occupational therapists facilitate peer support groups, connect patients with community resources, and foster social networks to provide emotional support and validation, which can positively impact pain perception and coping abilities. Support groups gives an opportunity to the patients to understand that they are not the only ones to experience pain but there are others who also experience pain. Similarly, the support group provides patient an opportunity to understand and learn the coping strategies adopted by others to deal with pain and also provide them a neutral place to express their pain experiences.

### Physical Interventions

*Postural corrections and ergonomics:* Patients often become fearful of experiencing pain while participating in activities and hence either avoid activity participation or participate assuming faulty posture to avoid pain which often leads to faulty postural habit and eventually the reason for more pain. By identifying the conditions or treatment interventions that may increase the risk of faulty posture and providing early education on correct posture, may prevent patients from experiencing pain. Occupational therapists often utilize various strategies, including audiovisual feedback to address postural issues and promote optimal musculoskeletal health. Similarly, they use ergonomics assessments to identify environmental factors causing or adding to pain and modify them to reduce or eliminate pain. Also, occupational therapist provides opportunities to practice safe and effective use of the body during routine tasks in natural environments like home, work or leisure. Instructions and rehearsal of proper body mechanics and postures during routine tasks becomes important.

*Activity tolerance:* Inactivity and immobility following the treatment of cancer can cause muscle weakness, joint stiffness, reduced endurance and generalized deconditioning. With the detrimental effects of inactivity, pain gradually sets in further leading to fear of movement and thus the vicious cycle of inactivity and pain entraps the patient. Increasing patient's activity level is thus the corner stone of subacute and chronic pain management. Occupational therapists provide individualized therapeutic activities and exercise programs are as per the patient's requirements, which are improved gradually as per the tolerance level of the patient, balancing with the right rest periods in between. Experience of pain before the rest period is avoided to prevent reinforcement of pain behavior.[25,26]

*Energy conservation and work simplification:* Prescription of energy conservation and work simplification techniques are essential for efficient functioning of the patients without exacerbating the pain experience. Occupational therapists regularly advise on work pacing, activity modification, ergonomical modifications and prescribe and train patients in use of assistive technology, in order to simplify work and improve work output.

*Environmental modifications:* Occupational therapists assess individuals' home, work, and community environments to identify factors that may contribute to pain or limit participation. They recommend environmental modifications, such as ergonomic adjustments, assistive devices, and home adaptations, to create supportive environments that promote comfort, safety, and accessibility.

*Supportive orthosis and adaptive equipment:* Occupational therapists play valuable role in deciding, prescribing and fabricating metal (hand), thermoplastic orthoses for patients with pain simultaneously trying to preserve patient functionality. The main function of any orthosis is to support the anatomical structures and offer pain relief without compromising on functions. They are also indicated in case of contractures and muscle imbalance. Spine is the commonest site for bony metastasis and frequently associated with pain. Various spinal orthoses are prescribed depending upon the location of lesion. Custom made plastic spinal braces are indicated for lesions at multiple levels and for the lesions located at the various spinal junctions.[27,28] Long bone metastasis and fractures are provided with different types of orthoses including functional cast braces. Conditions like radiation therapy induced brachial plexopathy or plexopathy in advanced cancer is supported with upper limb orthosis or shoulder sling offer considerable pain relief. Orthotic application ideally be balanced with active/active assisted/passive mobilization as total immobilization of the part (excluding spine) may lead to increased pain and dysfunction. Occupational therapist also prescribes adaptive equipment to increase functions and comfort. Proper bed positioning, pillow support and cushioning are used as comfort measures.[29] Patients having metastatic lesions in spine can be prescribed reachers, sock coolers, etc. Similarly, walkers and other ambulatory aids are prescribed for avoiding weight-bearing on the lower limb having metastatic lesions to avoid fractures and pain.

### Mirror Therapy

Mirror therapy is a relatively simple non-invasive intervention that offers promising results in the management of pain that originate in the amputated body part commonly known as 'phantom limb pain'.[30] It is often used as part of a comprehensive intervention strategy for individuals experiencing phantom limb pain following limb amputation surgery. Mirror therapy has demonstrated significant clinical effectiveness in managing phantom limb pain compared to many other treatments.[31,32] Research suggests that mirror therapy may be particularly effective for addressing 'deep somatic pain', including 'pressure sense' and 'proprioceptive pain' than the 'superficial pain'.[33] During mirror therapy, a mirror is placed in patients' sagittal plane, obliterating the view of the amputated limb, and patients are then instructed to perform various motor tasks or movements with the intact limb, such as rolling a ball or manipulating pegs, while observing the mirrored image of the unaffected limb in the mirror **(Fig. 22.1)**, with the mirrored image of the unaffected limb performing movements in the mirror, mirror therapy helps to bridge the gap between the brain's proprioceptive expectations and the visual feedback it receives. By creating the illusion of movement which is essentially pain-free, in the missing limb through the reflected image of the intact limb, mirror therapy helps to reorganize and integrate these sensory signals, reducing the perception of pain.

*Massage:* There are various types of massages practiced for pain relief. The most commonly used in clinical practice for patients treated for various cancer include scar tissue massage, myofascial release and manual lymphatic drainage. Scar tissue massage is recommended for releasing adherent surgical scar tissue. Occupational therapists take special training in myofascial release techniques and manual lymphatic drainage. Myofascial release is indicated not only for mobilizing scar tissue and adjoining adherent connective tissue but very widely used for treating myofascial trigger points. Manual lymphatic drainage is beneficial for reducing lymphedema, postoperative edema and associated pain. Massage techniques known to improve circulation and lymphatic and venous drainage, soft tissue elasticity, enhances parasympathetic activity and reduce sympathetic activity.[30,34] Similarly, massage biomechanically cause increased levels of serotonin and decreased levels of cortisol.[31,35] Massage is known not only for reducing pain experience but also is helpful in reducing anxiety, stress, muscular tension and fatigue.

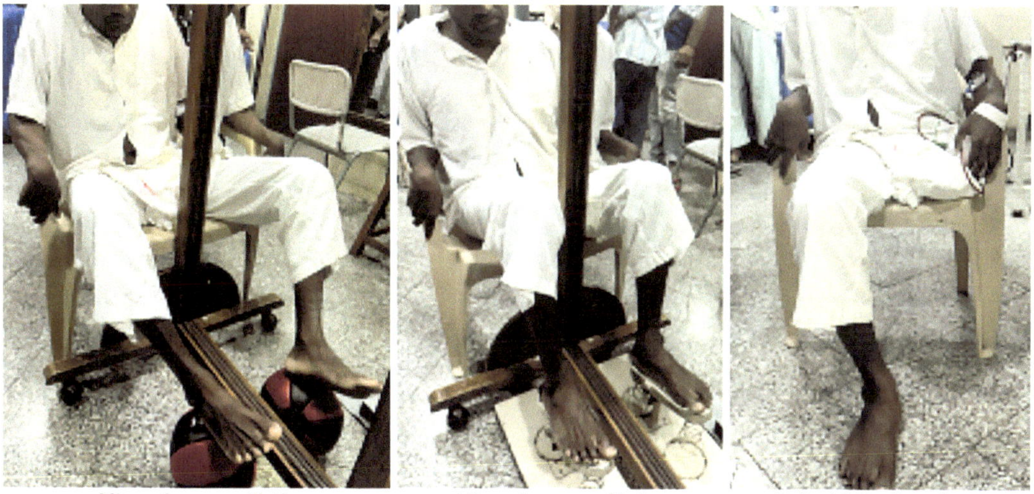

Mirror therapy with the medicine ball | Mirror therapy with the ankle exerciser | Patient following above knee ampulation surgery

**Fig. 22.1:** Mirror therapy for management of phantom limb pain

*Neuromuscular re-education:* EMG or electromyography is a method used to gauge the electrical impulses generated by muscles when they contract and relax. With EMG biofeedback, patients can visually or audibly monitor their muscle activity and learn strategies to modulate it. It helps to relax the tense muscles reducing (chronic) pain and allows to perform the required task avoiding abnormal movement patterns and postural deviations which contribute or exaggerate the pain experience. At the beginning, biofeedback training is given in a quiet, reclining situation allowing patients to focus on learning the techniques and gaining awareness of their physiological responses and as they become more proficient and comfortable with the techniques, it is gradually introduced into work-related activities.[36]

*Therapeutic modalities:* Occupational therapists (with appropriate post professional education) may use physical agent modalities as an adjunct to or in preparation for purposeful activities.[32,37] The physical agent modalities in treating cancer pain are not well studied due to the exacerbation of underlying disease. Application of 'cold packs', 'transcutaneous electrical nerve stimulation' (TENS), 'massage', 'biofeedback' is supposed to be safe and routinely prescribed for cancer patients.[33,38] Deep heating modalities are not advised in cancer pain management though the evidence stating it to be unsafe in cancer patients is lacking. Application of modalities irrespective of superficial or deep is contraindicated at the site of disease for the concerns of metastasis.

*Myofascial pain treatment:* Combination of manual therapy and pharmacological treatment for myofascial pain have potential for obtaining high patient satisfaction. Nonpharmacological and pharmacological treatment including myofascial release techniques, needling, stretching and flexibility exercises, scar tissue massage, exercises to improve posture, strengthening exercises, ergonomic modifications and ultrasound-guided myofascial trigger points injection were found effective.[34,35,39,40]

*Lifestyle management:* Occupational therapists teach lifestyle management to patients having cancer related pain by means of provision and training in use of assistive aids, orthotics, energy conservation, work simplification, counselling, reconstruction of occupational roles, modified environment, etc. to enable restoration of function without evoking pain experience or with reduced pain.[36,41]

## Conclusion

Nonpharmacologic interventions in cancer pain are important and routinely practiced though the evidence to support their effectiveness is still lacking. Occupational therapy interventions in pain management focus on relieving pain, empowering individuals with effective coping skills, and enhances their ability to participate in occupational performance.[32,37,42]

## References


1. Melzack R. The McGill Pain Questionnaire: major properties and scoring methods. Pain. 1975;1(3):277–99.
2. Bloch R. Rehabilitation medicine approach to cancer pain. Cancer Investigation, 2004;22(6), 944–48. doi: 10.1081/cnv-200039684
3. Hamdy RC. The decade of pain control and research (Editorial). Southern Med J. 2001;94:753–54.
4. US Department of Health and Human Services. Management of cancer pain. AHCPR: Rockville, MD; 1994
5. Houde RW. Methods for measuring clinical pain in humans. ActaAnaesthesiolScand 1982; 74(suppl.): 25–9.
6. Sriwatanakul K, Kelvie W, Lasagna L. The quantification of pain: an analysis of words used to describe pain and analgesia in clinical trials. ClinPharmacolTher. 1982; 32(2):143–48.
7. Pollard CA. Preliminary validity study of the Pain Disability Index. Index Percept Mot Skills. 1984;59:974.
8. Cheeland CS, Ryan KM. Pain assessment: Global use of the brief pain inventory. Annals of academy of medicine Singapore.1994;23(2):129–38.
9. Richards JS, et al. Assessing pain behavior: the UAB Pain Behavior Scale. Pain. 1982;14:393.
10. Fordyce WE. Behavioral methods for chronic pain and illness. Mosby: St Louis; 1976.
11. Follick MJ, Ahern DK, Laser-Wolston N. Evaluation of a daily activity diary for chronic pain patients. Pain. 1984;19:373–82.
12. Melzack R, Katz J. Pain measurements in persons with pain. In: Wall P D Melzack R (eds). Text book of pain. 3rd edition Churchill Livingstone New York.1994;33–51.
13. Herk R, Dijk M, Baar FPM, TibboelD, Wit R. Observational scales for pain assessment in older adults with cognitive impairments or communication difficulties. Nurs Res. 2007;56:34–43. DOI: 10.1097/00006199-200701000-00005
14. Jafari M, Bahrpeyma F, Mokhtari-Dizaji M, Nasiri A. Novel method to measure active myofascial trigger point stiffness using ultrasound imaging. Journal of Bodywork and Movement Therapies. 2018;22(2):374–78.
15. Cheatham SW, Kolber MJ, Mokha M, Hanney WJ. Concurrent validity of pain scales in individuals with myofascial pain and fibromyalgia. Journal of Bodywork and Movement Therapies. 2018; 22(2):355–60.
16. Sutton LM, Porter LS, Keefe FJ. Cancer pain at the end of life: a biopsychosocial perspective. Pain. 2002;99:5–10.
17. Keefe FJ, Abernethy AP, Campbell LC. Psychological approaches to understanding and treating disease related pain. Ann Rev Psychol. 2005;56:601–30.
18. Lapointe J. Cancer-related pain: the role of occupational therapy in prevention and management. Occup Ther Now. 2012; 14(5):10–2.
19. McCaffery M. Nursing management of the patient with pain. Philadelphia, JB Lippincott, 1979.

20. Turner JA, Romano JM. Cognitive behavioural therapy, In: BonicaJJ, (ed). The Management of pain, 2nd ed. Philadelphia, Lea&Fegiber, 1990;1711–21.
21. Engel JM, Rapoff MA. Biofeedback-assisted relaxation training for adult and pediatric headache disorders. Occupational Therapy Journal of Research. 1990a;10:283–99.
22. Strong J,Cramond T, Maas F. The effectiveness of relaxation techniques with patients who have chronic low back pain. Occupational Therapy Journal of Research. 1989; 184–192.
23. Heck SA. The effect of purposeful activity on pain tolerance. The American Journal of Occupational Therapy. 1998; 42 (9): 577–81.
24. Mohammadi A, Mehraban AH. Effect of Play-based Occupational Therapy on Symptoms of Hospitalized Children with Cancer: A Single-subject Study. Asia-Pacific Journal of Oncology Nursing.April2017https://www.researchgate.net/publication/316944739DOI: 10.4103/apjon.apjon_13_17
25. Fordyce WE. Behavioural methods for chronic pain and illness. Mosby, St Louis,1976.
26. Grzesiak RC. Cognitive and behavioural approaches to management. NY State J Med.1982;82:30–8.
27. Lee SH, Grant R, Kennedy C, Kilbride L. Positioning and spinal bracing for pain relief in metastatic spinal cord compression in adults. Cochrane Database of Systematic Reviews. 2015; (9).
28. Choo YJ, Chang MC. Effectiveness of orthoses for treatment in patients with spinal pain. Yeungnam University Journal of Medicine. 2020; 37(2), pp.84–89.
29. Dietz J. Rehabilitation oncology. New York, John Wiley & Sons, 1981.
30. Weinstein SM. Phantom limb pain and related disorders. Neurol Clin. 1998;16:919–36.
31. Weeks SR, Anderson-Barnes VC, Tsao JW. Phantom limb pain: theories and therapies. Neurologist. 2010;16:277–86.
32. McCabe CS, Haigh RC, Halligan PW, Blake DR. Simulating sensory-motor incongruence in healthy volunteers: implications for a cortical model of pain. Rheumatology (Oxford) 2005;44:509–16.
33. Sumitani M, Miyauchi S, McCabe CS, Shibata M, Maeda L, Saitoh Y, et al. Mirror visual feedback alleviates deafferentation pain, depending on qualitative aspects of the pain: a preliminary report. Rheumatology (Oxford) 2008;47:1038–43.
34. Field TM. Massage therapy effects. Am Psychol.1998; 53 (12):1270–81.
35. Field T, Hernandez-Reif M, Diego M, Schanberg S, Kuhn C. Cortisol decreases and serotonin and dopamine increase following massage therapy. Int J Neurosci.2005;115 (10):1397–13.
36. Hamilton AM. Electromyography: Potential Use in Occupational Therapy. Occupational therapy. November, 1983;316–18.
37. Engel JM. Pain management. Pendleton HM, Schultz-Krohn W. In Pedretti's occupational therapy: practice skills for physical dysfunction. ed 8. Mosby Elsevier: St Louis; 2018.
38. Watkins T, Maxeiner A. Musculoskeletal effects of ovarian cancer and treatment: a physical therapy perspective. RehabilOncol.2003;21:12–7.
39. Treaster D, Marras WS, Burr D, Sheedy JE, Hart D. Myofascial trigger point development from visual and postural stressors during computer work. Journal of Electromyography and Kinesiology. 2006;16: 115–124. doi: 10.1016/j.jelekin.2005.06.016. Epub 2005 Sep 16.
40. Hasuo H, Kanbara K, Abe T, Sakuma H, Fukunaga M. Factors Associated with the Efficacy of Trigger Point Injection in Advanced Cancer Patients. PhD Journal of Palliative Medicine. 2017; Volume 20, Number 20, 1-6. PMID: 28426271 DOI: 10.1089/jpm.2016.0541
41. Cancer pain. A monograph on the management of cancer pain. Ottawa, Health and Welfare Canada, Minister of Supply and Services Canada, 1986.
42. Engel JM. Evaluation and pain management. Pendleton HM, Schultz-Krohn W. In Pedretti's occupational therapy: practice skills for physical dysfunction. ed 6. Mosby Elsevier: St Louis; 2006.

Chapter 23

# The Role of Palliative Care in Pain Management at End-of-life

• Shamali Poojary • Anshita Sharma

## NEED FOR PALLIATIVE CARE

Caring for a loved one battling cancer can be physically exhausting and emotionally draining, and often, there is a sense of helplessness. As the disease progresses, the burden on the patient and the caregiver increases. The patients find themselves navigating different treatments and have frequent doctor appointments to attend to. Important decisions need to be made by the patient and or the immediate loved ones. Health-related suffering is serious when it cannot be relieved without medical intervention and when it compromises physical, social, spiritual and emotional functioning. Ninety percent of people who die from cancer globally experience serious health-related suffering. It is estimated that in India, the total number of patient require palliative care is likely to be 5.4 million a year. However, only 1% of patients have access to palliative care.

Palliative medicine emerges as a ray of hope during this challenging time, providing holistic support to improve the quality of life for patients and their families.[1]

Palliative medicine addresses the needs of individuals facing serious illnesses, such as cancer, by focusing on pain and other symptom management, psychosocial support, and spiritual care and empowers caregivers to take better care of the patient as well as themselves. It is integrated throughout cancer care, commencing from the time of diagnosis of advanced illness.

The palliative medicine team comprises doctors, nurses, psychologists, medical social workers, counsellors, rehabilitation specialists, and volunteers.[2] Compassion underpins all principles of palliative care. Some of the principles, according to the World Health Organization, are as follows:[3]

- *Pain and symptom management:* Palliative medicine emphasizes managing pain and other distressing symptoms associated with cancer and its treatment by combining pharmacological and non-pharmacological interventions. It includes disease and treatment-related symptoms like pain, breathlessness, vomiting, constipation, anxiety, depression, sleep, appetite, etc.
- *Betterment of quality of life for patients and their families:* Quality of life encompasses various dimensions, including physical and psychological well-being, social and spiritual needs. Palliative care aims to improve overall well-being and promote a sense of dignity.
- Affirming life and acknowledging death as a natural part of existence.
- Helping patients live as actively as possible.

- Neither hastens nor postpones death.
- *Providing holistic support:* Palliative medicine provides physical, emotional, social, psychological and spiritual aspects of care tailored to individual preferences and values. Counseling and support group meetings are some of the services provided
- Honouring patients' values, preferences, and beliefs, empowering them to make decisions that align with their goals and wishes.
- Communicating with patients and family-empathic and honest communication is essential in palliative care. Discussions about diagnosis and prognosis, treatment options, goals of care, preferred place of care, and end-of-life care and aligning them with patients' values and goals are important.
- *Advance care planning (ACP):* It helps in making important decisions about future preferences, place of care, decision-makers, and goals of care. Patients can document their wishes regarding resuscitation, life-sustaining treatments, and end-of-life care by having an open discussion with the team.
- *Promoting self-care:* In caring for the patients, caregivers often neglect themselves, sacrificing their physical and mental well-being. Palliative care emphasizes self-care, encouraging caregivers to prioritize their health and seek support when needed through respite care services, support groups, or individual counseling.
- Supporting the family during the bereavement.

## The Right Time to Involve Palliative Caregivers

Determining the appropriate time to involve palliative care providers can be challenging for caregivers. However, timely integration of palliative care into the cancer care continuum has been shown to have many benefits for patients and their families.

Identify the right time to engage palliative care providers can pose difficulties for caregivers. Yet, integrating palliative care into cancer treatment at the right time has proven to offer numerous advantages for both patients and caregivers. Early integration can be as soon as diagnosis of advanced malignancy.[4]

*Patient-triggered:* The commencement of palliative care support should be guided by the preferences and needs of the patient and their caregivers.[5, 6]

*Transition points:* Certain points in the cancer journey signal the need for palliative care involvement. These include transitions from curative to palliative treatment, progression or recurrence of disease, increase in symptom burden and decline in general condition.

Palliative care ought to be perceived as an essential element seamlessly integrated within the spectrum of cancer care services. Regular assessments of symptom burden and psychosocial needs enable timely referrals to palliative care providers.[7] Dispelling myths in palliative care.[8]

*Palliative care equals giving up:* Palliative care does not equare to relinquishing or halting treatment effort. It aims to integrate specialized support to reduce symptoms.

*Palliative care means no more treatment:* It can be provided along with cancer treatment. The palliative care team works with other healthcare providers to develop personalized care plans for individual patients.

*Palliative care is only for the last days of life:* While it is essential in supporting patients nearing the end of life, palliative care is not limited to this stage. It can be introduced early in the course of an illness alongside treatments.

*Palliative care is only available in hospitals:* Palliative care support can be provided in hospitals as well as other settings, including outpatient clinics, hospices, and even in the patient's own home.

*Palliative care hastens death:* There is a misconception that palliative care is linked to euthanasia. Palliative care does not aim to prolong life artificially or hasten death. Palliative care teams work ethically to secure that patients receive appropriate care that aligns with their preferences and goals.

*Palliative care is only for cancer patients:* It is not exclusive to cancer patients. Palliative care is beneficial for individuals facing a various serious illnesses, including but not limited to heart failure, advanced kidney disease, chronic obstructive pulmonary disease (COPD), dementia and Parkinson's disease.

*Palliative care is only for elderly:* There is a common misconception that palliative care is for older adults. Palliative care is appropriate for all ages, from children to the elderly.

*Palliative medicine is only about pain management:* While pain management is an essential component of palliative medicine, it is not the only focus. It addresses a wide range of symptoms and challenges associated with serious illness.

*Palliative care is solely provided by physicians:* Palliative care is a interdisciplinary approach that involves a team of healthcare professionals with diverse expertise.

*Death is painful, and pain is a part of dying:* Palliative care ensures dignified death, which is peaceful for the patient and emotionally acceptable by the caregivers.

In cancer care, palliative medicine provides compassion and support for patients and caregivers. Palliative medicine improves the quality of life by addressing the physical, emotional, psychosocial and practical needs of patients and caregivers. As caregivers navigate the challenges of cancer, palliative care offers comfort and guidance in the face of adversity.

## MANAGING PAIN AT TERMINAL STAGE

In the last days of life, a significant number of patients, ranging from 30 to 75% may experience pain.[9]

In end-of-life care, pain assessment is crucial for ensuring patients' comfort and quality of life. It involves regularly using validated tools to assess pain intensity, location, and impact. Patient self-report is preferred, but observational and proxy assessment may be necessary for patients unable to communicate. Pain assessment should be multidimensional, considering physical, emotional, social, and spiritual aspects. Accurate documentation and regular reassessment are essential for effective pain management. Evidence supports systematic pain assessment in improving patient comfort and overall quality of life during last days of life.

Opioids are the primary pharmacological agents used for managing pain in last days of life. Numerous studies and clinical guidelines support the effectiveness of opioids, e.g. morphine, hydromorphone, and fentanyl, in providing analgesia and improving life quality for patients with advanced illness or nearing the end-of-life. Opioids act on the central nervous system to relieve pain and are titrated based on the severity of pain and individual patient response.

End-of-life pain management requires a personalized approach that considers the unique needs and preferences of each patient. Comprehensive pain assessment, including evaluation of pain intensity, location, characteristics, and impact on physical and psychosocial functioning is essential for developing an individualized pain management plan. The choice of analgesics often depends on the individual needs, preferences and medical condition. These medications can be administered orally, intravenously, transdermally, or via other routes based on the patient's condition and the healthcare provider's assessment. The aim is to ensure the patient's comfort and alleviate suffering during this critical time. Additionally, non-pharmacological approaches for comfort and psychological support can be helpful. It is important to address reversible causes of pain, such as urinary retention, which can lead to discomfort and agitation in the final days of life. Regular reassessment of pain and adjustment of analgesic therapy are necessary to ensure optimal pain control and minimise adverse effects.

### Pharmacological Interventions

In end-of-life care, alternative routes of administration for analgesics, including opioids like morphine, are often utilized to effectively manage pain and provide comfort to patients. In addition to intravenous (IV) infusions and subcutaneous morphine administration, here are some alternative routes that may be employed:

1. *Transdermal route:* Transdermal opioid patches provide a convenient and non-invasive option for continuous pain management. Fentanyl patches are the most commonly used transdermal opioids during end of life, delivering a steady dose of medication through the skin over a 72-hour period. These patches can be particularly suitable for patients who have difficulty swallowing oral medications or who require long-term pain management.

2. *Intramuscular route:* Intramuscular injections of opioids can provide rapid pain relief when IV access is unavailable or difficult. While less commonly used than other routes, IM injections of opioids like morphine may be administered into large muscle groups for effective pain control.

3. *Rectal route:* Rectal administration of opioids can offer an alternative for patients who are unable to take medications orally or intravenously. Opioid suppositories or rectal solutions, such as of morphine, can be used to provide pain relief while minimizing discomfort to the patient.

4. *Sublingual/buccal route:* Sublingual or buccal administration of opioids allows for rapid absorption through the mucous membranes in the mouth. Opioid formulations, such as sublingual buprenorphine tablets or buccal fentanyl preparations, can provide effective pain relief for patients with difficulty swallowing or those requiring rapid onset of action.

5. *Nasal route:* Intranasal administration of opioids involves delivering medication through the nasal passages, where it is absorbed into the bloodstream. Nasal sprays containing opioids, such as tapentadol, offer a non-invasive option for pain management, particularly for patients who have difficulty swallowing or who require rapid relief.

Non-pharmacological interventions, including physical therapy, massage therapy, acupuncture, relaxation techniques, music therapy and guided imagery, may complement pharmacological approaches to pain management during last days of life.

These interventions help alleviate pain, promote relaxation, reduce anxiety, and enhance overall well-being for patients nearing final days of life. While the evidence for specific non-pharmacological interventions varies, they are generally considered safe and may offer additional benefits when used as part of a comprehensive pain management plan.

Integrating palliative care services into end-of-life pain management ensures holistic, patient-centric care that addresses physical, psychosocial, and spiritual needs. Interdisciplinary palliative care teams, comprising doctors, nurses, pharmacists, social workers, chaplains, and other healthcare professionals, collaborate to provide comprehensive pain assessment and management, psychosocial support, spiritual care, and symptom control for patients and their families. Research consistently demonstrates the advantage of interdisciplinary palliative care in improving pain control, enhancing quality of life, and promoting patient and family satisfaction with end-of-life care.

Overall, evidence-based pain management in end-of-life care emphasises a multimodal, interdisciplinary approach that prioritises individualized assessment and treatment, comprehensive symptom management, and patient-centered care to optimize comfort and quality of life for patients nearing the final days of life.[10]

## COUNSELING OF FAMILY MEMBERS OF PATIENTS WITH PAIN DURING END-OF-LIFE

Counseling for caregivers during pain in end-of-life care is essential to provide support and guidance during a challenging and emotionally taxing time.[11] Here's an overview of evidence supporting caregiver counseling:

1. *Psychological support:* Research shows that caregivers of terminally ill patients with pain often experience high levels of stress, anxiety, depression, and burnout. Counseling interventions, such as cognitive-behavioral therapy (CBT), supportive counseling, and psycho-education, have been shown to effectively reduce psychological distress among caregivers. These interventions help caregivers develop coping strategies, manage emotional challenges, and improve their overall well-being.

2. *Improved coping skills:* Counseling provides caregivers with an opportunity to learn effective coping skills and problem-solving techniques to navigate the complexities of end-of-life care. Evidence suggests that psychotherapeutic interventions aimed at enhancing coping mechanisms can lead to better adjustment and resilience among caregivers.

3. *Enhanced communication:* Effective communication is crucial for caregivers to express their needs, concerns, and emotions related to end-of-life care. Counseling interventions focus on improving communication skills, facilitating difficult conversations, and strengthening relationships within the care giving context. Studies have demonstrated that enhanced communication between caregivers and healthcare professionals leads to better care outcomes and increased satisfaction with end-of-life decision-making.

4. *Reduced caregiver burden:* Providing care for a terminally ill loved one can impose significant physical, emotional, and financial burden on caregivers. Counseling interventions targeted at addressing caregiver burden have been shown to alleviate stress, improve caregiver self-efficacy, and enhance overall quality of life. By addressing specific caregiver needs and concerns, counseling helps prevent caregiver burnout and promotes sustainable caregiving practices.

*5. Bereavement support:* Counseling services extend beyond the patient's death to provide bereavement support for caregivers. Grief counseling and support groups offer a safe space for caregivers to process their loss, express emotions, and receive validation from peers and mental health professionals. Research indicates that participation in bereavement counseling can facilitate the grieving process, reduce complicated grief symptoms, and promote psychological adjustment following the death of a loved one.[14,15]

Overall, evidence supports the efficacy of counseling interventions in addressing the multifaceted needs of caregivers during end-of-life care, ultimately enhancing their well-being and capacity to provide optimal care for terminally ill patients.

## LEGAL AND ETHICAL ASPECTS OF PAIN IN END-OF-LIFE

At the end-of-life, it is crucial to prioritise pain management, considering it as a patient's fundamental right and a moral obligation for clinicians, enforced by legal standards. The World Health Organization States that patients have a right to have their pain treated, as does the United States Supreme Court,[12,13] despite widespread misconceptions, opioids are deemed appropriate for pain relief, with risks like respiratory depression primarily affecting specific patient populations. The principle of double effect justifies aggressive pain treatment, ensuring that the intent is solely to alleviate suffering. When conventional methods fail, palliative sedation offers relief for those experiencing severe, unmanageable pain.[11]

Ethical issues in palliative care revolve around determining appropriate care for patients with limited life expectancy. Principlism, based on autonomy, beneficence, non-maleficence, and justice, guides ethical reasoning in the United States. Tensions may arise when working with surrogate decision-makers, especially in grave or irreversible situations. Health institutions should establish policies to address conflicts in medical decision-making.

Clinicians are not obligated to participate in care they find morally objectionable. Code status discussions should stem from comprehensive conversations about prognosis and care goals. Strategies are needed when families request to withhold distressing prognostic information. Clinicians must carefully consider how to respond to requests for assistance in dying, regardless of their ethical stance or legal permissibility.

The increasing number of older adults in the criminal justice system necessitates palliative care services within correctional settings. Incarcerated individuals face higher rates of chronic medical conditions and physical disabilities, often experiencing psychosocial palliative care needs and unique barriers to care. Despite incarceration, they maintain the right to a community standard of care, including access to palliative services. Ethical principles, including autonomy in medical decision-making, remain relevant. Challenges include limited access to medications and off-site care, necessitating timely advance care planning. Collaboration between medical and custodial administration is vital to ensure dignity in end-of-life care.

Advance care planning (ACP)[16] involves ongoing discussions among patients, their families, and healthcare providers to align medical care with the patient's goals, values, and beliefs. Clinicians inform patients about their prognosis and treatment options, helping them make decisions based on their values. Advance directives (ADs) like

Durable Power of Attorney for Health Care and Living Wills capture these preferences. Regular review of ADs is recommended, especially during health changes. While evidence on ACP's impact varies, it can improve outcomes for patients with serious illness. Clinicians assess decision-making capacity and designate surrogate decision-makers when needed. Physician orders are crucial for honouring patients' resuscitation preferences documented during ACP discussions.

Assessing end-of-life expectations and preferences is crucial for providing appropriate care, including discussions on CPR. Honouring patient preferences for the place of death is prioritised, with education provided to families about the dying process. Medication management focuses on discontinuing non-essential medications and administering necessary ones via non-oral routes. Recognizing signs of imminent death guides care, with emphasis on managing common symptoms like pain and dyspnea using integrated care pathways. Palliative sedation is considered for refractory symptoms after interdisciplinary assessment. Nursing care shifts towards comfort and emotional support, while guidelines for pronouncing death are followed.

In conclusion, palliative medicine and effective pain optimization are essential components of end-of-life care, providing holistic support to patients and their families. Through multidisciplinary approaches, including pharmacological and non-pharmacological interventions, and compassionate counseling, these services address physical, emotional, and spiritual needs while upholding ethical standards. Embracing early integration, dispelling myths, and navigating legal and ethical complexities ensure dignified and compassionate care for patients nearing the last days of life.

## References


1. Radbruch L, De Lima L, Knaul F, et al. Redefining Palliative Care—A New Consensus-Based Definition. J Pain Symptom Manage. 2020;60(4):754–764. doi: 10.1016/j.jpainsymman.2020.04.027
2. Hui D, Bruera E. Models of Palliative Care Delivery for Patients with Cancer. J Clin Oncol. 2020; 38(9):852–65. doi:10.1200/JCO.18.02123
3. World Health Organization. Palliative care. http://www.who.int/cancer/palliative/definition/en
4. Temel JS, et al. Effects of Early Integrated Palliative Care in Patients with Lung and GI Cancer: A Randomized Clinical Trial. JCO. 2017;35:834–841. doi:10.1200/JCO.2016.70.5046
5. Singh V, et al. Trigger-based pathways to increase utilization of palliative care services for cancer patients: A multi-disciplinary approach. JCO. 2022;40:e24007. doi: 10.1200/JCO.2022.40.16_suppl. e24007
6. Hui D, Hannon BL, Zimmermann C, Bruera E. Improving patient and caregiver outcomes in oncology: Team-based, timely, and targeted palliative care. CA Cancer J Clin. 2018;68(5):356–376. doi: 10.3322/caac.21490.
7. Crawford GB, et al. Care of the adult cancer patient at the end of life: ESMO Clinical Practice Guidelines. ESMO Open. 2021;6(4):100225. doi: 10.1016/j.esmoop.2021.100225.
8. IAPC. Palliative care. www.palliativecare.in
9. World Health Organization. Cancer Pain Relief and Palliative Care. Geneva: World Health Organization, 1990.
10. Coelho A, et al. Use of non-pharmacological interventions for comforting patients in palliative care: a scoping review. JBI Database System Rev Implement Rep. 2017;15(7):1867–1904. doi: 10.11124/JBISRIR-2016-003204.
11. Cherny NI, Ziff-Werman B. Ethical considerations in the relief of cancer pain. Support Care Cancer. 2023;31(7):414. doi: 10.1007/s00520-023-07868-3.
12. US. Supreme Court. Vacco v. Quill. Wests Supreme Court Report. 1997;117:2293–312.

13. Woodruff R. The Oxford Textbook of Palliative Medicine, 5th Edition. J Pain Palliat Care Pharmacother. 2016;30(4):335–6. doi: 10.1080/15360288.2016.1246509.
14. Bruera E, Higginson IJ, von Gunten CF, Morita T (Eds.). Textbook of Palliative Medicine and Supportive Care (3rd ed). CRC Press. 2021. doi: 10.1201/9780429275524.
15. Twycross R. Introducing Palliative Care 4th edn.
16. Morrison SR. Advance Directives/Care Planning: Clear, Simple, and Wrong. J Palliat Med. 2020; 23(7):878–79. doi: 10.1089/jpm.2020.0272.

Chapter 24

# Symptoms Associated alongside with Cancer Pain and their Management

• Prasun P • Dhanashri Kudal

This chapter explores the spectrum of symptomatology, alongside pain, encountered in patients with advanced malignancy. Specifically, it delves into dyspnea, nausea, emesis, constipation, fatigue, sleep disturbance, anxiety, loss of appetite and delirium. The subsequent section will provide a comprehensive analysis of these prevalent symptoms, including their pathogenesis and clinical presentation. Additionally, it will elucidate the diagnostic workup and therapeutic modalities employed in managing these clinical entities.

## DYSPNEA

Defined by American Thoracic Society as "a subjective experience of breathing discomfort that consists of qualitatively distinct sensations that vary in intensity. The experience results from interactions among multiple physiological, psychological, social, and environmental factors and may induce secondary physiological and behavioral responses".[1]

This is highly disabling symptom related to cancer which limits the biological and social functioning of an individual leading to an array of consequences from anxiety, isolation, withdrawal, depression to cardiovascular and muscular deconditioning and death.

It is a highly prevalent symptom with a prevalence more than 90% in cancers like lung and at the terminal phase of life. This symptom is not only distressing to the patient, but also to the carers to an equal extent.

### Pathophysiology

The pathophysiology of dyspnea is incompletely understood, in cancer patients it may be due to disruption of normal architecture of lungs, obstruction of airways by the tumor, lymphangitis carcinomatosis, effusion, thrombus formation, lung injury due to treatment, etc. or other non-cancerous cardiac or respiratory causes.

### Workup

Thorough history and examination. Apart from the routine history, it is important to know the genesis of the symptom, character, meaning to the patient, prior experience of dyspnea and relieving measures or maneuvers. Relevant investigations to establish the cause and rule out any reversible contributors.

### Management

Basic principles of management are:

1. Reversal of reversible/treatable causes like infection or effusion.
2. Non-pharmacological measures inclusive of breathing techniques.
3. Pharmacological measures to reduce the perception of breathlessness and anxiety.
4. An action plan for the crisis.

Common correctable causes are infections, effusions, pulmonary embolism and anemia. Conditions like superior vena cava obstruction may be promptly managed with stenting, radiotherapy (RT) or chemotherapy. Large tumors obstructing the airway may be considered for RT or steroids. Lymphangitis carcinomatosis could be given a trial of dexamethasone 8–12 mg/day.

Drug free approach includes airflow to face, acupuncture, relaxation exercises, cognitive behavioral therapy, music therapy, etc.[2]

Opioids are the mainstay of pharmacological treatment of dyspnea.[3] Multiple plausible mechanisms have been postulated for effectiveness of opioids. Systemic low dose morphine at 10 mg/day could be initiated in opioid naive patients and titrated upwards, with limited benefits seen beyond 30 mg/day. In patients on opioids for pain, a 25–50% increment is recommended for addressing dyspnea. Benzodiazepines are useful options when anxiety is predominantly associated with dyspnea. Oxygen supplementation should be considered whenever hypoxia is identified as the cause of dyspnea. A written crisis management plan can help reduce anxiety and emergency hospital visits.

## CONSTIPATION

Constipation in simple terms is when stools become hard, dry, infrequent, and difficult to pass. Its prevalence in palliative care varies from 40–90% depending on the diagnostic criteria.[4] There can be considerable variation in the frequency of defecation in the normal population.

### Pathophysiology

Constipation can be broadly categorized into two main causes: Primary and secondary. Primary constipation arises from problems within the colon or rectum itself, such as disruption of regular bowel movements or dysfunction of the rectal sphincter muscles. Secondary constipation, on the other hand, is caused by underlying diseases or medications that affect the digestive system, leading to issues like excessively dry stool or diminished rectal sensation.

### Workup

A good history on earlier bowel habits including frequency, consistency, changes in diet/medication, mobility and prior use of laxatives is the first step. Associated symptoms like vomiting, abdominal distension, abdominal colic, urinary continence can aid in arriving at cause diagnosis. Spurious or overflow diarrhea secondary to constipation needs to be carefully evaluated. Clinical examination should not miss per rectal and auscultation of the abdomen.

CECT would be the investigation of choice if suspecting malignant bowel obstruction (MBO).

A plain radiograph of the abdomen will help to distinguish constipation and obstruction. Blood levels of thyroid hormones and electrolytes should be checked if feasible.

### Management

Adequate hydration, a balanced diet and mobility should be encouraged as appropriate. Attention should be given to toilet preferences in inpatients. Drugs contributing to constipation should be revised whenever possible. The choice of laxative depends on the likely cause of constipation. The dose of laxatives should be titrated based on the individual's need. If constipation is secondary to spinal cord compression, spinal bowel regimen according to the type of bowel should be initiated. Surgical intervention or stenting may be considered in MBO for appropriate candidates.[5] Opioid related bowel dysfunction can be treated with a combination of stool softener and stimulant laxative providing the mush and push. PAMORA (Peripherally acting Mu (μ) Opioid Receptor Antagonists) like methylnaltrexone, naloxegol, and naldemedine are approved for OIC. These are currently not available in India.

## SLEEP DISTURBANCE

Sleep disturbances can be a problem in more than half of the patients with cancer.

It can be a cause or a result of symptoms like pain, anxiety, or depression. A comprehensive history on difficulty in sleeping or somnolence need to be taken focusing on sleep onset, staying asleep and patterns of awakenings. Other symptoms or medications contributing to the sleep disturbance must be elicited. Sleep pattern history including daytime sleeping or frequent naps are necessary for apt management. Insomnia in patients can also be exhausting to the caregivers who are deprived of it along with the patient.

Insomnia could be due to a variety of symptoms like pain, emesis, anxiety, depression, hiccups, cough, dyspnea, pruritus, stimulant beverages, or medications like dexamethasone at bedtime. Somnolence could be attributed to fatigue, electrolyte and hormonal imbalances, medications like opioids or antiepileptics.

Management of sleep disturbances include identification of underlying cause and its rectification. Sleep hygiene must be advised for all patients. Non-benzodiazepine Z drugs, benzodiazepines or melatonin could be prescribed as a pharmacological aid after correct diagnosis for short-term. Obstructive sleep apnea must be ruled out, especially in patients on opioids.

Nonpharmacological approaches include counseling, relaxation techniques, biofeedback, hypnosis, or cognitive behavioral therapy in appropriately selected patients.

## ANXIETY

Anxiety is another very prevalent symptom which occurs in clusters with pain. Anxiety may be experienced at different domains—emotional, physical, behavioral, and cognitive. It is important for the physician to identify and pick up the type by giving attention to the words of the patient while describing the symptom, e.g. "apprehensive," "frightened," "troubled," "on edge" which impart the experience of anxiety or fear.

Common anxiety disorders in patients with cancer include adjustment disorder with anxiety, generalized anxiety disorder, panic disorder, and post-traumatic stress disorder.

Details have been covered in Chapter 15.

## ANOREXIA

Anorexia, or loss of appetite, is a frequent and multifaceted challenge faced by cancer patients on palliative care. Patients have lack of desire to eat often which is due to multiple factors like changes in taste perception, nausea, and pain, particularly odynophagia. Bloating and constipation can further contribute to the problem. Anorexia often exists alongside cachexia, a wasting syndrome characterized by significant muscle loss.

Assessing the root cause of anorexia in these patients is crucial. A detailed history can reveal contributing factors like pain or nausea, allowing for targeted interventions to address them. For patients in advanced stages of cancer, it is equally important to recognize that diminished appetite may be a natural consequence of the disease progression. In such cases, forcing food or resorting to artificial nutrition and hydration can exacerbate existing symptoms and offer little benefit. While appetite stimulants like low-dose dexamethasone and megestrol can be used to some effect, they primarily increase appetite and weight, not muscle mass. Ultimately, a patient-centered approach that prioritizes quality of life and alleviate the anorexia is essential in palliative care.

## NAUSEA AND VOMITING

Nausea and vomiting is experienced by almost 6–68% of patients with advanced cancer.[6] Nausea can be "described as an unpleasant sensation of the need to vomit and having sick or uncomfortable feeling behind the throat or the stomach." Nausea can lead to vomiting. Vomiting is "forceful expulsion of the stomach contents due to contraction of the abdominal and chest wall musculature."

Causes of nausea and vomiting in palliative care include:[7]

- Cancer related—like bowel obstruction
- Cancer treatment related, e.g. chemotherapy or radiotherapy related nausea and vomiting
- Infections
- Complications like electrolyte imbalance, renal or hepatic failure, raised intracranial disease, etc.
- Medications related, e.g. opioids
- Vestibular disturbances.

*Risk factors include:* Young age, female, stress, multiple pregnancy.

*Classification of chemotherapy related nausea and vomiting:*[8]

- *Acute:* Within 24 h of administration of chemotherapy and is mediated by 5HT3
- *Delayed:* Occurs 24 h to 5 days after chemotherapy and is mediated by substance P binding to NK1 receptors
- Anticipatory nausea and vomiting occurs before chemotherapy treatment like a conditioned response

- Breakthrough—within 5 days of initiating chemotherapy despite the antiemetic prophylaxis
- Refractory—occurs after chemotherapy in subsequent treatment cycles after the failure of prophylactic antiemetics in previous chemotherapy cycles.

### Pathophysiology

Nausea is caused by activation of autonomic nervous system and vomiting is mediated through complex reflex. It results from activation of chemoreceptor trigger zone, cerebral cortex, vestibular apparatus and peripheral stimuli from visceral organs and vasculature which is related to exogenous stimuli like irritation, inflammation, etc.[9]

### Management

Non-pharmacological measures:

- *Food, drink and dietary modification:* Cold pleasant tastes decrease nauseating stimuli.
- Acupuncture and acupressure.
- Behavioral therapy helps in anticipatory nausea.
- Music therapy, and
- Visual imagery may reduce severity and duration of chemotherapy related nausea and vomiting.

### Pharmacological Measures

Choice of antiemetic depends on the etiology or empirical approaches have also been proven to be effective.[9]

#### *Dopamine antagonist*

- *Metoclopramide:* For example, bowel obstruction, opioids related delayed emptying of bowel
- *Haloperidol:* Chemical/metabolic etiology

#### *Serotonin (5HT3) antagonist*

- *Ondansetron and granisetron:* Chemotherapy/radiotherapy induced nausea, vomiting, metabolic etiology.

#### *Atypical antipsychotic*

- *Olanzapine:* Chemotherapy/radiotherapy induced nausea, vomiting, metabolic etiology, refractory nausea/vomiting

#### *NK1 antagonist*

- *Aprepitant:* Chemotherapy/radiotherapy induced nausea, vomiting, metabolic etiology.

## FATIGUE

Cancer fatigue mainly due to cancer or cancer treatment. In this patient feels exhausted or extremely tired despite enough sleep. In patients with extreme fatigue their activities of daily living get affected. Fatigue related to cancer is not improved with sleep or rest and may be present even during rest and without any activity. Symptoms related to cancer fatigue are as follows:

- Having no energy; feeling extremely tired, drained, or lethargic
- Having difficulty moving; feeling heavy or slow
- Having difficulty concentrating, remembering, or thinking
- Having a sense of physical, emotional, and/or mental exhaustion

Cancer cells may utilize more energy and nutrients depriving it from the normal cells, making patients feel fatigued. Cancer and its treatment also led to release of certain inflammatory mediators which causes fatigue. Cancer Cachexia is a wasting syndrome which leads to muscle and weight loss which may further cause more fatigue.

### Workup

History of fatigue and its impact on the functioning will be useful in tailoring the management to the individual patient. Hormonal-thyroid and androgens, vitamins and micronutrients levels, organ functions, electrolytes and hematological parameters must be evaluated. Functional assessment of chronic illness therapy (FACIT)-fatigue subscale, functional assessment of anorexia/cachexia therapy (FAACT) and the Edmonton symptom assessment system-revised can be used for assessment of cancer related fatigue.[10]

### Management

The basics of fatigue management include finding the cause and correcting all the correctable along with nutritional optimization, exercises, and energy conservation.

Correctable causes include:

- Management of anemia include dietary changes, blood transfusions, or hematinic.
- Correction of hormonal, electrolytes and vitamins derangements and deficiencies which contribute to fatigue.
- Treatment of pain can help in decreasing tired, but certain analgesics can itself cause tiredness.
- Cancer fatigue can be worsened by stress, fear, hopelessness, or depression. Mental health therapists may help patients by using cognitive behavioral therapy and talk therapy. This helps to manage their feelings and relieve fatigue. Antidepressants should be considered for patients with depression and fatigue.

### Fatigue Specific Pharmacological Measures

Short-term steroids are used in patients with advanced cancer but have limited effect. Corticosteroids effect lasts for 2–4 weeks only. Dexamethasone is a steroid that is used in such conditions, but risks outweigh benefits on prolonged use.[10,11] Psychostimulants like methylphenidate may help in opioid induced sedation and depression. These medications may increase energy and improve the ability to think and concentrate in patients with advanced cancer.

A recent Cochrane review confirmed that planning and pacing activities of the day, exercises like 30 minutes' walk, aerobics exercises helped in cancer related fatigue.[12] Mind–body practices like qigong, tai chi, yoga.[13] Relaxation techniques like guided imagery, hypnosis and acupuncture are other therapies which are studied for cancer fatigue.[14] Ginseng capsules of ground ginger root can be used to treat cancer related fatigue. Other dietary supplements example coenzyme Q10 and L-carnitine are also included in some clinical trials for treating cancer fatigue.

## DELIRIUM

Delirium is confusion which comes on suddenly, over days or hours.

Patients with delirium might experience restlessness and agitation, sleepiness, confusion, memory problems, disorientation, hallucinations, paranoia, poor concentration, reduced appetite, or a temporary change in personality.

The prevalence of delirium in palliative care is 13.3–42.3% and incidences of admission is 3–45%.[15]

A patient may have some or all these symptoms with diurnal variations. It may be transient for a few hours in some or may last days or weeks in others.

There are three types of delirium:

- Hyperactive delirium—patient may have restlessness, agitation, or may be aggressive.
- Hypoactive delirium—patient may be withdrawn, quiet and sleepy.
- Mixed delirium—the patient has mixed picture of hyperactive and hypoactive symptoms.

Hypoactive delirium is commonly seen in patients with a terminal illness and it is more difficult to recognize this type of delirium. It is sometimes misunderstood as depression, fatigue or dementia or may not get noticed at all. This can mean delirium goes undiagnosed and untreated or is diagnosed late.

### What is the difference between dementia and delirium?

The symptoms related to dementia present slowly and develop over months–years, whereas the symptoms of delirium develop over a few days, or hours. Some patients may have both dementia and delirium—delirium is common in people with advanced dementia.

### Causes of Delirium

Delirium can be multifactorial and patients may often have more than one. Most seen causes are electrolyte imbalance; medicines including opioids and steroids; withdrawal related to drugs like alcohol, nicotine, sedatives, antidepressants; infections; constipation; urinary retention; dehydration; organ failure; uncontrolled pain; hypoxia; hypoglycemia/hyperglycemia. It could also be due to new onset brain metastasis or worsening of existing metastasis or primary malignancies of the brain.[16]

By taking into consideration the causes of delirium it is easy to find potential ways to manage it.

### Workup

By early detection of delirium patient's quality of life will be improved. This will help for better communication and might help to notice subtle changes in their behavior early. Assessment tools helps to identify delirium quickly, by checking for orientation, attention, alertness. Blood and imaging investigations to identify the cause must be carried out on priority.

### Management

Delirium is managed depending on the cause of delirium, patient's care preferences, nature and stage of their illness, overall health condition. If patient is lacking decision making capacity, then any decisions made on behalf of patient should be in their best interests, and guided with advance care plans.

Identified cause must be treated with ethics guiding the treatment decision in terminally ill patients. Antibiotics, electrolyte correction or anticancer treatments must be considered in appropriate patients. Terminal delirium may not be reversible and develops in the last few days or hours of life. Treatment in these patients focuses on supporting the patient's comfort and relieving any distressing symptoms.

### Non-pharmacological Measures

- Help the patient to get reoriented to the surrounding.
- A clock and calendar are present within the sight of the patient.
- Functionality of hearing aids and glasses should be monitored closely.
- Clear communication with short sentences and simple language, easy to understand. To encourage patient to eat and drink safely.
- Ensure bladder bowel movements.
- Encourage a sleep cycle routine, limit noise at night.
- Check for signs of unmanaged pain, and treat accordingly.
- Help the patient mobility—provide support to walk and do other activities safely.

### Pharmacological Measures

Antipsychotics may be considered in patients refractory to non-drug measures despite correcting the correctable. Benzodiazepines may be considered if the delirium is irreversible and the patient poses a threat to self or others.[17] Melatonin is another drug which may be considered for delirium though the evidence is still mixed.

Delirium can be distressing for the caregivers as well. It is equally important to support them by describing about delirium, explaining regarding causes and risk factors, discussion regarding upcoming conditions and issues, explaining how to support the patient, help in coping.

In conclusion, effectively managing cancer symptoms alongside pain can significantly enhance a patient's holistic well-being. This can improve their satisfaction and quality of life, allowing them to function at their maximum capacity. By addressing accompanying symptoms, as discussed above, patients experience greater comfort and are better equipped to manage their pain and participate in their treatment plan.

## References

1. Parshall MB, Schwartzstein RM, Adams L, Banzett RB, Manning HL, Bourbeau J, et al. An Official American Thoracic Society Statement: Update on the Mechanisms, Assessment, and Management of Dyspnea. Am J Respir Crit Care Med. 2012;185(4):435–52.
2. Zemel RA. Pharmacologic and Non-Pharmacologic Dyspnea Management in Advanced Cancer Patients. Am J Hosp Palliat Care. 2022 Jul;39(7):847–55.
3. Takagi Y, Sato J, Yamamoto Y, Matsunuma R, Watanabe H, Mori M, et al. Opioids for the management of dyspnea in cancer patients: a systematic review and meta-analysis. Int J Clin Oncol. 2023;28(8):999–1010.
4. Larkin PJ, Cherny NI, La Carpia D, Guglielmo M, Ostgathe C, Scotté F, et al. Diagnosis, assessment and management of constipation in advanced cancer: ESMO Clinical Practice Guidelines†. Ann Oncol. 2018;29:iv111–25.

5. Henry JC, Pouly S, Sullivan R, Sharif S, Klemanski D, Abdel-Misih S, et al. A scoring system for the prognosis and treatment of malignant bowel obstruction. Surgery. 2012;152(4):747–56; discussion 756–757.
6. Solano JP, Gomes B, Higginson IJ. Comparison of symptom prevalence in advanced cancer, AIDS, heart disease, chronic obstructive pulmonary disease and renal disease. J Pain Symptom Manage. 2006;31(1):58–69.
7. Smith HS, Laufer A. Opioid induced nausea and vomiting. Eur J Pharmacol. 2014 Jan 5;722:67–78.
8. Gupta K, Walton R, Kataria SP. Chemotherapy-Induced Nausea and Vomiting: Pathogenesis, Recommendations, and New Trends. Cancer Treat Res Commun. 2021;26:100278.
9. Singh P, Yoon SS, Kuo B. Nausea: a review of pathophysiology and therapeutics. Ther Adv Gastroenterol. 2016;9(1):98–112.
10. Miura T, Okizaki A, Hasuo H, Satomi E, Tagami K, Imai K, et al. Dexamethasone 8 mg for Cancer-Related Fatigue in Inpatients with Advanced Cancer Undergoing Palliative Care: A Multicenter Phase II Trial. Palliat Med Rep. 2021;2(1):316–23.
11. Yennurajalingam S, Frisbee-Hume S, Palmer JL, Delgado-Guay MO, Bull J, Phan AT, et al. Reduction of cancer-related fatigue with dexamethasone: a double-blind, randomized, placebo-controlled trial in patients with advanced cancer. J Clin Oncol Off J Am Soc Clin Oncol. 2013;31(25):3076–82.
12. Jiang M, Ma Y, Yun B, Wang Q, Huang C, Han L. Exercise for fatigue in breast cancer patients: An umbrella review of systematic reviews. Int J Nurs Sci. 2020;7(2):248–54.
13. Hilfiker R, Meichtry A, Eicher M, Nilsson Balfe L, Knols RH, Verra ML, et al. Exercise and other non-pharmaceutical interventions for cancer-related fatigue in patients during or after cancer treatment: a systematic review incorporating an indirect-comparisons meta-analysis. Br J Sports Med. 2018;52(10):651–8.
14. Jang A, Brown C, Lamoury G, Morgia M, Boyle F, Marr I, et al. The Effects of Acupuncture on Cancer-Related Fatigue: Updated Systematic Review and Meta-Analysis. Integr Cancer Ther. 2020;19:1534735420949679.
15. Hosie A, Davidson PM, Agar M, Sanderson CR, Phillips J. Delirium prevalence, incidence, and implications for screening in specialist palliative care inpatient settings: a systematic review. Palliat Med. 2013;27(6):486–98.
16. Bush SH, Lawlor PG, Ryan K, Centeno C, Lucchesi M, Kanji S, et al. Delirium in adult cancer patients: ESMO Clinical Practice Guidelines. Ann Oncol Off J Eur Soc Med Oncol. 2018;29(Suppl 4):iv143–65.
17. Hui D, Frisbee-Hume S, Wilson A, Dibaj SS, Nguyen T, De La Cruz M, et al. Effect of Lorazepam with Haloperidol vs Haloperidol alone on Agitated Delirium in Patients with Advanced Cancer receiving Palliative Care: A Randomized Clinical Trial. JAMA. 2017;318(11):1047–56.

Chapter 25

# Nurses Role in the Management of Cancer Pain

• Sindhu Nair • Supriya Salunkhe

## INTRODUCTION

With increase in the global burden of cancer, oncology nursing is gaining importance. Though long recognized as a specialty, it is essential to understand the role of the nursing team in the cancer care continuum. Pain being the commonest presentation in patients with cancer, the need for integrating the nursing force in pain management is of utmost priority.[1]

Nurses' role in cancer pain management includes pain assessment and care planning. Controlling cancer pain includes assessment of pain, planning the care, administration of analgesics, evaluating effectiveness, monitoring the side effects of pain medications, and ensuring compliance to pharmacological and non- pharmacological treatments.

### Nurses Role in Assessment and Education of Pain

As the perception of pain is subjective, the nurse's key role in pain management is to believe and acknowledge patients pain. While assessing pain, the nurse must remain neutral and non-judgmental, be empathetic, show acceptance of pain and develop rapport with the patient. During assessment, patient must feel respected and believed. Absence of expression does not necessarily mean lack of pain. On the other hand, some patients may be reluctant to ask for pain relief due to socio-cultural beliefs. The nurse needs to anticipate the patient's pain needs, in such cases.[2] Nurses must educate patient about the importance of pain relief for physiological betterment like good sleep, rest, deep breathing, early ambulation and preventing complications of immobilization.

Pain assessment must include use of standardized, accepted pain assessment tools with the aim of recording and documenting patient self reported pain scores. Self-reported pain scores is the gold standard for pain assessment. Vulnerable patients' populations (e.g., children, patients with learning disabilities or who are cognitively impaired) require special considerations with pain assessment.[3]

As the nurses spend more time with patients, their observation and documentation regarding patient's physical signs related to pain and response to pain relieving measures will help in better pain management. While controlling cancer pain, nurses need to understand the emotional state of the patient diagnosed with cancer, pathophysiology of cancer pain, pain management therapies, patients' socio-cultural background and hazardous effects of persistent unrelieved pain.[1] In surgical patients pain score is assessed at various occasions like pain score at rest, at movement, while doing deep breathing exercises. The tools used for pain assessment are as follows (explained in detail in previous chapters)

- Numeric rating scale/universal pain assessment tool
- Wong Baker FPS–R scale (age faces pain rating scale)
- *FLACC scale:* Face, leg activity, cry and consolability scale
- Neuropathic pain scale

Patient should be explained how to use relevant scales and importance of reporting pain at its onset rather than waiting until it becomes severe.

## Nurses Role in Patient Care

While providing nursing care, every effort should be made to prevent pain by careful handling of drainage tubes, invasive line, during transfer/movement of critical patients. It is advisable to give an analgesic well in advance before initiating procedures that are expected to be painful. For good pain control, analgesics are to be given at right dose, right time and at the right intervals. Nurses must evaluate effectiveness of pain medication based on repeated assessment and report to physician regarding need for changes inclusive of drug change, dose or route to ensure optimum pain relief.

## Specialized Role of Nurses

*Nurses as part of the acute pain service (APS):* A nurse led model has been advocated in many centers across the globe. This makes the concept more sustainable and viable. Under the direction of the pain physician, APS nurses conduct following activities: Preoperative counseling, ensure smooth conduct and care of regional based pain relief techniques, monitoring of side effects and lastly educate patient and families about non-pharmacological techniques.[4]

1. *Preoperative counseling:* Preoperative counseling of patients about pain management is essential for better management of postoperative pain as the patients are in a better state to understand the concept of pain scales and need for mobilization post-surgery. Surgery can be physically and psychologically stressful for patients. Providing education to the patients about the procedure before surgery reduces anxiety and enhances postoperative outcomes. Preoperative counseling includes:
   - Understanding patient's and family members attitude, expectation, understanding and previous experiences about postoperative pain.
   - Explanation to patient and family regarding options available for postoperative pain management and emphasize on the benefits to comply with the institutional rehabilitation protocols.
2. *Nurses' role in pharmacological pain management interventions:* Pain management involves collaborative approach to treat patients with pain. Every pain management intervention involves meticulous nursing care.
   - *Nursing care of patient receiving bolus dose through epidural catheter*. Vital signs including oxygen saturation needs to be checked before and after the bolus dose through epidural catheters. Careful monitoring for side effects including hypotension and motor blockade is mandated.
   - *Nursing care of patient receiving medication through regional catheters:* Assessment of pain score before and after the medication administration. Maintain adequate

sterility barrier during drug administration. Ensuring intact dressing and remain viligant for possible catheter site infection. Nurses must check for leakage and pain while administering medication.

- *Nursing care of patient while removing epidural and regional catheter:* One needs to check coagulation profile of patient. In case of derangement, report to physicians as removal of epidural catheter is contraindicated in presence of any coagulopathy. The nursing team must ensure that the removal of neuraxial catheters is timed with prophylactic doses of low molecular weight heparin formulations which are commonly used in postoperative period to prevent deep vein thrombosis. It is essential to educate the patient about rare but serious complications like epidural infection and hematomas. Knowledge of the early signs which include altered sensation, lower limb weakness, pain and the contact details of healthcare providers should be provided to all patients and relatives.
- *Administration of pain medication through patient controlled analgesia (PCA):* Nurse taking care of patient with PCA need to check the patency of intravenous line. There should be one IV access which should be used solely for the IVPCA and without any stop-cock/three way attached to it. The nursing team must be well versed with monitoring for potential side effects of opioids and initial management of the same. Trouble-shooting equipment problems inclusive of alarms given by PCA like air accumulation, high pressure, low battery, cassette empty is expected from the nursing team.

3. ***Monitoring of patient for side effects of treatment:*** It is essential to monitor the patient's vital signs pre- and post-drug administration, watch for any respiratory distress, hypotension, tachypnea or any other side effects. The patient's level of alertness, oxygen saturation needs careful monitoring. Table 25.1 enlists the side effects of pain infusions that need to be addressed immediately.
4. ***Nonpharmacological nursing interventions to relieve pain:*** Nurses play an important role in relieving pain by their gentleness in handling the patient; and promoting comfort and support to painful areas. Massage with emollient oil especially on pressure points can relax tense muscles and relieve musculoskeletal pain. Distraction strategies like reading books, performing religious rituals listening to music, allowing family visit, watching television and use of other relaxation techniques can help in minimizing pain.[5] Performing passive and active range of motion exercises to stretch muscles is beneficial.

| Table 25.1: Side effects of pain infusion to be addressed immediately[4] |
|---|
| • Shortness of breath<br>• Difficulty swallowing<br>• Dizziness or light headedness<br>• Patient expression of impending doom<br>• Nausea and vomiting<br>• Pruritus<br>• Redness, warmth, tenderness or discharge at site of catheter insertion<br>• Catheter dislodgment or leak from catheter site |

## Home Care of Patients with Pain

Cancer patients and caregivers are often apprehensive about pain control at home. Nurses can play a significant role at home in ensuring patient comfort by providing consistent care, 24-hour access, and working in collaboration with other healthcare professionals. Nurses intervention has shown to prevent re-hospitalization for pain issues.[6]

Pain control can improve quality of life of patients with advance cancer. Although cancer pain cannot always be fully relieved, there are ways to make it less severe and aid patients with their daily activities.

Home care team can visit the patient at their house to see the compliance of medication, overall physical health of patient. Apart from pain other aspects of cancer care such as nutrition, wound care, stoma care can be instituted by the nurses to optimize patient care.

Education of patients and relatives on narcotic medications about doses, frequency and side effects to be monitored is essential. Patient receiving transdermal patch must undergo a brief training inclusive of a demonstration on application of patch.

## Care of Patient in Hospice

Hospice care includes physical comfort, emotional, social and spiritual support for people nearing the end of life. Hospice care focuses on relieving pain and ease of other symptoms as per the disease condition of patient. The hospice nurse aims to assess the patient's needs and provide individualized care. The pain nurse works closely with the medical team for the pain management plan. This may involve the use of medications, physical therapy and complementary therapies. Hospice nurses are trained experts to handle symptoms especially pain effectively, to ensure that the patient is as comfortable as possible.[7]

## Challenges and Barriers in Nursing Management of Patient with Pain

The inadequate education of staff specific to pain and its management is a major and persistent barrier to effective pain management. Despite development of pain management guidelines by numerous professional bodies, core pain management competencies for entry level nursing staff have not yet been established.[8]

To address these barriers, following interventions can be undertaken for effective pain policies in hospital.

- Pain assessment and management training to be made as integral and compulsory competency of induction training for newly recruited nursing staff.
- Pain assessment and pain management to be included as mandatory yearly in-service education topic.
- Standard operating protocols related to nurses role in pain assessment and pain management to be made available for all the nurses as ready reference.
- Regular audits related to pain assessment and of pain procedures to be conducted using standard pain audit checklist.
- Motivate pain team nurse to undertake quality improvement project (QIP) based on findings of audit.
- Short-term course with planned syllabus to be prepared and conducted.

- Training of ward staff in pain care course to be done on regular basis so that nurses working in ward are sensitized toward pain assessment and management.
- Encourage pain team nurses to attend conferences and workshop nationally and internationally related to advances in pain management.
- Encourage pain team nurse to conduct nursing oriented research related to pain management.
- Encourage and motivate pain team nurse to present research related papers at conferences.

## Conclusion

The role of nurses in pain management is multifaceted. They act as assessors, advocates, educators, coordinators contributing to a patient centered and comprehensive approach to pain care. Recognizing the significance of their role ensures optimal pain relief and improved quality of life for patients.

## References

1. Young AM, Charalambous A, Owen RI, Njodzeka B, Oldenmenger WH, Alqudimat MR, So WKW. Essential oncology nursing care along the cancer continuum. Lancet Oncol. 2020;21(12):e555–e563. doi: 10.1016/S1470-2045(20)30612-4. Epub 2020 Nov 16. PMID: 33212045.
2. Mahfudh SS. Nurse's role in controlling cancer pain. J PediatrHematolOncol. 2011;33 (Suppl) 2:S146-8. doi: 10.1097/MPH.0b013e318230dfd8. PMID: 21952573.
3. Fink R. Pain assessment: the cornerstone to optimal pain management. Proc (BaylUniv Med Cent). 2000 Jul;13(3):236–9. doi: 10.1080/08998280.2000.11927681. PMID: 16389388; PMCID: PMC1317046.
4. Acute Pain Nursing in the Field, pages 125–128., downloaded from site https://www.dvcipm.org/site/assets/files/1083/chapt31.pdf on 19.3.2024
5. Zeleke S, Kassaw A, Esthetie Y. Non-pharmacological pain management practice and barriers among nurses working n Debre Tabor Comprehensive Specialized Hospital, Ethiopia. PLoS One. 2021;15;16(6):e0253086. Doi:10.1371/journal.pone.0253086.PMID:34129616;PMC8205171.
6. Magrum, Lynn C, et al. "Pain Management in Home Care." Seminars in Oncology Nursing. 1996;12(3):202–18. https://doi.org/10.1016/s0749-2081(96)80038-6. Accessed 5 Mar. 2021.
7. Hagan TL, Xu J, Lopez RP, Bressler T. Nursing's role in leading palliative care: A call to action. Nurse Educ Today. 2018;61:216–19. doi: 10.1016/j.nedt.2017.11.037. Epub 2017 Dec 8. PMID: 29245101; PMCID: PMC5859921.
8. Fishman SM, Young HM, Lucas Arwood E, Chou R, et al. Core competencies for pain management: results of an interprofessional consensus summit. Pain Med. 2013;14(7):971–81. doi: 10.1111/pme.12107. Epub 2013 Apr 11. PMID: 23577878; PMCID: PMC3752937.

Chapter 26

# Opioid Policies at Tata Memorial Hospital

• Chhaya Dhanve • Bharti Veer

## INTRODUCTION

Narcotic drugs and psychotropic substances (NDPS) have many essential medical and research uses. However, these substances can be abused and illegally transported. India's approach towards NDPS is summarized in Article 47 of the Constitution of India, which states that the "state shall endeavor to bring about prohibition of the consumption except for medicinal purposes or intoxicating drinks and of drugs which are injurious to health."[1]

Contributors to poor access and narcotic availability for medical use in India.[3]

- The initial legislature for narcotics traces to the British era when narcotics were essentially a trade crop. Heavy restrictions were implanted to safeguard the commercial interests of the British. The NDPS Act, 1985 reflected the same restrictive tone and language.
- The state NDPS rules were non-uniform and prevented distribution of legitimate opioids for medical use across the country.
- The mandates given to government offices were prohibitory. All efforts were made to ensure that any medical or scientific use of narcotics was met with strict rules and regulations.
- There was no system in place to ensure consistent supply from official sources of raw material to manufacturers producing oral morphine.
- Medical institutions faced stringent regulations, inclusive of the need to maintain multiple license for acquiring, stocking, prescribing and using opioids.
- Strict punishments were laid down in the NDPS Act, 1985 (e.g. possible 10 years of rigorous imprisonment even for clerical errors). This discouraged institutions and pharmacist from stocking the narcotics.
- Attitude and knowledge of professionals towards use of opioids were negative.
  - Professionals had limited exposure to use of opioids and this was restricted only to acute or emergency situations. They had exaggerated fear of opioid addiction and respiratory depression with the use of these drugs.
  - Limited and restricted availability of opioid medication like oral morphine at medical colleges and hospitals, prevented exposure and training of professionals with the use of these medications in the treatment of chronic pain. A fear of opioids (opiophobia) developed amongst medical care providers.

The public associated with opioid addiction or a terminal medication and were unwilling to use the formulations at the cost of inadequate pain relief and suffering. The physicians due to above reasons failed to reassure deserving patients.

### Need for Opioid Policy

- Opioid are efficacious, cost effective and preferred analgesics for managing severe pain in selected group of patients.
- It is essential to establish a system which permits the use of these medication for medical use while ensuring that there is no misuse or diversion of these medication for illegal purpose.
- The paperwork essential for procuring and storing of these medications for medical reasons should be simplified.

NDPS Act has created statutory authorities such as Narcotics Commissioner (Section 5). Central Bureau of Narcotics is a chief organization headed by the Narcotics Commissioner. The Narcotics Control Bureau was created, in addition, though a notification under Section 4 of the Act. Each of these authorities have specified functions. Ministry of Health and Family welfare, Government of India, Health Department of states, state drug controllers and chief controller of factories are authorized to provide access to morphine/opioid for cancer pain relief and palliative care.

National policy on NDPS has been prepared in consultation with the concerned ministries, organizations and state governments. It aims to:

a. Draw the Indian Policy with respect to Narcotic Drugs and Psychotropic substances.
b. Serve as a quick reference guide to various ministries and government organizations inclusive of NGOs and relevant international bodies.
c. Re-enforce the nations stand to deal with the menace of drug trading in a holistic manner.

### Glimpse of Amended NDPS Act, 2014[4]

1. Expanded the scope of the act to include medical and scientific use.
2. Prepared a notified list of essential narcotic drugs (END), i.e. the opioid identified for medical use, approved by the Drug Controller General of India.
3. The notified list of ENDs currently includes: Morphine, methadone, codeine, hydrocodone, oxycodone and fentanyl.
4. Transferred the power to regulate ENDs to the central government.
5. Regulations are applicable uniformly across India.
6. It defined 'Recognized Medical Institution' (RMIs) with criteria for stocking and dispensing opioids for medical use.
7. Conferred the powers for authorizing medical institutions as RMIs for stocking and dispensing ENDs to a single state agency—State Drug Controller/Commissioner, Food and Drug Administration (FDA).
8. Those institutions fulfilling the criteria that is the RMIs, may apply to the State Drug Controller/Commissioner, FDA to procure and dispense END.
9. The authorization of RMIs is for the period of 3 years and can be renewed from the same agency.

## DISPENSING AND ADMINISTRAITON OF NARCOTICS

Narcotic and psychotropic drugs are potential for abuse or addiction which needs to be held under strict control. The common narcotics used are morphine sulfate, fentanyl citrate and buprenorphine. Nurses in health care institution need to ensure appropriate access and convenience for patients who require them. The following policy guides nurse on safe and effective narcotic drug management including indenting, procuring, storing, transporting, administering, recording and disposing these drugs safely.

### Guidelines for Management of Narcotic Drugs

1. It is the responsibility of the health institution to provide a detailed document pertaining to essential narcotics drug (END) procedures including; indenting, issue, administration, storage, receipt, transfer and reporting of incidents.
2. All information and procedures of this document are based on the national guide to management of narcotics in health institutions.
3. Nursing staff need to follow the list of approved narcotics to be used in the institution.
4. Each health institution dealing with narcotic drugs is obligated to keep separate registers for narcotic drugs.
5. All ENDs are considered high alert medications where they need special consideration in collection, storing in special cabinets/vaults with labeling.
6. All ENDs are administered following the "management of medication" policy.
7. Verbal or telephone orders for Narcotic medications should not be acceptable.
8. Borrowing ENDs from any other unit/ward (within the institution) is limited to emergency, when pharmacy services are not available.
9. Injectable ENDs are limited to inpatients and emergency room only and not to be dispensed by outpatient pharmacy and not to be given to patients for use outside the hospital.
10. ENDs prescription should only be written by the physician.
11. Ensure the compliance with ENDs prescription and administration guidelines during inter- or intra-hospital transfer of patient.

### ENDs Supply, Collection, Receiving from Medical Store and Record Keeping

*1. Receiving from the medical store/pharmacy to the wards/units/outpatient clinics*

a. Request for ENDs stock should be made by the nurse in-charge of the ward, unit or clinic and counter signed by the other nursing officer. In the absence of the nurse in-charge the shift senior nurse may sign the form.

b. The requisition form is sent to the medical store/pharmacy by the nurse in-charge. The pink prescription pad and the ward narcotic drug register is carried along with the requisition form (Form 26.1).

c. The pharmacist in-charge of the medical store/pharmacy checks the request and issues the ENDs.

d. The nurse in-charge checks and receives the ENDs issued and makes appropriate entry in the narcotics drug register (Form 26.2).

**Form 26.1:** Narcotic indent form

| Hospital Name: | | | |
|---|---|---|---|
| | **Narcotic Indent Form** | | |
| | | | Date: |
| Case No. | Name | Age | Sex |
| | | | |
| | | | |
| | | | |
| | | | |
| | | | |
| Ward and essential narcotic drug (END) No | Diagnosis/Indication | Doctor/Unit Administering the Narcotic Drug | |
| | | | |
| | | | |
| Name of drug | Dose | Route | Date/Time |
| | | | |
| | | | |
| Administered by | | Sister In-charge | |
| Signature: | | Signature: | |
| Name: | | Name: | |
| C.C.No: | | C.C.No: | |
| | | | |
| Prescribed by | | Dispensed by | |
| Signature: | | Signature: | |
| Name: | | Name: | |
| C.C.No: | | C.C.No: | |
| Quantity prescribed: | | Quantity dispensed: | |
| | | | |
| Prescription ID: | | | |

Unused/Broken glass ampoule should be handed over to the pharmacist for necessary replacement
Note: This form is in duplicate: Pink is dispensary copy and white is indenter's copy

e. Where electronic system for the requisitioning of ENDs is introduced, protections in the software is essential to be in place to ensure that:
   - Only nursing in-charge is authorized to place requisition for indent.
   - Protection is incorporated in the software to ensure each entry is identifiable.
   - Entries should not be altered at a later date.
   - A log of all date entered is saved and can be recalled for audit purposes.

*2. Narcotic drugs' stock, storage and count in ward/unit/outpatient clinic.*

When nursing in-charge receives the narcotic drugs:

**Form 26.2:** Narcotic register format

| Date | Stock qty | Indent date | Indent no. | Indent qty | Patient name | Patient case file no. | Doctor's name | Reg/ employ no. of doctor | Qty used | Batch no. | Expiry date | Memo no . | Transac-tion ID | Qty balance | Broken am-poule | Dose wastage amt | Remark | Sign & CC no. of Nurse (1) | Sign & CC no. of Nurse (2) |
|---|---|---|---|---|---|---|---|---|---|---|---|---|---|---|---|---|---|---|---|
| 15.3.24 | 20 | 15.3.24 | 5 | 10 | --- | ----- | ------ | ---- | --- | A1234 | March 26 | --- | --- | 30 | | | ----- | ABC/ 12345 | DEF/ 45632 |
| 16.6.24 | 30 | --- | ----- | ----- | Mr. XYZ | CU/12345 | Dr. FYZ | II/1245 | 1 | A1234 | March 26 | M7896 | 745632 | 29 | | | ---- | LOP/ 78534 | PAI/ 45213 |
| | | | | | | | | | | | | | | | | | | | |
| | | | | | | | | | | | | | | | | | | | |
| | | | | | | | | | | | | | | | | | | | |
| | | | | | | | | | | | | | | | | | | | |
| | | | | | | | | | | | | | | | | | | | |
| | | | | | | | | | | | | | | | | | | | |
| | | | | | | | | | | | | | | | | | | | |
| | | | | | | | | | | | | | | | | | | | |
| | | | | | | | | | | | | | | | | | | | |
| | | | | | | | | | | | | | | | | | | | |
| | | | | | | | | | | | | | | | | | | | |
| | | | | | | | | | | | | | | | | | | | |
| | | | | | | | | | | | | | | | | | | | |

a. Check the ENDs against the requisition including the name of the drug, number ordered, batch number, expiry date, intactness of the ampoule and discoloration. If this is correct, then the duplicate sheet in the END requisition form is signed in the "received by" section.
b. Place the ENDs in appropriate vault/cabinet with dual lock system.
c. Enters the ENDs in ward END register. Checks the register for current balance quantity and tallies with the quantity physically present.
d. The cabinet/vault should be always double locked when not in use.
e. The END cabinet/vault keys should always be with the two senior most nursing staff on duty.
f. The cabinet/vault should be used only to store narcotic drugs.
g. A logbook should be maintained to write the time of taking and returning the keys in between shifts (Form 26.3).
h. The END registers to be stored securely.
i. END counts/handing over:
   - Inventory of ENDs to be taken every shift and ensure it is documented in inventory sheet (Form 26.4).
   - If an inaccuracy is found in filled or empty ampoules, immediately notify nurse in-charge and fill up incidence report. Report to nursing administration and pharmacy in-charge.
   - In case END vault/cabinet key is missing, the concerned institution will have its own internal procedure for handling missed keys.

*3. Prescription, administration and documentation of narcotic drugs.*

a. END should be dispensed to a patient in the ward/unit/clinic only with a written prescription by the physician.
b. Narcotic drugs prescription in capital letters should contain date, name of the patient, age, sex, case number, diagnosis, indication, doctor's unit administering END, dose, route, frequency, drug form and strength of the preparation. It also contains name, sign and employment number of staff prescribing, dispensing, administering and nurse in-charge (physician should mention his/her state medical council registration number).

**Form 26.3:** Logbook for narcotic drug key handover between shifts

| S. no. | Date | Name of the staff | Time taken | Time return | Signature |
|---|---|---|---|---|---|
| | | | | | |
| | | | | | |
| | | | | | |
| | | | | | |
| | | | | | |
| | | | | | |
| | | | | | |
| | | | | | |
| | | | | | |

**Form 26.4:** Format for daily inventory of narcotic drugs

| S. no. | Generic name | Trade name | Dose | Stock | Expiry date | | DD/MM/YYYY | | | DD/MM/YYYY | | | DD/MM/YYYY | | | DD/MM/YYYY | | | DD/MM/YYYY | | | DD/MM/YYYY | | | DD/MM/YYYY | | |
|---|---|---|---|---|---|---|---|---|---|---|---|---|---|---|---|---|---|---|---|---|---|---|---|---|---|---|---|
| | | | | | | | M | E | N | M | E | N | M | E | N | M | E | N | M | E | N | M | E | N | M | E | N |
| 1 | Inj. Fentanyl Citrate | | | | | Full | | | | | | | | | | | | | | | | | | | | | |
| | | | | | | Empty | | | | | | | | | | | | | | | | | | | | | |
| | | | | | | Total | | | | | | | | | | | | | | | | | | | | | |
| | | | | | | | | | | | | | | | | | | | | | | | | | | | |
| 2 | Inj. Morphine Sulfate | | | | | Full | | | | | | | | | | | | | | | | | | | | | |
| | | | | | | Empty | | | | | | | | | | | | | | | | | | | | | |
| | | | | | | Total | | | | | | | | | | | | | | | | | | | | | |
| Name of the staff | | | | | | | | | | | | | | | | | | | | | | | | | | | |
| Sign of the staff | | | | | | | | | | | | | | | | | | | | | | | | | | | |

c. Prescription must not be altered or changed using correcting fluid.
d. Nursing in-charge should check prescription for its correctness and completeness.
e. Details of the prescribed narcotic drug (dose, route, duration, frequency) should be entered in the medication chart by the treating physician.
f. Follow the rights of drug administration:
   - Right patient-identify patient by two identifier-patient's full name and case file number
   - Right drug, right dose, right route, right time
   - This has to be done by two nurses' independently.
g. Document the drug administered along with needed information in narcotic register.
h. First nurse who administers the medication, makes the entry in END register and second nurse ensures that:
   - Patient and drug information is accurate.
   - The balance of drug tallies with the quantity physically present.
   - The remaining stock is returned to the END vault/cabinet.
   - The dose wastage to be documented in the END register.
   - Sign the patient's medication chart.
i. Each narcotic drug should be single prescription and single dose for single patient.
j. After administering the narcotic dose, the remaining balance should be immediately discarded with another nurse witness.
k. Treatment with narcotic drug to be discontinued by treating doctor with signature and date.
l. Ensure a clear documentation of drug discontinued in the patient's medical file and prescription form, which makes it invalid for further doses.
m. If a END is prescribed for outpatient, it should be administered in the treatment room of the hospital.

For hospitals with computerized data system.

a. Complete one narcotic module entry for each narcotic order used.
b. Enter one entry in the narcotic register along with transaction ID (to show consumption in the narcotic module) and Memo number (to charge for narcotics). Steps to generate transaction ID and Memo number **(Flowcharts 26.1 and 26.2)**.

*4. Monitoring patients with END administration*

a. Assess patient's vital signs and oxygen saturation pre- and post-drug administration to prevent any respiratory distress, hypotension, tachypnea or any other physiological side effects.
b. Assess patient for any adverse events. These side effects include but not limited to: Respiratory distress, tachypnea, urinary retention, nausea, vomiting and constipation.
c. Educate the patient about drug side effects and assess patient frequently.
d. Assess level of alertness, drowsiness, confusion, agitation or sedation.
e. Assess patient's pain score periodically to understand effectiveness of drug.
f. Make sure to keep the bed rails up to avoid risk of fall.
g. To follow "fall prevention protocol" as per hospital policy.

**Flowchart 26.1:** Process to generate transaction ID

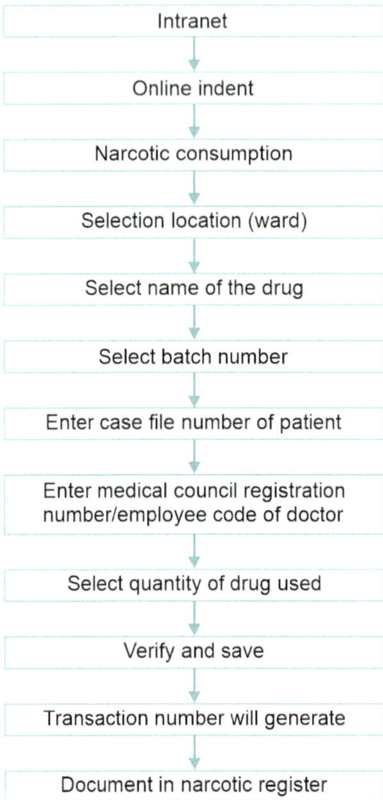


**Flowchart 26.2:** Process to generate memo

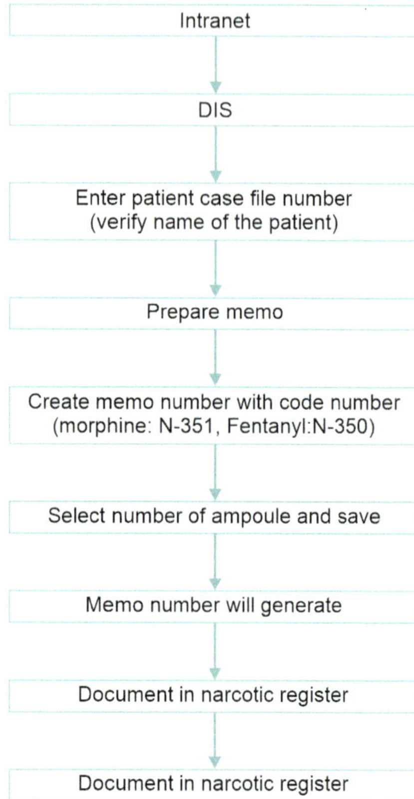


*5. Narcotic drug wastage*

a. Medication, which are left over or unused, should be discarded in the wash basin after diluting with water and witnessed by another senior nurse.

b. Document the reason of wastage in the remark column of the narcotic register against the name of the patient.

*6. Narcotic drug breakage or spillage, loss of ampoule*

a. In case of accidental breakage, spillage or loss of ampoule, notify to the nurse in-charge, pharmacist and fill an incident report form.

b. The incident report along with the broken ampoule to be handed over to the pharmacist.

c. Complete the incident report form and forward it to the nursing administration and then office of the medical superintendent for further action.

*7. Expired narcotic drug in the ward/unit/outpatient clinic*

a. Nurse in-charge should regularly check expiry date of the available stock.

b. If narcotic drug with near expiry date within 3 months is available in vault/ cabinet should be returned to pharmacy in-charge as per hospital policy and to be documented in narcotic register.

*8. Narcotic drugs brought in the hospital by patient on admission*

a. Notify the pharmacy in-charge regarding NDs brought by the patient at the time of admission.
b. In the event of discharge or death of patient, return the unused narcotic drug as per hospital policy to the pharmacy.
c. Document in the narcotic register.

*9. Patient receiving oral form of narcotics:*

a. Narcotic tablet should be procured by hospital personnel from the dispensary with a valid prescription.
b. On receiving the medication from the dispensary it should be checked for the correct medication, correct dose and expiry date.
c. The medication should be entered in a narcotics register in which patients medicines will be entered.
d. Tablet strip should be labeled with patient name, case number and date of procurement.
e. Narcotics tablet strip/bottle should be kept in the narcotic vault/cabinet.
f. The narcotic tablet kept in narcotic vault, should be removed and given by senior nurse on duty when required by the patient to the assigned nurse.
g. At the time of discharge, ensure patient gets correct prescription filled by the treating physician.
h. Quantity of the prescribed medication should be as per the patient's medical requirement and the hospital policy for discharge.
i. Narcotic medication should be properly explained to the patient and relatives before discharge, and document clearly the information in the patient's file.
j. The signature of patient's relative should be taken on the oral form narcotic register at the time of keeping the medicine in the vault and also at the time of returning it to them.

## Specific Staff Education

Staff needs to given periodical education on narcotic policy and importance of avoiding and reporting medication error related to narcotics. Narcotics policy and pain management is to be included as a part of an induction for newly recruited staffs.

## Compliance Check Using Narcotic Audit Tool (Form 26.5)

- Narcotics audit to be done every quarterly using audit checklist.
- Audit team includes pharmacy in-charge, representative from nursing administration, and the nurse in-charge of the specific area.
- During audit physical stock of narcotics drugs (filled and empty ampoules) should be checked against the narcotic register entry and narcotic consumption module.
- The report of audit including recommendations should be forwarded to nursing and medical superintendent for corrective actions.

## Conclusion

Narcotic medications are safe and effective in managing cancer pain. To meet the requirements of NDPS Act, we need to strictly adhere to the procedures as per narcotic

**Form 26.5:** Narcotic audit tool

Audit checklist for narcotic drugs

Audit objective: To ensure safe storage of narcotic drugs — Date:

| S. no. | Audit criteria | Method | Ward/ Dept/ Clinic: | | | |
|---|---|---|---|---|---|---|
| 1. | Is narcotics drugs stored in double lock vault/ cabinet? | O | | | | |
| 2. | Is the narcotic drugs vault/cabinet locked? | O | | | | |
| 3. | Is the narcotic drugs vault/cabinet keys available with two senior nurse on duty? | O/ I | | | | |
| 4. | Is the list of narcotic drugs available as per the requirement of department? | O | | | | |
| 5. | Are the numbers of ampoules as per the stock? | O | | | | |
| 6. | Is the expiry date of medication checked? | O-C | | | | |
| 7. | Is the inventory of narcotic drug maintained in every shift? | O-C | | | | |
| 8. | Is the narcotic register record maintained? | O-C | | | | |
| 9. | Is logbook of key hand over between shifts maintained? | O-C | | | | |
| 10. | Are all the details of patient filled in pink narcotic indent form? | O | | | | |
| 11. | Are entries in narcotic drug register signed by two nurses? | O | | | | |
| 12. | Is the reason for discarding leftover drug written in the remark column of narcotic register? | O | | | | |

**Note:** O: Observation, I: Interview, C: Checklist

Auditor 1: Name and sign — Auditor 2: Name and sign

drug policy regulations for stocking, dispensing and maintaining proper record. Also we need to develop our professional competency by training staffs to identify patients in pain, therapeutic benefits, adverse effects and misuse of narcotic drug.

## References


1. National Policy on Narcotics Drugs and Psychotropic Substances. Downloaded from http://www.dor.gov.in
2. NDPS Act, 1985.
3. Mr Rajgopal, et al. India: Opioid availability—An update, Journal of pain and Symptoms management, Nov 2006.
4. Guidelines for stocking and dispensing essential narcotics drugs downloaded from http://wwwtmc.gov.in
5. Management of Medication, Nursing manual, Tata Memorial Hospital, Pages 51–55.
6. Nursing Guidelines in the Management of Narcotics and Psychotropic Drugs. MoH/DGN/GUD/003/vers.01. June 2023.

# Index